The Sociology
of Human Fertility

AN ANNOTATED BIBLIOGRAPHY

BY RONALD FREEDMAN

A POPULATION COUNCIL BOOK

NEW YORK IRVINGTON PUBLISHERS, INC.

Halsted Press Division
JOHN WILEY & SONS

NEW YORK LONDON SYDNEY TORONTO

Library of Congress Cataloging in Publication Data

Freedman, Ronald, 1917-
The sociology of human fertility.

(Population and demography series)
"A Population Council book."
1. Fertility, Human—Bibliography. I. Title.
DNLM: 1. Demography—Abstracts. 2. Fertility—
Abstracts. Z7164.D3 F853s 1961-70,
Z7164.D3F7   016.30132'1   73-12272
ISBN 0 470-27732-7

Printed in the United States of America

Distributed by Halsted Press,
a Division of John Wiley & Sons, Inc., New York.

CONTENTS

PREFACE

In 1961 the author prepared "The Sociology of Human Fertility: A Trend Report and Annotated Bibliography" under the auspices of the International Sociological Association (*Current Sociology* 10, 11, no. 2, 1961-1962). That bibliography, consisting of only 636 items, has been cited extensively and has been translated into several languages. The present work consists mainly of an annotated and classified bibliography of the literature on fertility published since 1961. It also includes a reworking of that portion of the original essay which dealt with the basis for the recent interest in the sociology of human fertility and a descriptive model of the classes of variables that affect fertility.

An analytical discussion regarding the sociological factors related to fertility is not included. Any synthesis of the trends in fertility research would have to cope with the explosion of research literature published during the past decade. The recent literature draws on an enormous range of disciplines and demands a great deal of those who aspire to summarize the status of the field. For example, biologists, epidemiologists, and public health workers have become involved in the biosocial aspects of fertility through their analyses of such phenomena as fecundability, fetal mortality, lactation, postpartum amenorrhea, and age at menarche and menopause. An adequate sociology of human fertility must take into account not only the work of such medical and health scholars, but also that of ecologists, economists, anthropologists, geographers, political scientists, agronomists, and others. Clearly, the emergence of the population field—and specifically fertility analysis—as an important part of public policy making has helped to arouse the interest of a growing number of specialists from many fields.

As a result of the new research, we know more in the absolute sense about fertility than we did a decade ago, yet we probably know much less relative to our improved perception of the total system to be investigated. The reproductive processes and the social causes and consequences are more complicated than we had imagined. Detailed empirical work has made increasingly suspect some of the historical generalizations of an earlier day. Simplistic statements of the modern "demographic transition" for Europe simply do not fit the emerging body of historical data. The diversity of the historical record may require several different theories for different circumstances or a revised general theory quite different from that which has been accepted for many years.

The trend in fertility research has been to break apart relationships and analyze the component elements in the complex fertility model. While such analysis is undoubtedly useful, because it has produced new and more precise measurements of analytical relationships, we still do not have working models that enable us to put the specific elements back together in such a way as to reconstruct the dynamics of population as a whole.

The enlarged scope and the complexity of the field made it difficult to complete a comprehensive analytical review without delaying unduly the publication of this bibliography. Fortunately, Geoffrey Hawthorne's *Sociology of Fertility* (London: Collier-Macmillan, 1970) provides a useful discussion of many of the topics. While the author differs with Hawthorne on some points, Hawthorne's work is stimulating and covers important substantive issues.

To provide the reader with further indication of works published since compilation, classification, and annotation ended in mid-1970, a selected listing of publications is given in the appendix.

The author owes a special debt to Richard Cohn for extensive assistance in preparation of the bibliography and in developing the final version of the classification system. At earlier stages the assistance of Rhea Kish and Lolagene Coombs was appreciated. Miss Susan Robbins and her staff at the Population Council were very helpful in reading proof, editorial review, and making detailed arrangements for publication. Financial support was provided by the Population Council. The bibliography was completed during a period of residence as a Fellow at the Center for Advanced Study in the Behavioral Sciences, Stanford, California.

INTRODUCTION

AN HISTORICAL PERSPECTIVE

Public concern and debate about population and fertility control in the decade of the 1960s increased at a rate far exceeding the growth of either research on fertility or of fertility control programs. Early in the 1960s, in a review of research since World War II, this writer noted that "Interest ... has increased greatly among social scientists, administrators, political leaders, and the informed public in many countries" (113).[1] Since then, public figures have made many more frequent and stronger pronouncements about the seriousness of "the population problem." According to a recent summary:[2]

> In 1960 only three countries had anti-natalist population policies (all on paper), only one government was offering assistance, no international organization was working on family planning. In 1970 nearly 25 countries on all three developing continents, with 67 percent of the total population, have policies and programs; and another 15 or so, with 12 percent of the population, provide support in the absence of an explicitly formulated policy ... five to ten governments now offer external support (though only two in any magnitude); and the international assistance system is formally on board (the UN Population Division, the UNDP, WHO, UNESCO, FAO, ILO, OECD, the World Bank).

Fertility and birth control, mentioned only cautiously a decade ago, now are topics that appear often in the mass media and as subjects for political debate and legislation in many countries. They have become a part of both pop and high-brow culture, appearing in slogans on bumper stickers and psychedelic posters, as well as in countless symposia, forums, and in the solemn deliberations of the United Nations agencies. "The population problem" and "fertility control" commonly are rated among the two or three most important problems facing the world.

If reducing the birth rate is that important and urgent, then the results of the expanded research during the 1960s are still pathetically inadequate. There are serious proposals for social programs on a vast scale to change reproductive institutions and values that have been central in human

[1] Numbers in parentheses refer to items in the bibliography.
[2] B. Berelson, "Where Do We Stand," paper prepared for Conference on Technological Change and Population Growth, California Institute of Technology, May 1970, p. 1.

society for millenia. While the increase in knowledge about fertility in the 1960s probably has been greater than in any preceding decade in man's history, the sound research base for the far-reaching population policies being proposed is still small. The likelihood is that research and knowledge will have to grow partly as a by-product of the administrative needs of population policies based largely on the best available wisdom and judgments and a process of trial and error.

A kaleidoscopically changing set of social movements for "family planning," "fertility control," and "ecology" have brought fertility research into the public arena recently. Understandably, the mixed results are difficult to assess at this early point. There is more access to money and sites for research. The demands of the population programs and the debates about public policy have stimulated work on scientific problems previously receiving little attention. Further, the mass media have created such a demand for instant, capsule information that research workers are under pressure to produce early reports, to concentrate on what seems urgently useful, and to draw implications that may be premature. In presenting fertility data to the innumerable conferences of concerned laymen and leaders with a wide variety of interests, the cautious, detailed qualifications of background reports may become parenthetical or be regarded as nitpicking by the new audiences. Emotional involvement in the issues seems greater. Under the direct pressure of greater public scrutiny of results, social scientists are likely to become more committed and involved, either in connection with the social movements to which their studies are related or in defense of their own hypotheses and policy views. It is a mistake to assume that the scholar who remains aloof from the social movement also does not have a self-interested stake in the fate of his own point of view about the problem and policy. Discussion and research from a variety of bases probably is necessary in a field such as this, which is an inextricable mixture of social policy, values, and quantifiable facts. In this field, as in others, open publication of results and methodology is probably the best way to maximize reasonable objectivity.

Such problems affect every scientific field with important practical applications. The impact in population studies in the last decade has been unusually great, partly because laymen can project generalizations from their own experience in this field, partly because the public interest has expanded so rapidly, and partly because in previous decades the professional experts were a small group whose careful statistical analyses were of interest mainly to each other.

There has been more research on social aspects of human fertility by workers from disciplines not previously much involved (e.g., economics, biology, anthropology, epidemiology). There has also been much more reporting, writing, and research by persons with little scientific training in this field, who have a primary interest in applications (e.g., administrators, practicing medical workers, publicists). There is, then, a much wider range of publication, which is much harder to cover and to assess. Some publications by persons who are not population research specialists contain useful and unique data, even if analysis is lacking. The publications themselves are among the social facts deserving of scientific analysis.

This bibliography aims to classify important work from a scientific point of view. It would be a gross distortion, however, not to acknowledge from the outset that the development of the field has been heavily influenced by nonscientific persons and movements. It would also be a distortion not to include in the review consideration of the social movements, policies, and programs as an element of the scientific problem area under study.

The bibliography lists 1567 English-language publications. In a rough way, this number indicates a large field of research and publication, but progress in answering crucial research questions has been modest.

The background for the rapid increase in interest in human fertility is an interrelated complex of changes in society and in knowledge about population. Various factors in the interrelationship are described below.

1. *A growing realization that the problematic factor in population is the fertility rate.* Growth rates in most countries depend mainly on mortality and fertility levels and are little affected by international migration. In the developing countries, mortality either already has fallen to low levels or is expected to decline following the application of known technology. Fertility rates, however, are expected to remain high for at least a time, with the result that the overall rate of growth will reach new highs—to the point where most development experts regard population growth as a threat to programs of economic and social development (1386, 1391, 1409). Obviously, then, many people concerned with these aspects of development are eager for knowledge that can be used in action programs aimed at accelerating fertility decline.

Research also shows with increasing precision that population growth rates in the developed countries, too, now depend mainly on fertility trends (1466). Mortality is so low in the developed countries that future increases in life expectancy will have relatively small effects on population growth, because only modest mortality decreases are likely. The important fact is that almost everyone in developed societies now lives through the child-bearing years, and only mortality gains in the child-bearing years would significantly affect population growth. Greater life expectancy for older

5

people would not have nearly the comparable (opposite) effect that any change in fertility would. In 1959, Coale[3] illustrated these consequences dramatically by calculating that the attainment of immortality for the entire population of the United States would have less effect on its long-run population growth than a 20 percent increase in fertility! It is now commonly accepted that if families in countries with low mortality rates have an average of three children—historically a moderate number—a rapid rate of population growth results.

Before World War II, most demographers simply expected a continued decline in fertility rates or at least a stabilization at very low levels, probably because of the contraceptive information available. Because prewar population projections erred mainly in failing to allow adequately either for the possibility of higher fertility rates or for their volatility, demographers have turned to more broadly based social research on fertility for better predictions of this element in population growth. The dynamic and problematic character of fertility rates in the developed countries has come to be emphasized by a series of oscillations. Immediately after World War II, fertility rates rebounded from the all-time lows of the 1930s to levels above replacement in most Western countries, with still higher rates and larger families in the non-European Western countries (a long postwar "baby boom"). It became clear that families could be planned to be larger as well as smaller, and such planning appears to have happened in many countries during the fifteen years after 1945. The sharp declines of birth rates in many non-European Western countries in the 1960s was partly a predicted (e.g., 461, 1506) result of temporary demographic abnormalities and of variations in the timing of the family cycle (324). However, it now appears very likely that in the United States, at least, the families started in the early 1960s will continue to be smaller than those of the postwar era.[4]

Spectacularly rapid fertility declines following legalization of induced abortion in Japan and in some Eastern European countries have been followed by a leveling off once net reproduction rates reached replacement levels. On the other hand, in Romania, where as a result of legalized abortion birth rates fell from 24.2 per 1000 in 1956 to 14.3 per 1000 in 1966,

[3] A.J. Coale, "Increases in Expectation of Life and Population Growth," in *Population Conference, Vienna 1959* (Vienna: International Union for the Scientific Study of Population, 1959), pp. 36–41.
[4] For example, *see* U.S. Bureau of the Census, *Current Population Reports,* Series P-20, No. 203, 6 July 1970, "Fertility of the Population, January 1969."

the withdrawal of abortion facilities in 1966 caused the birth rate to rise in one year to 27.4—perhaps the most rapid fertility rise on record.[5]

That fertility may move up or down in relation to political, social, and economic conditions means that bulges or gaps may be created at the bottom of the age structure that may seriously affect many aspects of society at some later time.

2. *The age structure of a population appears to depend much more on fertility than on mortality trends.* Until recently, most social scientists did not know that the "aging" of Western population resulted mainly from the decline in the birth rate rather than from lower mortality. In the developing areas, a decrease in mortality without a decrease in fertility creates a younger rather than an older population and greatly increases the size of the dependent child population, for which costly social services must be provided (1385, 1406, 1466).

Social-policy interest in stopping population growth must deal with the fact that even if age-specific birth rates are at zero growth-replacement levels, substantial growth may continue for as long as 50–60 years (1469). The effect of past fertility in creating a young population with many couples of prime reproductive age inflates crude birth rates and deflates crude death rates for generations afterward. Japan's net reproduction rate has averaged about 1.0 (the replacement level) since the 1950s, but even if this continues, the population of Japan will not stop growing until after the year 2000. The fact that mortality rates are substantially higher for males than for females in most societies means that variations in the fertility rates will affect both the sex as well as the age composition of populations. So, the fertility and the basic demographic structures of population interact in ways that pose problems both for research and social policy.

3. *A reemphasis on the essential functions of the family in an industrial urban society.* Writings about the urban family in the two decades before World War II stressed its loss of functions to other specialized institutions and used the decline in family size as an important index of this trend. A logical extension of this orientation were projections of very low fertility and many intentionally childless families. Special social incentives to child bearing were widely discussed at that time as means of achieving the reproductive needs of the society. In the early postwar period sociologists rediscovered

---

[5] Following this increase, the birth rate declined to 19.6 by 1971. This episode in Romanian demographic history is a dramatic example of the kinds of "natural experiments" occurring in the field of human fertility, most of which are not studied systematically in order to observe causes and consequences.

the persistent strength of primary groups, and especially of the family.[6] It is difficult to judge how much this change in point of view reflected major social trends inconsistent with the prewar interpretation of disintegrating familial institutions: higher birth rates and larger families, an increasing proportion married and a decrease in the age at marriage, increased expenditures on single-family homes in some countries and on family-oriented consumer durables in almost all of them.

In the international youth culture of the present day, some observers again see a weakening of family ties in such phenomena as more open sexual relationships, the generation gap, communal living arrangements, illegitimacy, a decrease in the percentage married, and an increase in the age at marriage. But even in this new generation, almost everyone still gets married (if somewhat later) and has children, so the long-term trends in family and fertility are still uncertain.

By the early months of 1972 the birth rate in the United States had declined to low levels comparable to the lowest levels of the 1930s. While it is still uncertain that completed family size will return to the very low levels of the 1930s, that is possible. However, in view of the uncertainty about why these changes have occurred, most informed observers would not be surprised to find another rise in basic fertility rates sometime during this decade.

In general, these short-run episodic changes in fertility and family life make basic long-run research on fertility so important. For the entire period from about 1920 to 1970, we are uncertain about what is secular trend and what is short-term variation. What happened and why are still questions that stimulate inquiry.

4. *Methodological developments have created more possibilities for many kinds of fertility study.* In recent years the technique of the sample interview survey has been used to study important variables closely related to fertility but formerly thought too personal and intimate for systematic study. "Sensitive subjects," such as contraception, abortion, and fecundity, are now studied in a variety of cultural settings. Researchers have had enough success to demonstrate the feasibility of such investigations, although major problems of reliability and validity in measurement do exist. Another technique that has increased the resources for fertility studies is the

---

[6] For example, E. Shils, "The Study of the Primary Group," in D. Lerner and H. Lasswell, eds., *The Policy Sciences* (Stanford: Stanford University Press, 1951); M. Young and P. Willmot, *Family and Kinship in East London* (London: Routledge & Kegan Paul, 1957); R. Firth, *Two Studies of Kinship in London,* London School of Economics Monographs on Social Anthropology, No. 15 (London: University of London, Athlone Press, 1956); R. Freedman et al., *Principles of Sociology* (New York: Holt, Rinehart and Winston, 1956), Chaps. 11 and 12.

census—now taken by many countries—and the resultant sophistication in statistical reporting systems. Comparative studies are at least made possible by the efforts of the United Nations to standardize definitions and procedures. A variety of techniques and models have been developed and partially tested to make estimates from the incomplete and inaccurate data available for most developing countries. Unfortunately, what is known has not been applied to provide minimal demographic measures for most of the world's population, and this failure limits the chances for improvement of the methodology that comes from its use. Nevertheless, the new methodology increases greatly the potential for research. Judging by past work in fertility study, however, much has been done, but the need is enormous.

5. *People have come to believe that fertility above optimum levels causes major social and personal problems.* It is commonly believed that the development of poor countries is impeded by high fertility and low mortality, although some scholars are skeptical and dissent from this view (for example, *see* 1410 and 1541). The development issue has stimulated a growing amount of population research by economists. The popular interest in ecology has made the question of fertility above replacement level—even in affluent countries—a major factor in discussing pollution, crime, congestion, and, ultimately, survival itself (13, 1567). Some of the problems attributed to population growth may be more plausibly related to the growth of urban concentration and technology at rates far exceeding the rates of population growth. There seems to be general agreement that in the long run a zero growth rate for population is inevitable. In highly industrial countries such as the United States, there appear to be great controversies about the urgency of attaining zero or even negative rates of growth (*see* 13, 654, 656). The international public has demanded both pertinent information and allocation of funds for research and action programs about fertility.

LEVELS OF FERTILITY ANALYSIS

The unit for fertility analysis may be the whole society, the strata or groups within a society, or a reproducing couple classified in terms of psychological characteristics that cut across social categories. Comparative studies of different societies or of one society at different cultural stages are probably essential in order to answer many of the most interesting sociological questions about fertility: Why is fertility high in most developing countries and relatively low in the developed industrial societies? Does a high rate of social mobility in a society lead to low fertility even in nonmobile strata? Statistics for answering such questions may be based on data for millions of couples. The problem is not why one couple rather than another is at a particular place in the frequency distribution of births in a society, but why the society as a whole has the particular fertility distribution that distinguishes it from another.

Intrasocietal sociological analyses usually involve cross-section comparisons of fertility rates and distributions for major social strata or groupings or types of families at a moment in time. Most fertility studies have been of this type, where the ultimate sociological problem should be to explain why one social grouping rather than another has a particular fertility level or distribution. But most of the empirical work has involved descriptions of the differences; the explanations are usually more or less unsystematic speculations. Intrasocietal studies are valuable, but they cannot substitute for intersocietal comparisons. For example, the relationship of income levels to fertility for individuals within a society depends on other characteristics of the society and may be quite different when societies are the units. Similarly, a society with a dominant joint family system may have higher fertility than one with a dominant nuclear family system, but within the first society joint families may be smaller than nuclear families.

Interindividual fertility comparisons cutting across social categories usually introduce social-psychological variables to explain why particular couples conform to or deviate from the norm for a society or a group. Social-psychological variables are also introduced as "intervening" between the social setting and the individual to explain how a particular social situation motivates individual behavior. The studies using psychological variables on a systematic empirical basis are still few and, so far, have been rather unsuccessful in adding much to the variance explained by social and demographic variables (see 1512, 1534), although informal speculation about the psychology of human fertility has a very long history.

The systematic use of aggregate and individual data simultaneously is a promising approach not used very often, because the appropriate data often are not available and their use involves special methodological problems. Duncan (498), for example, found in a reanalysis of data from the Indianapolis fertility study, that both aggregate area rent measures and individual rent are related to fertility, that having both measures predicts more than having either alone, and that significant effects of areal measures persist after allowing for several other pertinent individual measures.

Srikantan[7] compared neighborhood and individual effects in responses to a family planning program and also in prior use of birth control. Obviously, numerous questions of this kind may be asked: Are levels of fertility different for illiterates who live in neighborhoods of higher rather than lower educational status? Is the effect on fertility of living in an extended family unit different when the number of such units in the local community is few rather than many? Does living in neighborhoods with high average economic aspiration levels affect fertility differently for individuals from population strata characterized in the aggregate by low or high aspiration levels? This method of research does not require inferring correlations for individuals from areal or other aggregate measures (the so-called ecological fallacy). Instead, the assumption here is that the aggregate indexes measure aspects of the individual's social environment or of collectivities that influence his behavior. In this sense, the aggregate measures refer to social facts that can be used along with individual measures to assess the total set of influences on behavior. Presumably, the aggregate measures are useful only insofar as they relate to approximations of real units of social interaction. The use of such "contextual" data about the whole unit as well as about the individual has become well known through educational studies in which the characteristics of the school and the individual students both enter into assessments of achievement and other outcomes.[8] The computer has increased the possibility of using the mass population data for joint analyses of both family and personal characteristics in relation to fertility and other demographic variables (285).

The comparative sociological study of fertility is less developed than might be expected from the nature of the problem and available methodological resources. It is obvious that every society must maintain a particular minimum fertility level appropriate to its mortality and migration level if it is to survive at all. In this sense, the study of fertility levels clearly is part of the analysis of the essential functions of any society. It probably is also true that every society tends to develop a characteristic fertility level that affects the rate of reproduction, the growth rate, age structure, and other vital aspects of the society. A variable that is at once universally observable and relevant to important structural variables deserves a high priority for comparative study.

---

[7] K. Srikantan, *Effects of Neighborhood and Individual Factors on Family Planning in Taichung,* Ph.D. dissertation in sociology, University of Michigan, 1967 (published in microfilm by University Microfilms Xerox).

[8] For example, J. Coleman, E. Q. Campbell, and C. F. Hobson, *Equality of Educational Opportunity* (Washington, D.C.: U.S. Office of Education, 1966).

There appears to be immediately at hand a considerable body of data for comparative studies in the rapidly growing collections of censuses and vital statistics, from which can be derived not only direct and indirect measures of fertility but also a variety of other characteristics of the population. There is also available a growing collection of fertility studies based on sample surveys that are a potential basis for comparative analyses involving a wider range of variables. Data characterizing whole populations are probably available for larger samples of societies on such demographic characteristics as fertility than for any other class of sociological variable.

The systematic comparative study of fertility is more a promise than a reality. The vast majority of studies still are limited to a particular society and are comparative only by implication.

Most studies, whether for one society or many, are not yet consciously oriented to sociological concepts and problems, which is not surprising since most statistical data on fertility and its correlates are collected for the administrative needs of a particular country by persons without sociological training or interests. While the sociologically relevant data being collected are increasing in quantity and quality, the comparability of the variables covered and their definitions leave much to be desired, despite the significant efforts of the United Nations to standardize procedures and concepts. The lack of data is much more obvious if historical series are required, since census taking or other statistical operations are very recent for most of the world. In any case, no official statistical system has ever collected data regularly on most of the variables that immediately affect fertility (e.g., the use of contraception or abortion) or on most of the important structural variables believed to affect fertility.

This is not to deny the great importance of the existing statistical resources for the ingenious investigator. Fortunately, the statistical needs of the administrator and the sociologist converge at a number of important points: For example, both are interested in such stratification variables as education and occupation. But for much of the world at present, reliance must be placed on scattered ethnographic and documentary materials that do not deal with essential demographic variables. These data are only now being supplemented by an increasing number of sample surveys that may be a basis for future comparative studies.

In view of the scarcity of the data on many crucial variables, much of the comparative work is necessarily speculative, with empirical data used for illustration rather than for systematic validation of theories. In this respect, the sociology of human fertility is not unusual, but deficiencies are more obvious, because poor demographic predictions about fertility can be checked more easily than in most other fields.

VARIABLES THAT AFFECT FERTILITY

Fertility levels are part of a complex system of social, biological, and environmental interactions, as is any phenomenon dependent on such central and universal human concerns as sex, marriage, and kinship. Because most studies concentrate on only a small part of the complex interacting whole, a gross initial classification of all the major sets of variables can place these individual studies in a larger perspective. A classification may explain or condition a particular relationship by reference to other classes of variables. Demographic research has been more distinguished by the systematic use of reliable data for a small number of variables than by efforts to place many excellent explicit research findings in the larger context. Few of the research studies listed in the bibliography deal with much of this larger system, and many scholars might contest its utility. However, in recent years the use of multivariate analysis has increased, as has the development of data systems covering more variables simultaneously. While no research has yet established a set of data for all of the identified major variables for any population at any moment in time, recognition of the existence of the broader system may help to guide future research. Different investigators probably will continue to work on different parts of the system, and the integration of results may be the work of others with still different skills and interests.

Our suggested model for the sociological analysis of fertility levels is shown in Figure 1 on page 15 and described below. This model works backward from measures of fertility to classes of variables affecting the fertility levels of a society or of strata or groups within a society. The classes of variables are as follows:

I. *The means of fertility control that fall between the social organization and the social norms on the one hand and fertility on the other.* Davis and Blake (81) have provided a very useful classification of these means, called "intermediate variables," which are:
  A. Factors affecting exposure to intercourse (the "intercourse variables")
    1. Those governing the formation and dissolution of unions in the reproductive period
      a. Age of entry into sexual unions
      b. Permanent celibacy: proportion of women never entering sexual unions

    c. Amount of reproductive period spent after or between unions
        (1) When unions are broken by divorce, separation, or desertion
        (2) When unions are broken by death of husband
  2. Those governing the exposure to intercourse within unions
    a. Voluntary abstinence
    b. Involuntary abstinence (from impotence, illness, unavoidable but temporary separations)
    c. Coital frequency (excluding periods of abstinence)
B. Factors affecting exposure to conception (the "conception variables")
  1. Fecundity or infecundity,[9] as affected by involuntary causes
  2. Use or nonuse of contraception[10]
    a. By mechanical or chemical means
    b. By other means
  3. Fecundity or infecundity, as affected by voluntary causes—sterilization, subincision, medical treatment, etc.
C. Factors affecting gestation and successful parturition (the "gestation variables")
  1. Fetal mortality from involuntary causes
  2. Fetal mortality from voluntary causes

As Davis and Blake indicate, different combinations of values for these intermediate variables may produce identical fertility levels. On the other hand, societies or groups with very different fertility levels may have similar values for some of the intermediate variables. It is unnecessary, and often incorrect, to assume that the intermediate variables always are used deliberately to limit fertility. The effect on fertility is often an unintended

---

[9] Infecundity refers here to any physiological impairment to a normal rate of reproduction; it is not restricted to complete sterility. The term fecundity refers in standard demographic usage to the capacity for bearing children, as distinguished from fertility—the actual bearing of children. Clearly, any of the other intermediate variables may affect the correspondence between fecundity and fertility. For most individuals as well as for most societies and social strata, fertility is below the maximum biological potential. In recent years a more precise term, fecundability, has been used to denote the probability of conceiving during any observed monthly period. This operational definition facilitates research in which fecundability is observed to vary not only as between individuals but also at different times in the life history of an individual. For example, fecundability tends to be substantially below average for an individual woman during periods of amenorrhea following the birth of a child.

[10] Contraception refers here to any means for avoiding conception, including prolonged or periodic abstinence, coitus interruptus, and any mechanical or chemical methods.

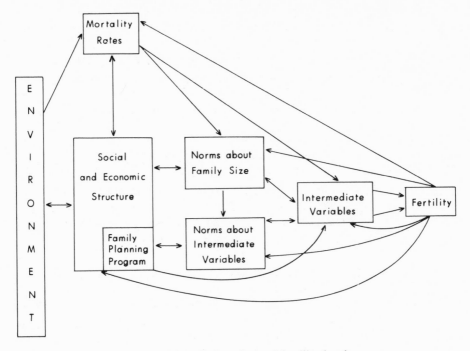

Figure 1. A model for the sociological analysis of fertility levels.

consequence of cultural patterns with no explicit connection to fertility. Other factors can affect fertility only through one or more of these intermediate variables. Figure 1 is drawn to make this point. The only direct causal influences involve lines of connection through the intermediate variables rather than directly to fertility.

II. *Social norms about family size.* The number of children a couple should have is a problem so universal and so important in every society that it would be a sociological anomaly if normative cultural solutions were not developed to meet this problem in most cases. The norm about what family size ought to be is likely to specify a range of permissible or desirable numbers of children, perhaps as vague as "at least three or four" or "as many as possible."

III. *Social norms about each of the intermediate variables.* Although most of the intermediate variables are controlled by the norms of the society, some (e.g., contraception) may be unknown and therefore not subject to cultural prescription. It is possible in research to assign a value (if only zero) to the actual effect of each intermediate variable even if no norm operates. Presumably, the norms controlling the intermediate variables tend to produce a fertility level consistent with the norms about family size, but a continuing inconsistency is possible, especially since the effects of the intermediate variables on fertility frequently are not intended or understood by members of the society. Moreover, the norms governing the intermediate variables may develop to meet problems only remotely related to fertility. Recent discussions about developing countries have been concerned with an apparent discrepancy between the norms about family size-contraception and other intermediate variables that affect the implementation of small family norms. Norms about various aspects of sex, reproduction, and marriage are found in all societies and profoundly affect fertility, but because they may be based on either superstition or sound scientific knowledge, such norms are not easily identified.

IV. *Aspects of the social organization that function to support the norms about family size by providing social rewards and punishments that depend on the numbers of children in the familial unit.* Will having particular numbers (or ranges of numbers) of children affect the ability of the reproducing unit to attain socially valued goals? This question centers on the division of labor between the familial unit and other social institutions and the extent to which the family's important personal and social functions depend on the number of children. The assumption here is that family-size norms will tend to correspond to a number that maximizes the net utility to be derived from having children in the society or stratum. Obviously, different aspects of the society may exert pressures in opposite directions on the norms. For example, if the state has a higher or lower fertility objective than would be realized by the existing balance of social rewards and punishments, population policy may exert a counterpressure on the norm and the practice. Having many children may be valued by the parents as a source of security in their old age, but, on the other hand, many children may impose difficult burdens on the parents during the period of child dependency.

V. *Other aspects of the social organization that affect fertility by influencing the norms or actual values for the intermediate variables, either independent of or in relation to the effect on the norms about fertility.* While results inconsistent with the fertility norms may be produced by any of these organizational elements, presumably such social practices have the greatest chance of surviving if they are not too inconsistent with the reproductive optimum specified in the norms. Inconsistent pressures and results are possible, and even probable, especially during periods of rapid social change.

A large variety of social practices or organizations may affect the norms about or the actual values of the intermediate variables in ways that are more or less consistent with the social norms about family size. This may or may not involve awareness of the ultimate effect on fertility. It may involve organizations specializing in the control of one or more intermediate variables (e.g., the family planning movement). It may involve the organization and effectiveness of the familial unit itself for implementing the family size norms (e.g., the internal communication pattern needed for consensus about family planning). It may involve organizations whose activities have quite different objectives (e.g., a religious organization that prescribes periods of abstinence for ritual purposes). It may involve indirect and unintended effects without explicit reference to the norms for either the intermediate variables or for family size (e.g., the economic organization as a whole may serve to reduce the fecundity of the lowest stratum by supplying inadequate nutrition).

The intermediate variables should produce the number of living children considered normatively desirable for the society. By definition, a social norm operates to control behavior in appropriate situations. If there are mass discrepancies between the norm and behavior, the social reality of the norm about family size may be in question.

Organized programs to affect fertility or the intermediate variables or the norms about them are a part of the social organization, of course. They are as designated in Figure 1, only a small element of the large social organization complex, recent and limited interventions in an ongoing set of changing organizational controls that have determined fertility levels in various ways for millennia.

The two immediately preceding classes of variables (IV and V) together encompass a very wide range of social and economic variables. Significant social and economic variables may be sought wherever there is an observable functional connection between some element of the social organization and the norms for family size, the norms for the intermediate variables, or the intermediate variables themselves. The fact that we do not specify the organizational variables concretely should make it clear that the model is not a substantive theory; it is a classificatory framework, with theoretical implications. We provide some *ad hoc* substantive classifications in the bibliography itself.

VI. *Mortality level, which determines how large a surplus of births is required to produce the normative number of children.* Most of the social and economic consequences of different fertility levels probably are related to number of living children rather than to number of births. A norm specifying "three or four children" as desirable is quite consistent with a much larger average number of live births per woman in a society with high and variable mortality levels. This may account in part for the apparent discrepancy between a stated desire for three or four children and much higher fertility levels in underdeveloped areas. Infant mortality also may affect fertility by decreasing the period of temporary sterility following a birth brought about by breast feeding. The death of a child and the cessation of breast feeding will shorten the period of reduced fecundability. If a child lives and is breast fed, the probability of a conception is reduced for a limited but significant period of time.

VII. *Net migration level, which determines the number and ages of persons available to the families and to the society as a whole.* At most times and places, migration is relatively unimportant in the reproductive balance of the whole society, but in the form of physical and social mobility within a society it may have a very important effect on the reproductive balance, or fertility, of societal subgroups.

VIII. *Other factors in the environment that affect the intermediate variables in ways inconsistent with the fertility norms.* Venereal diseases introduced from the outside, a weather-induced famine, or any other variable exogenous to the social system may reduce fertility below desired levels.

In brief, this model specifies that the fertility of any social collectivity tends to correspond with a level prescribed by the social norms, which are in turn an adjustment to the way in which varying numbers of children affect the achievement of socially valued objectives. In the long run, the net effect of the intermediate variables affecting fertility should produce approximately the normative reproductive level. In a complex and changing society, however, the other organizational and environmental factors may affect the intermediate variables in ways that are inconsistent with the family-size norms. It is not necessary to assume an equilibrium model to use this classification.

The order of the preceding listing of classes of variables was intentionally reversed; it ran from fertility through the intermediate variables to the much wider range of social, demographic, and other environmental influences that ultimately affect fertility. This strategy is consistent with the demographic tradition of working with variables that are or can be "hard" facts. It is also consistent with the idea that the facts about what is to be explained should be clear before the construction of elaborate theories to explain them. The suggested strategy is to begin near the end of the causal chain, where all relevant factors must have their effects on fertility through the limited number of intermediate variables. The much more numerous, diffuse, and elusive variables that are farther back in the causal process necessarily converge and are funneled through the intermediate variables. By analogy, we can visualize this as working backward from the narrow neck of a funnel to the broadening opening, where we are likely to find that we cannot deal simultaneously with all the important variables in the foreseeable future. But, an inventory of the number and complexity of the variables puts our work in perspective and helps to explain why current studies account for only a small part of the total variance in fertility.

The funnel approach is especially relevant here, because all other factors affecting fertility must have their influence through the limited number of intermediate variables. One test of a hypothesized causal connection between variable x and fertility is to specify the intermediate variables through which x affects fertility. For example, in many populations a normative preference for sons is believed to keep fertility higher than it otherwise might be. In a number of studies there is evidence of a stated preference for sons. In fewer studies there is empirical evidence that, among couples with similar numbers of living children, those without a son are more likely to have another child. Even fewer studies have an additional explanatory link: evidence that the couples without a son are less likely than others to use contraception or to practice abortion or to limit the frequency of coitus. The pertinent question is: How are those with and without sons differentiated by practices that could have the observed effects in subsequent fertility? Differentials in group fertility should be associated with corresponding differentials in one or more of the intermediate variables.

While we are considering fertility mainly as the dependent variable to be explained, it can interact with other socioeconomic variables both as a cause and as an effect. For example, there is a considerable body of literature on how family size affects intellectual development and educational attainment of the children. Likewise, educational attainment of parents or their perception of the educational advantages of a small family can be seen as the independent variables affecting their fertility. Similarly, economic status may affect or be affected by family size. These are not contradictory propositions. The observation over time by many people that varying family sizes have differing consequences for socially valued goals affects the development of social norms about family size and motivates appropriate behavior. The study of the consequences of differing fertility levels is indispensable for understanding their causes.

Apart from the fact that fertility itself has feedback effects on all aspects of the system, there may be a considerable series of interactions and feedback loops between other sets of variables prior to any effect on fertility. For example, under conditions of high mortality, if the survival of a few sons is regarded as essential the culture is likely to reward high fertility, even if this often means an "excess" of surviving sons. If mortality declines, the survival of a much larger number of sons puts a strain on housing arrangements, inheritance customs, and other aspects of culture developed on the long-term assumption of high mortality. If the resulting strains reduce the number of sons desired, greater use of birth-control methods to limit fertility may ensue. Lower fertility may further decrease infant mortality—and the set of repercussions begins again after having gone full-circle through many way-stations.

RELATION OF THE CLASSIFICATION SYSTEM TO THE FERTILITY MODEL

Most elements of the classification system of the bibliography can be related to the model shown in Figure 1. One series of classifications relates elements of the social structure to the norms about fertility or fertility itself: stratification variables (IV)[11]; family structure variables (V); nonfamilial institutions with specific programs to affect fertility, the intermediate variables or the norms about them (VI); other general characteristics of the society or subgroup (VII)—for example, density, urbanization, migration, economic structure, and so on; and social-psychological variables (VIII).

Since the impact of social variables on fertility is through the intermediate variables, a specific category (IX) is concerned with the effect of social and demographic factors on the levels and the norms for the intermediate

[11] Roman numerals in parentheses refer to the major headings of the classification.

variables. Biomedical studies of fertility control (XIII) provide essential sociobiological linkages on which the effects of intermediate variables depend. The relation between the intermediate variables and fertility (XIV) is the final link in the chain of influences running from the social system to fertility.

In recognition of the feedback influences from fertility, another category (X) deals with the effects on other specific aspects of society of the norms and actual levels of fertility and the intermediate variables. In a more general sense, fertility is interdependent with migration and mortality in producing some kind of demographic balance in relation to resources broadly defined. That broad interdependence and such theories about it as "the demographic transition" and "optimum population" are the subject matter of category XII.

Other parts of the classification system list types of studies that provide the material or methods required for research on fertility. One set of publications deals with measurement techniques for fertility, the intermediate variables, or the norms about them (II). In view of their special importance in the field, a separate classification (XI) refers to major intensive sample surveys that deal simultaneously with norms and levels of fertility and the intermediate variables. Historical and descriptive studies (III) provide data and perspective for many of the substantive research categories.

Finally, there are categories of publications that are general in the sense that they cut across many aspects of the field (I): general works or collections of papers, discussions of important theoretical issues or review of the literature, bibliographies, and multivariate analyses.

THE BIBLIOGRAPHY

A NOTE ON THE BIBLIOGRAPHY

The 1657 items included in this bibliography are a selection of pertinent English-language publications that came to the attention of the author-compiler up until June 1970. (The appendix provides an unannotated listing of works on fertility published from mid-1970 to 1 April 1972.) The compilation was carried on sporadically over a period of years, which means that the detail and character of the annotation varies. The bibliography suffers from the irregularities often found in hand-crafted products. A list based on computer search and analysis would probably have been more complete and consistent. However, this bibliography has the advantage of being organized in relation to a conceptual scheme, with annotations and classifications reflecting the compiler's 25 years of work in this field.

The compiler's 1961 bibliography (113) covered 636 items that appeared approximately during the 15 years after World War II. From among these, 146 English-language items were selected because they were believed to be of special historical or analytical value. These retained items are indicated by an asterisk (*) placed before the author's name.

Publications in languages other than English are omitted, despite their growing volume and importance. The obvious magnitude of this literature, together with the difficulties of access to the journals and of dealing with many languages, resulted in a decision to restrict the bibliography to publications in English.

The basic source from which selections were made is the *Population Index*, the remarkably useful and complete bibliographic journal for the population field. The great majority of the items cited in this bibliography are in *Population Index*, although we do not include all its listings about fertility. In addition, items were found in other bibliographies (*see* 112–127) and in footnotes or bibliographies cited in other books or periodicals. The literature more or less connected to this field is now so voluminous that no claim for inclusiveness can be made.

The objective was to include as a central core all publications considered important, but not all included items are considered equally important or of high quality. Then, too, many items were intentionally omitted. In fact, about 500 final-stage listings (25 percent of the total) were not included for the following major reasons:

1. The material represents a partial report covered more completely in a later publication.
2. The subject is peripheral to the field, and similar items are adequately represented in the bibliography.
3. The report is not published in a form available to the public (e.g., mimeographed papers).
4. The item is brief, not available for reading, and from the limited information available does not appear to be important.
5. The item presents basic statistics about fertility with little analytical discussion.

There was less intentional omission for those topics represented by fewer publications, and some works on little-studied topics have been retained to highlight research lacunae.

We were able to read some of the publications and to scan most others. For the classification and annotation of many items, we relied on the brief abstracts in the *Population Index*. No annotation is made where (1) the title itself is an adequate indication of the main theme of the article, or (2) we had insufficient information to prepare an annotation, although on the basis of author and title the item seemed important enough to include.

Many studies relevant to two or more of the topics have their primary listing under the topic for which they seem most pertinent, but are listed also by number under the headings for other relevant topics. In some cases, therefore, the *see also* listings by number include the most important publications in a particular class. For example, a major sample survey (listed in Class XI) may have a secondary listing for educational fertility differentials (IVC), which is more important than some of the primary listings under that topic.

The classification system in this volume reflects the changing research emphases since the 1961 bibliography. Some changes here include the following:

1. A category (ID) covers the increasing number of pertinent bibliographies, indicative both of more publication and more interest.

2. A category (IE) covers some of the multivariate analyses that cut across other classifications, and are more prevalent in many fields as a result of the computer and the increase in complex data systems.

3. Many of the types of items classified as descriptive or historical (III) in the 1961 bibliography have here been given primary classification in an analytical or methodological category. This result is partly a recognition of the growing importance, analytical substance, and methodological sophistication of historical demography. It also reflects an ambivalence about what distinguishes historical from social science analysis.

4. A set of detailed categories (VIB) covers the voluminous literature about "programs specifically concerned with affecting the practice of birth control." The items now cited in the VIB category are less than half of those considered for inclusion. It seemed desirable to represent the considerable range of publications in this area. With increasing numbers of countries and organizations involved in birth-control programs, analyses and reports of their activity, origins, and effects are an essential part of the sociology of human fertility. We have cited illustratively only a small proportion of the large number of reports describing or making detailed recommendations about program operations (VIB1 and VIB2). We have cited more completely those which analyze the programs, their clients, and effects in some systematic way (VIB3). However, even in this category we have omitted a large number of reports where data or statistics appear with little analysis.

5. There has been a large number of publications in recent years dealing with religious views (particularly the Roman Catholic) and the effect of various aspects of religion on fertility and population. Many of these publications are statements of doctrine, moral belief, or argumentation rather than empirical studies of the relation of religious affiliation, belief, or practice to fertility variables. Therefore, a selection of the publications that are primarily statements of belief or doctrine (VID1) is separated from empirical studies (VID2). Many of the studies listed under VID2 cannot properly be said to refer to "nonfamilial institutions with explicit programs to affect fertility" (the major heading for VI). However, it seemed more practical to keep all religious studies together than to create several different classifications in other places in the bibliography.

6. In view of the substantially greater number of studies involving economic variables, these have been divided on the basis of their major emphases into micro and macro studies (VIIC1–VIIC2 and XB1–XB2).

7. The number of studies dealing with the social and demographic factors affecting intermediate variables (IX) has increased greatly since 1961. In addition, a major set of new classifications (XIV) has been added for studies of the effect of intermediate variables on fertility—the last and indispensable link in the model we are using.

8. The interrelations between vital rates (fertility, mortality, and migration) and their interaction with resources raise very broad issues about the demographic transition, optimum populations, and man's place in the general ecosystem. The great upsurge of popular interest in the population problem and in the ecology problem is reflected in the larger number of entries under this topic (XII). Since many of the discussions of these issues involve only incidental mention of fertility, we have listed only an illustrative selection.

Items are listed alphabetically by author's name. Where more than one article by the same author appear in the same category the items are chronological, beginning with the earliest work. If more than one monograph by one author was published in the same year, the internal order is again alphabetical by title.

OUTLINE OF THE CLASSIFICATION SYSTEM

consequences, effects, etc. Studies dealing with the field acceptance of various contraceptives by various social groups represent quite a different set of studies with social components, classified elsewhere.) *1585–1609*

XIV. The Effects of Various Intermediate Variables on Fertility

A. Nuptiality status and age at marriage *1610–1629*
B. Child-spacing patterns *1630–1632*
C. Fecundability (including postpartum amenorrhea and coital frequency) *1633–1637*
D. Fetal mortality *1638–1642*
E. Contraception *1643–1646*
F. Combinations of intermediate variables as they affect fertility *1647–1657*

I. GENERAL

I.A General works or collections of papers on population that include treatments of fertility or the intermediate variables

See also: 119.

1

Agarwala, S.N.
Some Problems of India's Population.
Bombay: Vora, 1966; 152p.

Chapters on population growth, nuptiality patterns, widow remarriage and length of fertile union, fertility, sterility, migration and urbanization, population policy, and demographic training and research.

2

American Academy of Arts and Sciences.
"Historical Population Studies". *Daedalus* 97(2), Spring 1968: pp. 353-681.

Articles from two conferences on historical demography; pertinent articles cited separately.

3

Benjamin, B.
Demographic Analysis. New York: Frederick A. Praeger, 1969; 160p.

Manual of demographic methods for the general reader; also relates population trends to social change.

4

Bogue, D.J.
Principles of Demography. New York: John Wiley & Sons, 1968; 917p.

Sections on methodological and descriptive aspects of fertility.

5

Bose, A., ed.
Patterns of Population Change in India, 1951-61. Institute of Economic Growth. Bombay: Allied Publishers, 1967; 403p.

Conference papers, includes some treatment of fertility.

6

Bourgeois-Pichat, J.
Population Growth and Development. International Conciliation, No. 556. New York: Carnegie Endowment for International Peace, 1966; 81p.

Summarizes fertility and population trends in relation to development on basis of papers of 1965 World Population Conference.

7

Brass, W. et al.
The Demography of Tropical Africa. Princeton: Princeton University Press, 1968; 540p.

A monumental work on African demography bringing together data from a wide variety of sources, evaluating them, and developing and applying techniques for making estimates from defective data; includes major methodological contributions in the analysis of fertili-

ty as well as important estimates of levels of fertility and nuptiality.

8
Caldwell, J.C. and Okonjo, C., eds.
The Population of Tropical Africa. A Population Council book. New York: Columbia University Press; London: Longmans, Green, & Co., 1968; 457p.

Forty-seven papers from the First African Population Conference covering fertility, family planning, and their demographic and social correlates.

9
Carr-Saunders, A.M.
World Population: Past Growth and Present Trends. London: Frank Cass, 1964; 336p.

New edition, original published in 1936; reviews world population history up to the 1930s.

10
Drake, M., ed.
Population in Industrialization. London: Methuen, 1969; 200p.

A reader dealing almost entirely with Great Britain.

11
Dublin, L.I.
Factbook on Man, from Birth to Death. 2nd ed. New York: Macmillan, 1965; 465p.

General work on demographic characteristics and health of the American people; chapters on fertility, nuptiality, and the family.

12
Durand, J.D., ed.
"World Population." *The Annals of the American Academy of Political and Social Science* 369, Jan. 1967: pp. 1-140.

Special issue with articles on fertility and its consequences.

13
Ehrlich, P.R. and Ehrlich, A.H.
Population Resources Environment, Issues in Human Ecology. San Francisco: W.H. Freeman, 1970; 383p.

Emphasizes the idea that the world is over-populated and growing at a dangerous pace in relation to the broad ecology of population-resources-environment; demographic analysis is relatively minor.

14
European Population Conference, Strasbourg, 30 Aug.–6 Sept. 1966. *Official Documents of the Conference.* 3 vols. Strasbourg: Council of Europe, 1966. [Papers are in English or French with summaries in the other language.]

Section on fertility.

15
Farmer, R.N. et al., eds.
World Population—The View Ahead: Proceedings of the Conference on World Population Problems held at Indiana University on May 3-6, 1967. International Development Research Center Series, No. 1. Bloomington: Bureau of Business Research, Indiana University 1968; 310p.

Various aspects of population growth, the demographic-economic relationship, and population control.

16
Freedman, R., ed.
Population: The Vital Revolution. Garden City: N.Y., Doubleday, Anchor, 1964; 274p.

Essays originally part of the radio forum series of the U.S. information service.

17
Glass, D.V.
Population Policies and Movements in Europe. 1st ed. 1940. Reprints of Economic Classics. New York: A. M. Kelley, 1967; 490p.
  Reissue of a classic work; new introduction.

18
Heer, D.M., ed.
Readings on Population. Readings in Modern Sociology Series. Englewood Cliffs, N.J.: Prentice-Hall, 1968; 234p.
  Fifteen readings, several on fertility and population policy.

19
Heer, D.M.
Society and Population. Foundations of Modern Sociology Series. Englewood Cliffs, N.J.: Prentice-Hall, 1968; 118p.
  A short introductory text; sections on fertility.

20
Hutchinson, E.P.
The Population Debate: The Development of Conflicting Theories Up to 1900. Boston: Houghton Mifflin, 1967; 466p.
  Review of early theories about socioeconomic consequences of population growth.

21
International Union for the Scientific Study of Population.
Contributed Papers. Sydney Conference, Australia, 21–25 Aug. 1967. Canberra: Australian National University Press, 1967; 1099p.
  Many papers on fertility and related topics.

22
Kammeyer, K.C., ed.
Population Studies: Selected Essays and Research. Chicago: Rand McNally, 1969; 481p.

23
Karl Marx University. Institute of Mathematical Statistics.
First International Demographical Symposium of the Institute of Mathematical Statistics of the Faculty of Economic Sciences, 20–24 Sept. 1966, Leipzig: 1966.
  Thirty-eight leaflets.

24
*Milbank Memorial Fund.
The Interrelations of Demographic, Economic and Social Problems in Selected Underdeveloped Areas. New York: 1954; 200p.
  Articles on fertility.

25
Milbank Memorial Fund.
Emerging Techniques in Population Research. Proceeding of a Round Table at the Thirty-Ninth Annual Conference of the Milbank Memorial Fund, 1962. New York: 1963; 307p.
  Papers on the methodology of fertility measurement and analysis; relevant articles are cited separately in this bibliography.

26
Milbank Memorial Fund.
"Demography and Public Health in Latin America." *Milbank Memorial Fund Quarterly* 42(2, Part 2), Apr. 1964; 359p.
  Papers on data evaluation, demographic research, demographic training, and the relation of demographic changes to health and welfare.

27
Milbank Memorial Fund.
Components of Population Change in La-

tin America. Edited by C.V. Kiser. New York: 1965; 384p.

28
Myrdal, G.
Asian Drama: An Inquiry into the Poverty of Nations. A Twentieth Century Fund Study. New York: Pantheon, 1968; 3 vols.

Extensive study of economic and social development in South and Southeast Asia; includes sections on demographic problems and policies.

29
Nam, C.B., ed.
Population and Society: A Textbook of Readings. Boston: Houghton Mifflin, 1968; 708p.

General reader on population; sections on fertility trends and differentials, the relation of demographic changes to social and economic forces.

30
Petersen, W.
Population. 2nd ed. New York and London: Macmillan, 1969; 735p.

Revision of basic undergraduate text; expanded sections on non-Western countries.

31
Price, D.O., ed.
The 99th Hour: The Population Crisis in the United States. Chapel Hill: University of North Carolina Press, 1967; 130p.

Brief papers on U.S. population, trends, optima, policies, emphasing social problems generated by growth.

32
Royal Society of London.
"A Discussion on Demography." Proceedings of the Royal Society of London, Series B. *Biological Sciences* 159(974), Mar. 1964: pp. 1-255.

Conference papers, many on fertility and the intermediate variables.

33
Sauvy, A.
Fertility and Survival: Population Problems from Malthus to Mao Tse-Tung. New York: Criterion Books, 1961; 287p.

Deals broadly with the role of fertility trends and fertility control as part of a sweeping assessment of the implications of current population trends and policy.

34
Sauvy, A.
General Theory of Population. Translated by C. Campos. Cambridge Group for the History of Population and Social Structure, No. 2. London: Weidenfeld & Nicolson; New York: Basic Books, 1969; 551p.

Major treatment of many aspects of population.

35
Schlesnyak, M.C.
Growth of Population: Consequences and Controls. New York: Gordon and Breach, 1969; 458p.

Verbatim transcript of a 1968 conference of experts from a variety of fields on the consequences of potential population growth and influences that might reduce fertility.

36
Spiegelman, M.
Introduction to Demography. Rev. ed. Cambridge, Mass.: Harvard University Press, 1968; 514p.

A basic text on general demography, with special reference to the United States and Canada.

37

Stockwell, E.G.

Population and People. Chicago: Quadrangle Books, 1968; 307p.

Causes and consequences of major population trends in the United States.

38

Stycos, J.M. and Arias, J., eds.

Population Dilemma in Latin America. Washington: Potomac Books, 1966; 249p.

Conference papers on demographic problems in Latin America; some relevant papers cited separately below.

39

Szabady, E. et al., eds.

Studies on Fertility and Social Mobility. International Demographic Symposium, Budapest, 20-30 Nov., 1962. Budapest: Akadémiai Kiadó, 1964; 331p.

Papers mainly about Central and Eastern Europe on fertility, nuptiality, stratification, and social and geographic mobility.

40

Szabady, E. et al., eds.

World Views of Population Problems. Demographic Committee of the Hungarian Academy of Sciences and Demographic Research Institute. Budapest: Akadémiai Kiadó, 1968; 447p.

English texts of 35 papers first published in the quarterly, Demográfia 10 (2,3,4), 67.

41

Thomlinson, R.

Population Dynamics: Causes and Consequences of World Demographic Change. New York: Random House, 1965; 576p.

Treatment of most of the topics in the present outline.

42

Thomlinson, R.

Demographic Problems: Controversy over Population Control. Belmont, Calif.: Dickenson, 1967; 117p.

Introductory text; discussion of fertility trends and population control programs.

43

Thompson, W.S. and Lewis, D.T.

Population Problems. 5th ed. New York: McGraw-Hill, 1965; 593p.

Revised, updated, and expanded edition.

44

United Nations. Department of Economic and Social Affairs.

Proceedings of the World Population Conference, Belgrade, 30 Aug.-10 Sept. 1965. 4 vols. New York: 1966.

Vol. II is concerned with fertility and family planning.

45

*United Nations. Population Division

The Determinants and Consequences of Population Trends: A Summary of the Findings of Studies on the Relationships between Population Changes and Economic and Social Conditions. ST/SOA/Ser. A/17. New York: 1953; 404p.

Comprehensive treatise on population; considerable discussion—both historical and analytical—of fertility.

46

Vielrose, E.

Elements of the Natural Movement of Population. Translated by I. Dobasz. New York: Pergamon Press, 1965; 288p.

Chapter on births.

47

Wrigley, E.A.

Population and History. World University Library. New York: McGraw-Hill; London: Weidenfeld & Nicolson, 1969; 256p.

> Chapters on historical demography, population and demographic change in preindustrial societies, and on the relation of population changes to the industrial revolution.

48
Young, L.B.
Population in Perspective. New York: Oxford University Press, 1968; 460p.

> Readings on social and biological aspects of population growth.

I.B General texts, histories, or collections of papers concerned mainly with fertility or the major intermediate variables that affect fertility

See also: 758.

49
Agarwala, S.N.
Attitudes toward Family Planning in India. Institute of Economic Growth Occasional Papers, 5. Bombay: Asia Publishing House, 1962; 55p.

> Summarizes main findings of 26 family planning attitude surveys.

50
Barnes. AC., ed.
The Social Responsibility of Gynecology and Obstetrics. Baltimore: Johns Hopkins Press, 1965; 224p.

> Symposium papers covering a wide range of social and medical aspects of fertility and family planning; directed to medical community.

51
Behrman, S.J. et al., eds.
Fertility and Family Planning: A World View. Ann Arbor: University of Michigan Press, 1969; 503p.

> Conference papers on fertility trends, biological aspects of fertility, socioeconomic determinants, and consequences and family planning.

52
Berelson, B., ed.
Family-Planning Programs: An International Survey Study. New York: Basic Books, 1969; 310p.

> Essays describing specific national family planning programs, originally presented as part of the international radio forum series of the U.S. information service.

53
Berelson, B. et al., eds.
Family Planning and Population Programs: A Review of World Developments. Proceedings of the International Conference on Family Planning Programs, Geneva, Aug. 65. Chicago and London: University of Chicago Press; Toronto: University of Toronto Press, 1966; 848p.

> Sixty-one papers and reports comprehensively cover family planning programs with respect to organization, evaluation, research, etc.; specific papers classified under detailed categories of the bibliography.

54
Bogue, D.J., ed.
Sociological Contributions to Family Planning Research. Chicago: Community and Family Study Center, University of Chicago, 1967; 409p.

Papers based on University of Chicago dissertations.

55
Chilman, C.S. and Liu, W.T., eds.
"Family Planning and Fertility Control." *Journal of Marriage and the Family* 30(2), May 1968: pp. 189-366.
Special issue of 20 articles, many of which are cited separately in this bibliography.

56
***Grabill, W. et al.**
The Fertility of American Women. New York: John Wiley & Sons, 1958; 448p.
Comprehensive summary of historical trends and differential fertility in the U.S. based on official census and vital statistics.

57
Greep, R.O., ed.
Human Fertility and Population Problems. Proceedings of the seminar sponsored by the American Academy of Arts and Sciences. Cambridge, Mass.: Schenkman, 1963; 278p.
Biological, economic, medical, and sociological aspects of fertility.

58
Hankinson, R.K.B. and Soewondo, N., eds.
Family Planning and National Development. Proceedings of the Conference of the International Planned Parenthood Foundation, Banding, June 69. London: International Planned Parenthood Foundation, 1969; 260p.
Many organizational aspects of family planning programs.

59
International Planned Parenthood Federation.

Proceedings of the Third Conference of the Region for Europe, Near East and Africa of the International Planned Parenthood Federation. Warsaw, 5-8 June, 1962. Edited by K.V. Earle. International Congress Series, 71. The Hague: Excerpta Medica, 1963; 232p.
National reports, a survey of the demographic situation of the region, and a study group's reports on contraception.

60
International Planned Parenthood Federation.
Proceedings of the Seventh Conference of the International Planned Parenthood Federation. Singapore, 10-16 Feb., 1963. International Congress Series, 72 Amsterdam: Excerpta Medica, 1964; 748p.

61
International Planned Parenthood Federation. Europe and Near East Region.
Preventive Medicine and Family Planning: Proceedings of the Fifth Conference of the Europe and Near East Region of the IPPF. Copenhagen, 5-8 July, 1966. London: 1967; 293p.

62
International Planned Parenthood Federation.
Proceedings of the Eighth International Conference of the International Planned Parenthood Federation. Santiago, Chile, 9-15 Apr. 1967. London: 1967; 537p.
Medical aspects of reproduction, evaluation of family planning programs and contraceptive methods.

63
International Planned Parenthood Federation.

The Role of Family Planning in African Development. Hertford, Eng.: 1968; 72p.

Medical and community welfare development needs in Africa and papers on family planning programs.

64
Kiser, C.V. et al.
Trends and Variations in Fertility in the United States. Vital and Health Statistics Monographs, American Public Health Association. Cambridge, Mass.: Harvard University Press, 1968; 338p.

Comprehensive report on factors associated with fertility on basis of 1960 U.S. census, earlier censuses, and some reference to other sources; treats many factors in varying depth.

65
Liu, W.T., ed.
Family and Fertility. Notre Dame, Ind.: University of Notre Dame Press, 1967; 257p.

Papers of the fifth Notre Dame conference on population; intended to emphasize the relationship of family structure and reproductive behavior.

66
*Milbank Memorial Fund.
Approaches to Problems of High Fertility in Agrarian Societies. New York: 1952; 171p.

Papers presented in the early 1950s dealing with origins and consequences of high fertility in agricultural societies.

67
*Milbank Memorial Fund.
Current Research in Human Fertility. New York: 1955; 164p.

From the 1954 conference of the Fund, papers on then-current research issues in the U.S. and other countries.

68
*Milbank Memorial Fund.
Thirty Years of Research in Human Fertility: Retrospect and Prospect. New York: 1958; 158p.

Papers from the 1958 conference of the Fund.

69
Milbank Memorial Fund.
Current Research on Fertility and Family Planning in Latin America. Proceedings of the Forty-Second Conference of the Milbank Memorial Fund. New York, 17-19 Oct. 1967. Edited by C.V. Kiser. *Milbank Memorial Fund Quarterly* 46(3, Part 2), July 1968; 294p.

Papers on levels and on social and demographic correlates of fertility, abortion, and contraception.

70
Muramatsu, M. et al.
Japan's Experience in Family Planning; Past and Present. Tokyo: Family Planning Federation of Japan, 1967; 124p.

Important papers on Japan's fertility trends, differential fertility, abortion, contraception, and other factors affecting postwar fertility and family planning.

71
*National Bureau of Economic Research.
Demographic and Economic Change in Developed Countries. Princeton: Princeton University Press, 1960; 536p.

Some important papers on fertility in developed countries.

72
Rainwater, L., ed.
"Family Planning in Cross-National Perspective." *Journal of Social Issues* 23(4), Oct. 1967: pp. 1-194.

Short essays and studies on various aspects of family planning in several different countries.

73

Sheps, M.C. and Ridley, J.C., eds.

Public Health and Population Change: Current Research Issues. Pittsburgh: University of Pittsburgh Press, 1966; 557p. [Many of the articles are reprinted in *Journal of Chronic Diseases* 18, Nov. 1965.]

> *Symposium papers from 1964 about fertility, birth control, and related population trend and policy issues.*

74

Stycos, J.M., ed.

Family Planning in Modernizing Societies. Menasha, Wisc.: Marriage and Family Living, 1963; 80p.

> *Special issue devoted to family planning in selected developing societies.*

75

Stycos, J.M., ed.

Human Fertility in Latin America: Sociological Perspectives. Ithaca, N.Y.: Cornell University Press, 1968; 318p.

> *Papers first published between 1955 and 1967; many aspects of social and demographic contexts of fertility.*

76

Thailand. National Research Council.

National Seminar on Population Problems in Thailand. 1st, Bangkok, 1963. Bangkok: 1963; 510p. [In Thai and English.]

> *Papers presented at the seminar concerning population problems and methods of population control in Thailand; for a review of the studies see Gille (399).*

I.C Discussions of important theoretical issues and general reviews of fertility research and research on the major intermediate variables

See also: 113, 377, 429, 656, 712, 937, 1544, 1551, 1653.

77

Berelson, B. and Steiner, G.A.

Human Behavior: An Inventory of Scientific Findings. New York: Harcourt, Brace & World, 1964; 712p.

> *An inventory of behavioral science findings, including references to tested findings about fertility.*

78

Beshers, J.M.

Population Processes in Social Systems. New York: Free Press; London: Collier-Macmillan, 1967; 207p.

> *An attempt to provide a theoretical framework for predicting and understanding fertility and migration behavior, with emphasis on decision theory at the micro level, differentiating rationalistic planners and others; reviews some of important fertility literature and creates a research agenda for further work.*

79

Brackett, J.W.

"The Evolution of Marxist Theories of Population: Marxism Recognizes the Population Problem." *Demography* 5(1), 1968: pp. 158-173.

80

Coale, A.J.

"The Decline of Fertility in Europe

from the French Revolution to World War II." In Behrman et al., eds. (see 51): pp. 3-24.

An important progress report on the Princeton study of the course and correlates of modern Western European fertility decline; challenges conventional views about initiating causes.

81
*Davis, K. and Blake, J.
"Social Structure and Fertility: An Analytic Framework." *Economic Development and Cultural Change* 4(3), Apr. 1956: pp. 211-235.

Classifies the intermediate variables that immediately affect fertility; discusses their level and relation to selected social factors in preindustrial society.

82
Dubey, D.C. and Devgan, A.K.
Family Planning Communications Studies in India. A Review of Findings and Implications of Studies on Communications. Monograph Series, 8. New Delhi: Central Family Planning Institute, 1969; 96p.

Analysis of the role of program and medical personnel, mass media use, personal and group contacts, the goals and effects; annotated bibliography.

83
Easterlin, R.A.
"Towards Socioeconomic Theory of Fertility: A Survey of Recent Research on Economic Factors in American Fertility." In Behrman et al., eds. (see 51): pp. 127-156.

Reviews pertinent research as a basis for developing a theory of fertility in which economic variables are stressed but the role of social variables is made explicit in determining levels of demand for children.

84
*Eversley, D.E.C.
Social Theories of Fertility and the Malthusian Debate. Oxford: Clarendon Press, 1959; 313p.

85
*Freedman, R.
"American Studies of Family Planning: A Review of Major Trends and Issues." In Research in Family Planning. Edited by C.V. Kiser. Princeton: Princeton University Press, 1962: pp. 211-227.

86
Freedman, R.
"Norms for Family Size in Underdeveloped Areas." *Proceedings of the Royal Society* Series (B), 159, 1963: pp. 220-245.

A framework for the concept that norms about family size depend on the functional value of children in the society; illustrative data.

87
Freedman, R.
"The Transition from High to Low Fertility: Challenge to Demographers." *Population Index* 31(4), Oct. 1965: pp. 417-429.

Suggests research issues in current changes in fertility and speculates about trends, taking population policy into account.

88
Glass, D.V.
"Population Growth and Population Policy." In Sheps and Ridley, eds. (see 73): pp. 3-24.

Reviews facts and theories about population growth history in the West as a basis for considering problems of population policy.

44

89

Goldberg, D. and Litton, G.
"Family Planning: Observations and an Interpretive Scheme." In Shorter and Güvenc, eds. (*see* 357): pp. 219-240.

Develops a model in which open access to modern ideas is the crucial intervening variable between socioeconomic and other background variables and contraceptive use; tests this with Turkish data; suggests the objective of a family planning program is to overcome such access barriers in traditional strata.

90

Hawthorn, G.
"Explaining Human Fertility." *Sociology* 2(1), Jan. 1968: pp. 65-78.

Critique of the theoretical framework of current fertility surveys and discussion of desiderata for future research.

91

Hill, R.
"Research on Human Fertility." *International Social Science Journal* (Paris) 20(2), 1968: pp. 226-262.

Survey of changes in the problem and methodological orientations of fertility research; short multilingual bibliography.

92

Kiser, C.V.
"The Growth of American Families Studies: An Assessment of Significance." *Demography* 4(1), 1967: pp. 388-396.

Reviews purpose, methods, and predictive success of the GAF studies.

93

Kozlov, V.I.
"Some Causes of the High Fertility of the Population of Developing Countries." *Proceedings of the World Population Conference, 1965 (see* 44*):* pp. 155-159.

A Soviet demographer's general view that the causes of high fertility come initially from the social and economic conditions of life which in turn affect the desire for children, age at marriage, and other intermediate variables; basic analysis and theory is similar to that of Western demographers, although the rhetoric is different.

94

Levine, A.L.
"Economic Science and Population Theory." *Population Studies* 19(2), Nov. 1965: pp. 139-154.

Reviews the treatment of the relation between economic and demographic phenomena in British and American literature since World War II.

95

Mauldin, W.P.
"Fertility Studies: Knowledge, Attitude and Practice." *Studies in Family Planning* 7, June 1965: pp. 1-10.

General survey of results of many KAP studies on fertility rates, ideal family size, family planning; section on validity of attitude responses.

96

Mohanty, S.P.
"A Review of Some Selected Studies on Abortion in India." *Journal of Family Welfare* (Bombay) 14(4), June 1968: pp. 39-48.

97

National Academy of Sciences. Committee and Public Policy.
The Growth of World Population: Analysis of the Problems and Recommendations for Research and Training. National Research Council Publication 1091. Washington: Government Printing Office, 1963; 38p.

A summary review of trends and broad policy recommendations.

98
Pohlman, E.
The Psychology of Birth Planning. Cambridge, Mass.: Schenkman, 1969; 496p.
Extensive review of the psychological aspects of actual and desired fertility, unwanted fertility, and birth control; general survey of the literature and an extensive bibliography.

99
Robinson, W.C.
"The Development of Modern Population Theory." *American Journal of Economics and Sociology* 23(4), Oct. 1964: pp. 351-392.
A review of modern population theories and their historical predecessors.

100
Robinson, W.C. and Horlacher, D.E.
"Evaluating the Economic Benefits of Fertility Reduction." *Studies in Family Planning* 1(39), Mar. 1969: pp. 4-8.
Reviews recent literature in the context of two major trends in economic analysis of fertility control.

101
*Ryder, N.B.
"Fertility." *The Study of Population: An Inventory and Appraisal* Chicago: University of Chicago Press, 1959: pp. 400-436.

102
Ryder, N.B.
"Notes on the Concept of a Population." *American Journal of Sociology* 69(5), Mar. 1964: pp. 447-463.
Theoretical framework of a population for both micro- and macroanalysis of social change.

103
Ryder, N.B.
"The Character of Modern Fertility." In *Annals of the American Academy of Science* 369, Jan. 1967: pp. 26-36.
An attempt to characterize in general terms the varying paths to low fertility in urbanized and industrialized countries, with emphasis on the normative change in the relation between children and parents.

104
Sadvokasova, E.A.
"Birth Control Measures and Their Influence on Population Replacement." In *Proceedings of the World Population Conference, 1965 (see 44):* pp. 110-114.
Urbanization, development, and especially involvement of women in the economy leads to lower fertility with birth control as a means, which will otherwise be ineffective; argues that lower fertility in some Western countries is due to unemployment not found in socialist countries.

105
Sheps, M.C. and Ridley, J.C.
"Emerging Research Issues." In Sheps and Ridley, eds. *(see* 73): pp. 501-517.
Review of major research issues emerging from a conference on public health and population change.

106
Spengler, J.J.
"The Economist and the Population Question." *American Economic Review* 56(1), Mar. 1966: pp. 1-24.
Historical review of the intellectual interest of economists in demographic change.

107
Spengler, J.J.
"Values and Fertility Analysis." *Demography* 3(1), 1966: pp. 109-130.

How norms and values effect fertility, with reference to economic value theory.

108
Stycos, J.M.
"Needed Research on Latin American Fertility: Urbanization and Fertility." *Milbank Memorial Fund Quarterly* 43(4, Part 2) Oct. 1965: pp. 299-323.
Survey of areas for further research: urbanization patterns, fertility, nuptiality, and contraception use and attitudes.

109
Tien, H.Y.
"The Intermediate Variables, Social Structure, and Fertility Change: A Critique." *Demography* 5(1), 1968: pp. 138-157.
Critique of the intermediate variables concept; suggests that demographic, institutional, and information variables are of great importance in studying the sociology of fertility.

110
Yasukawa, M.
"The Population Problem of Japan and the Trend of Its Study." *Keio Economic Studies* 4, 1966-67: pp. 94-107.
Review of selected studies published mainly in Japan between 1933 and 1967; bibliographical footnotes.

111
Yaukey, D.
"On Theorizing about Fertility." *American Sociologist* 4(2), May 1969: pp. 100-104.
Suggests new research approach to intermediate variables and the variables that affect them.

I.D Bibliographies dealing with fertility and related variables

See also: 82, 98, 270, 620, 977, 985.

112
Aldous, J. and Hill, R., compilers.
International Bibliography of Research in Marriage and the Family, 1960-1964. Minneapolis: University of Minnesota Press for Minnesota Family Study Center and the Institute of Life Insurance, 1967; 508p.
About 13,000 items with many references pertinent to fertility and family planning.

113
Freedman, R.
"The Sociology of Human Fertility: A Trend Report and Bibliography." *Current Sociology* 10-11(2), 1961-1962: pp. 35-121.
Major review of the sociological research in human fertility since World War II, with an annotated bibliography; the earlier bibliography and trend report on which this bibliography is based.

114
Fuguitt, G.V.
Dissertations in Demography 1933-1963. Madison: College of Agriculture, Department of Rural Sociology, University of Wisconsin, 1964; 72p.
Lists doctoral dissertations from U.S. universities.

115
Geijerstam, G.K.
An Annotated Bibliography of Induced Abortion. Ann Arbor: Center for Population Planning, University of Michigan, 1969; 359p.
Bibliography of studies covering all aspects of induced abortion.

116
Hill, R.
"A Classified International Bibliography of Family Planning Research 1955-68 and Commentary." *Demography* 5(2), 1968: pp. 973-1001.

117
Kapil, K.K. and Saksena, D.N.
A Bibliography of Sterilization and KAP Studies in India. Bombay: Demographic Training and Research Centre (Chembur), 1968; 38p.

> *Extensive bibliography, including 202 sterilization studies and 241 KAP studies; reports listed are in mimeographed form; represents the large number and wide variety of Indian studies, which range from news notes to detailed scientific treatises.*

118
Kasdon, D.L.
International Family Planning 1966-1968: A Bibliography. Chevy Chase, Md.: National Institute of Mental Health, 1969; 62p.

119
Marsh, R.M.
"Comparative Sociology, 1950-1963: A Trend Report and Bibliography." *Current Sociology* 14(2), 1966: pp. 1-152.

> *Comparative sociological studies: a review of the literature and a classified, annotated bibliography including items on demography and the family.*

120
Meier, G.
"Research and Action Programs in Human Fertility Control: A Review of the Literature." *Social Work: Journal of the National Association of Social Workers* 11(3), July 1966: pp. 40-55.

> *Lists recent reports on birth control programs.*

121
Population Reference Bureau.
"A Sourcebook on Population." *Population Bulletin* 25(5), Nov. 1969; 51p.

> *Annotated bibliography of demographic literature; lists of population training centers, libraries, and private and government organizations.*

122
Tietze, C., ed.
Selected Bibliography of Contraception: 1940-1960. New York: National Committee on Maternal Health, 1960; 76p.

123
Tietze, C., ed.
Bibliography of Fertility Control 1950-1965. New York: National Committee on Maternal Health, 1965; 198p.

124
Tietze, C. and Neumann, L., eds.
Surgical Sterilization of Men and Women: A Selected Bibliography. New York: National Committee on Maternal Health, 1962; 38p.

125
United Nations.
Family Planning, Internal Migration and Urbanization in ECAFE Countries. New York: 1968; 66p.

> *Bibliography of available studies on Asian population trends and family planning.*

126
University of Lucknow. Demographic Research Center.
Demography and Development Digest 1(1), 1967; 168p.

Annotated bibliography and current news of demographic development topics; the first volume of a continuing series.

127
University of North Carolina. Carolina Population Center. Educational Materials Unit.
Family Planning Educational Materials: An Annotated Bibliography of Selected Items. Chapel Hill: University of North Carolina, 1968; 89p.
Bibliography of education and training materials used in family planning programs.

I.E Multivariate analyses of the relation to fertility or to intermediate variables or sets of other variables cutting across the basic categories of the bibliography

See also: 303, 507, 966, 1310.

128
Adelman, I.
"An Econometric Analysis of Population Growth." *American Economic Review* 53(3), June 1963: pp. 314-339.
Regression analysis of fertility rates on indexes of industrialization using international data for the period 1947–57.

129
Adelman, I. and Morris, C.T.
"A Quantitative Study of Social and Political Determinants of Fertility."

Economic Development and Cultural Change 14(2), Jan. 1966: pp. 129-157.
Using factor analysis for cross-sectional analysis of a large number of variables for 1957-62, proposes a set of four underlying factors to explain variations in the crude birth rate in developing countries; suggests important hypotheses but sources and validity for some key sets of data not clear.

130
Collver, A. et al.
"Local Variations of Fertility in Taiwan." *Population Studies* 20(3), Mar. 1967: pp. 329-342.
Multivariate analysis of socioeconomic and demographic factors in areal fertility and nuptiality rates.

131
Friedlander, S. and Silver, M.
"A Quantitative Study of the Determinants of Fertility Behavior," *Demography* 4(1), 1967: pp. 30-70.
A cross-national regression analysis of socio-economic, political, and cultural determinants of fertility.

132
Hathaway, D.E., et al.
People of Rural America. Washington: Government Printing Office, 1968; 289p.
1960 U.S. census monography with two chapters (IV and V) on fertility trends and differentials involving rural-urban-metropolitan classifications in multivariate relations to region, race, education, wife's labor-force status, occupation, income, and demographic control variables.

133
Heer, D.M.
"Economic Development and Fertility." *Demography* 3(2), 1966: pp. 423-444.

Factor analysis used on cross-sectional data to study relationship of fertility to economic growth and associated factors such as functional literacy, infant mortality, energy consumption and population density.

134
Heer, D.M. and Turner, E.S.
"Areal Differences in Latin American Fertility." *Population Studies* 18(3), Mar. 1965: pp. 279-292.

Uses census data (circa 1950) for local areas within 18 Latin American countries to measure relationship of certain development indexes to fertility.

135
Liu, P.K.C.
"Socio-economic Development and Fertility Levels in Taiwan." *Industry of Free China* (Taipei) 24(2), Aug. 1965: pp. 2-17.

Multivariate analysis using as the basic unit Taiwan's 361 local administrative units; overlaps with analysis by Collver et al. (see 130).

136
Mazur, P.
"Birth Control and Regional Differentials in the Soviet Union." *Population Studies* 22(3), Nov. 1968: pp. 319-333.

Multivariate anaylysis of differences in child-woman ratios related to male and female literacy, female dependency, and proportion married for areas differing in contraceptive use and urbanization.

137
Paydarfar, A.A.
"Modernization Process and Demographic Changes." *Sociological Review* 15(2), July 1967: pp. 141-153.

Data from 10 countries and 13 provinces of Iran used to analyze the relation of indexes of industrialization, education, and urbanization to age-sex composition, marital and occupational fertility, and migration patterns.

138
Schultz, T.P.
A Family Planning Hypothesis: Some Empirical Evidence from Puerto Rico. Memorandum RM-5405-RC/AID. Santa Monica, Calif.: RAND Corporation, 1967; 76p.

Hypothesis that inferences about desired family size can be made from knowledge of mortality conditions, inferences about uncertainty in the family life cycle and environmental factors; regression analysis of data from 1890s and 1950s of the relation of mortality-level changes, education, female labor-force participation, percent married, and urbanization to fertility.

II. MEASUREMENT TECHNIQUES AND PROBLEMS

II.A Fertility or family size

See also: 80, 101, 261, 264, 270, 318, 337, 338, 352, 378, 397, 424, 430, 500, 508, 533, 738, 794, 809, 1133, 1365, 1470, 1515.

139
Acsádi, G.
"Fertility Forecasts on Basis of Cohort Numbers of Children." In Szabady et al., eds. (*see* 39): pp. 83-94.
Illustrates from the Hungarian experience, superiority of cohort to period rates in projections.

140
Acsádi, G.
"Measuring Fertility Trends: Cohort Fertility in Hungary." In Szabady et al., eds. (*see* 40): pp. 365-386.

141
Arretx, G. et al.
"Survey Methods, Based on Periodically repeated Interviews, Aimed at Determining Demographic Rates." *Demography* 2, 1965; pp. 289-301.
Describes survey method to estimate vital rates that claims to be only slightly affected by data omission.

142
Bogue, D.J. and Palmore, J.A.
"Some Empirical and Analytic Relations among Demographic Fertility Measures, with Regression Models for Fertility and Estimation." *Demography* 1(1), 1964: pp. 316-338.
Develops regression equations with which one set of fertility paramaters can be used to estimate others.

143
Choldin, H.M. et al.
"Cultural Complications in Fertility Interviewing." *Demography* 4(1), 1967: pp. 244-252.
Description of interviewing process in Pakistani area of low literacy and little experience with social research.

144
Coale, A.J.
"The Use of Fourier Analysis to Express the relation between Time Variations in Fertility and the Time Sequence of Births in a Closed Human Population." *Demography* 7(1), Feb. 1970: pp. 93-120.

145
Collver, O.A.
Birth Rates in Latin America: New Estimates of Historical Trends and Fluctuations. Institute of International Studies,

Research Series, 7. Berkeley: University of California Press, 1965; 187p.

Estimates birth rates for 20 countries after discussing problems of adjustment and estimation.

146
Coombs, L. and Freedman, R.
"Use of Telephone Interviews in a Longitudinal Fertility Study." *Public Opinion Quarterly* 28(1), Spring 1968: pp. 112-117.

Methodology of obtaining data at low cost and high response rate, via telephone in the U.S.

147
Dandekar, K.
"Standard Errors of Age-Specific Fertility Rates." *Artha Vijñāna* (Poona) 4(4), Dec. 1962: pp. 343-346.

Standard errors of fertility rates may be so large as to make trends indeterminate.

148
Demeny, P.
"A Minimum Program for the Estimation of Basic Fertility Measures from Censuses of Population in Asian Countries with Inadequate Demographic Statitics." In 1967 I.U.S.S.P. (*see* 21): pp. 818-825.

Important statement of how censuses can be used for obtaining key fertility paramaters in the absence of adequate vital statistics (for a more complete statement see 338).

149
El-Badry, M.A.
"An Evaluation of the Parity Data Collected on Birth Certificates in Bombay City." *Milbank Memorial Fund Quarterly* 40(3), July 1962: pp. 328-355.

Tests accuracy of information on birth certificates with information from detailed survey interviews; shows that fetal and child mortality is a principal cause of error.

150
Grabill, W.H. and Cho. L.J.
"Methodology for the Measurement of Current Fertility from Population Data on Young Children." *Demography* 2, 1965: pp. 50-73.

Procedures for deriving period measures of fertility from child-woman ratios and survival rates.

151
*Hajnal, J.
"The Analysis of Birth Statistics in the Light of the Recent International Recovery of the Birth Rate." *Population Studies* 1(2), Sept. 1947: pp. 138-164.

Important Methodological discussion of the relation of period and cohort rates for both nuptial and total fertility.

152
Henry, L.
"The Verification of Data in Historical Demography." *Population Studies* 22(1), Mar. 1968; pp. 61-81.

Methods of checking accuracy of registration records.

153
*Hyrenius, H.
"Reproduction and Replacement, A Methodological Study of Swedish Population Changes during 200 Years." *Population Studies* 4(2), Mar. 1951: pp. 421-431.

154
India. Office of the Registrar General. Vital Statistics Division.
Sample Registration in India. Report on

Pilot Studies in Urban Areas 1964-67. New Delhi: 1969; 24p.

Methodological history of the pilot studies to measure vital rates by matching results of sample surveys and continuous registration agents.

155
*Karmel, P.H.
"An Analysis of the Sources and Magnitudes of Inconsistencies between Male and Female Net Reproduction Rates in Actual Populations." *Population Studies* 2(2), Sept. 1948: pp. 240-273.

156
Keyfitz, N. et al.
"On the Interpretation of Age Distributions." *Journal of the American Statistical Association* 62(319), Sept. 1967: pp. 862-874.

Describes unified method of inferring birth rates and other vital rates from age distributions.

157
Khan, M.R.
"Estimation of Fertility in Pakistan." *Pakistan Economic Journal* (Dacca) 15, 1965: pp. 32-45.

Fertility estimates based on quasi-stable population models in relation to population estimates by a combination of registration and survey procedures.

158
Khan M.R. and Bean, L.L.
"Interrelationships of Some Fertility Measures in Pakistan." *Pakistan Development Review* (Karachi) 7(4), Winter 1967: pp. 504-518.

Evaluates several fertility measures obtained in Population Growth Estimation project, their interrelationships, and the possible impact on fertility of a rise in the age at marriage.

159
Krotki, K.J. and Ahmed, N.
"Vital Rates in East and West Pakistan: Tentative Results from the PGE Experiment." *Pakistan Development Review* (Karachi) 4(4), Winter 1964: pp. 734-759.

Description of method and presentation of estimates of vital rates derived from Population Growth Estimation experiment.

160
Kusukawa, A.
"A Demographic Model of Fertility Related to Coitus for Populations Not Practicing Family Limitation." *Kyushu Journal of Medical Science* (Fukuoka) 14(6), Dec. 1963: pp. 369-378.

Develops intrinsic crude birth rates and net reproduction rates according to level of sexual activity in terms of coital frequency, controlled for age and whether coitus is spaced.

161
Liu, P.C.
The Use of Household Registration Records in Measuring the Fertility Levels of Taiwan. Translated by W.L. Parish. Economic Papers, Selected English Series, No. 2. Taipei: Academia Sinica, Institute of Economics, 1967; 70p.

Survey results used to examine errors in estimation of fertility indexes from registration data.

162
Mauldin, W.P.
"Estimating Rates of Population

Growth." In Berelson et al., eds. (*see* 53): pp. 635-653.

Use of various combinations of sample surveys and registration schemes for estimating fertility and other population paramaters.

163
Mazur, D.P.
"A Demographic Model for Estimating Age-Order Specific Fertility Rates." *Journal of the American Statistical Association* 58(303), Sept. 1963: pp. 774-788.

Methods of estimating age- and order-specific birth rates from other parameters.

164
Mazur, D.P.
"The Graduation of Age-Specific Fertility Rates by Order of Birth of Child." *Human Biology* 39(1), Feb. 1967: pp. 53-64.

165
Mitra, S.
"Model Fertility Tables." *Sankhyā* (Calcutta) (Series B) 27(1-2), Sept. 1965: pp. 193-200.

Constructs a set of model age-specific fertility tables from general fertility rates.

166
Mitra, S.
"The Pattern of Age-Specific Fertility Rates." *Demography* 4(2), 1967: pp. 894-906.

Graduated equation model for age-specific fertility rates and application to data from 50 countries.

167
Mosley, H. et al.
Demographic Studies in Rural East Pakistan. Dacca: Pakistan-S.E.A.T.O. Cholera Research Laboratory, 1968; 26p.

Preliminary analysis of results of daily registration of vital events in vaccine field trial area in Comilla District.

168
Myers, G.C. and Gibson, J.R.
"Cohort Disaggregation Analysis of Fertility Data from a Sample Survey." *Demography* 6(1), Feb. 1969: pp. 17-26.

169
Naeem, J.
"Factors Affecting Vital Rates and Their Estimation in a Limited Geographic Area of a Developing Country." In 1967 I.U.S.S.P. (*see* 21): pp. 884-895.

Case-study exposition of the problems that affect both the level and the measurement of vital rates where normal registration is deficient; illustrates how health services may affect what is being measured.

170
Ravenholt, R.T. and Frederiksen, H.
"Numerator Analysis of Fertility Patterns." *Public Health Reports* 83(6), June 1968: pp. 449-457.

Outlines a technique for obtaining birth ratios when numerators and denominators that match in time and place are lacking.

171
Rele, J.R.
Fertility Analysis through Extension of Stable Population Concepts. Institute of International Studies, Population Monograph Series, 2. Berkeley: University of California Press, 1967; 91p.

Exposition of the rationale of quasi-stable population theory and its application to estimating reproductive levels in countries with incomplete statistics.

172
Rosenberg, H.M.
"Recent Developments in Seasonally

Adjusting Vital Statistics." *Demography* 3(2), 1966: pp. 305-318.

"Ratio-to-moving-average" method used to eliminate seasonal fluctuations in monthly marriage and vital rates.

173
Sagi, P.C. and Westoff, C.F.
"An Exercise in Partitioning Some Components of the Variance of Family Size." *Emerging Techniques in Population Research.* Proceedings of the 1962 Annual Conference of the Milbank Memorial Fund. New York: Milbank Memorial Fund, 1963: pp. 130-140.

174
Seltzer, W.
"Some Results from Asian Population Growth Studies." *Population Studies* 23(3), Nov. 1969: pp. 395-406.

Review of 19 studies in five Asian countries in which two independent collection systems can be compared as to completeness of reporting births and deaths; an important collection of results of such estimation techniques.

175
Sengupta, J.M.
"On the Validity of Fertility Data Collected through Interviews." *Sankhyā* (Calcutta) (Series B) 28(3-4), Dec. 1966: pp. 259-268.

Examines the problems of interview recall over varying time periods, in India.

176
Sengupta, J.M.
"Sampling Errors in the Estimation of Fertility Rates." *Sankhyā* (Calcutta)(Series B) 30(3-4), Dec. 1968: pp. 447-454.

177
Singh, R.P.
"On a Model for Couple Fertility." *Sankhyā* (Calcutta) (Series B) 29(3-4), Dec. 1967: pp. 319-320.

Outlines procedure for application of probability distribution derived by S.N. Singh (see 178).

178
Singh, S.N.
"Probability Models for the Variation in the Number of Births per Couple." *Journal of the American Statistical Association* 58(303), Sept. 1963: pp. 721-727.

Describes procedure for estimating parameters and applies model to two examples.

179
Singh, S.N.
"A Chance Mechanism of the Variation in the Number of Births per Couple." *Journal of the American Statistical Association* 63(321), Mar. 1968: pp. 209-213.

Derives and tests a probability distribution for the variation in the number of births per couple.

180
Sirken, M.G. and Sabagh, G.
"Evaluation of Birth Statistics Derived Retrospectively from Fertility Histories Reported in a National Population Survey: United States, 1945-64." *Demography* 5(1), 1968: pp. 485-503.

Evaluates retrospective estimates of births from the U.S. current population survey in 1965, by comparison with adjusted birth registration data controlled for race, age of mother, and birth order.

181
Srinivasan, K. and Muthiah, A.
"Problems of Matching of Births Inden-

tified from Two Independent Sources."
Journal of Family Welfare (Bombay)
14(4), June 1968: pp. 13-22.

182
Starovskii, V.N.
"The Technique of Studying the Components of Population Growth." *Soviet Soçiology* 6(1-2), Summer-Fall 1967: pp. 34-44.

Includes international comparison of crude birth rates and of expectation of life at birth.

183
Tekse, K.
"On Demographic Models of Age-Specific Fertility Rates." *Statistisk Tidskrift* (Stockholm) (3rd Series) 5(3), 1967: pp. 189-207.

Empirical models for age-specific fertility rates, based on 1961 data for Hungary.

184
United Nations. Department of Economic and Social Affairs.
"National Programmes of Analysis of Population Data as an Aid to Planning and Policy-Making." *Population Studies* 36, ST/SOA/Ser.A/36, New York: 1964; 67p.

Methodology and case-study analyzes of utilization of census data, including fertility measures.

185
Van de Kaa, D.J.
"The Estimation of Fertility from Census or Survey Data: As Exemplified by a Quasi-Stable Estimate of Papua and New Guinea's Birth Rate." *Tijdschrift voor Economische en Sociale Geografie* 59, Nov.-Dec. 1968: pp. 313-325.

186
Wells, H.B. and Agrawal, B. L.
"Sample Registration in India." *Demography* 4(1), 1967: pp. 374-387.

Description of sample registration project in rural areas.

187
*Whelpton, P.K.
"Reproduction Rates Adjusted for Age, Parity, Fecundity, and Marriage." *Journal of the American Statistical Association* 41(236), Dec. 1946: pp. 501-516.

An early analysis emphasizing the decomposition of fertility rates into factors that help to explain discrepancy between period and cohort rates.

188
*Whelpton, P.K.
Cohort Fertility, Native White Women in the United States Princeton: Princeton University Press, 1954; 492p.

Important early development and application of the cohort approach for analyzing fertility trends.

189
Whelpton, P. K.
"Cohort Analysis and Fertility Projections." *Emerging Techniques in Population Research.* Proceedings of the 1962 Annual Conference of the Milbank Memorial Fund. New York: 1963: pp. 39-64.

190
*Whelpton, P.K. and Campbell, A.A.
Fertility Tables for Birth Cohorts of American Women. Washington: U. S. Office of Vital Statistics, 51(1), 1960; 129p.

Important set of data on cohort fertility trends in the U.S. with illustrations of their utility and methodological discussions.

191
Yaukey, D. et al.
"Husbands' vs. Wives' Responses to a Fertility Survey." *Population Studies* 19(1), July 1965: pp. 29-43.
Analyzes discrepancies between husband and wife responses on a fertility survey in Pakistan.

II.B Important intermediate variables

II.B.1 Fecundity and its biological correlates
See also: 210, 220, 270, 1253, 1360, 1365, 1500, 1578, 1633, 1655, 1657.

192
Ebanks, G.E.
"Users and Non-Users of Contraception: Regression Analysis and Tests of Stationarity Applied to Members of a Family Planning Program." *Population Studies* 24(1), Mar. 1970: pp. 85-91.
Markov-chain analyses used to test the stationarity of the transition probabilities from user to nonuser and nonuser to user state over the program period; data from a survey of clients from Barbados.

193
Eckland, B.K.
"Genetics and Sociology: A Reconsideration." *American Sociological Review* 32(3), Apr. 1967: pp. 173-194.
Discusses relevance of demography and sociology in genetic studies.

194
Henry, L.
"Some Comments on W.H. James's Article." *Population Studies* 18(2), Nov. 1964: pp. 175-180.
Critical evaluation of estimates of fecundability by indirect methods in the study by James (see 195).

195
James, W.H.
"Estimates of Fecundability." *Population Studies* 17(1), July 1963: pp. 57-65.
Methods of estimating fecundability from distributions of completed family size.

196
James, W.H.
"Fecundability Estimates: Some Comments on L. Henry's Paper." *Population Studies* 18(2), Nov. 1964: pp. 181-186.
Rejoinder to comments by Henry (see 194).

197
Mooney, H.W. et al.
"Use of Telephone Interviewing to Study Human Reproduction." *Public Health Reports* 83(12), Dec. 1968: pp. 1049-1060.
Report on a U.S. study to collect information about resumption of menstruation and related data; from telephone interviews.

198
*Potter, R.G., Jr.
"Length of the Fertile Period." *Milbank Memorial Fund Quarterly* 39(1), Jan. 1961: pp. 132-162.

199
Potter, R.G., Jr.
"Birth Intervals: Structure and Change." *Population Studies* 17(2), Nov. 1963: pp. 155-166.

Estimates total length and component parts of birth intervals for samples not using contraception; has both methodological and substantive importance.

200
Potter, R.G., Jr. et al.
"Delays in Conception: A Discrepancy Re-examined." *Eugenics Quarterly* 10(2), June 1963: pp. 53-58.

An attempt to determine by survey interviews the basis for discrepant reports from different sources on birth intervals without contraception.

201
Potter, R.G., Jr. and Parker, M.P.
"Predicting the Time Required to Conceive." *Population Studies* 18(1), July 1964: pp. 99-116.

Waiting-time model used to estimate expected time to conception following specified past delays in conception.

202
Sheps, M.C.
"On the Time Required for Conception." *Population Studies* 18(1), July 1964: pp. 85-97.

An extension of models of distributions of fecundability, with emphasis on the time required for conception under various conditions.

203
Wolfers, D.
"Determinants of Birth Intervals and Their Means." *Population Studies* 22(2), July 1968: pp. 253-262.

Method for analyzing birth intervals to derive fecundability estimates.

II.B.2 Contraception and family planning
See also: 799, 806, 809, 816, 834, 920, 979, 1021, 1107, 1236, 1500, 1657.

204
Allingham, J.D. et al.
"Time Series of Growth in Use of Oral Contraception and the Differential Diffusion of Oral Anovulents." *Population Studies* 23(1), Mar. 1969: pp. 43-51.

Data from Toronto, Canada, used to illustrate possible sources of bias in reporting of educational, ethnic, and religious differential of oral contraception use.

205
Bailar, J.C., III and Gurian, J.
"The Medical Significance of Date of Birth." *Eugenics Quarterly* 14(2), June 1967: pp. 89-102.

Reviews the literature since 1937 to clarify problems in relating seasonality of births to medical conditions.

206
Bardis, P.D.
"A Pill Scale: A Technique for the Measurement of Attitudes toward Oral Contraception." *Social Science* 44(1), Jan. 1969: pp. 35-42.

207
de Bethune, A.J.
"Rhythm-Mathematical Probability of Success and Failure." *Journal of the International College of Surgeons* 43, Mar. 1965: pp. 327-333.

208
Enke, S. and O'Hara, D.J.
"Estimating Fertility Changes from Birth Control Measures." *Studies in Family Planning* 1(46), Oct. 1969: pp. 1-5.

Uses model based on proportion of women exposed and use-effectiveness as a basis for analysis of the economic efficiency of contraception and abortion programs.

209
Green, L.W.
"East Pakistan: Knowledge and Use of Contraceptives." *Studies in Family Planning* 1(39), Mar. 1969: pp. 9-14.

Model for estimating underreporting in contraception survey responses, by age, socioeconomic status, and family growth patterns.

210
James, W.H.
"Parameters of the Menstrual Cycle and the Efficiency of Rhythm Methods of Contraception." *Population Studies* 19(1), July 1965: pp. 45-64.

Criticism and review of theoretical models.

211
James, W.H.
"A Note of Correction with Reference to Parameters of the Menstrual Cycle and the Efficiency of Rhythm Methods of Contraception." *Population Studies* 22(2), July 1968: pp. 281-282.

Correction of data presented in an earlier article (see 210), with additional conclusions and comments.

212
James, W.H.
"The Mathematics of the Menstrual Cycle." *Population Studies* 22(3), Nov. 1968: pp. 409-413.

Rejoinder to comments by Potter (see 220) on James' studies of the rhythm of menstrual cycles and its relation to fertility control.

213
Kantner, J.F. and Zelnik, M.
"United States: Exploratory Studies of Negro Family Formation—Common Conceptions about Birth Control." *Studies in Family Planning* 1(47), Nov. 1969: pp. 10-13.

A report on an attempt to explore Negro attitudes and vocabulary in this field by use of videotaped small-group discussions.

214
Lasagna, L.
"The Quantification of Desired and Undesired Effects of Reproductive Controls: Some Principles and Problems." In Sheps and Ridley, eds. (*see* 73): pp. 450-459.

A critique of experimental designs used in evaluating contraceptive control methods.

215
*Poti, S.J. et al.
"Reliability of Data Relating to Contraceptive Practices." In *Research in Family Planning.* Edited By C.V. Kiser, Princeton: Princeton University Press, 1962; pp. 51-65

216
Potter, R.G., Jr.
"Length of the Observation Period as a Factor Affecting the Contraceptive Failure Rate." *Milbank Memorial Fund Quarterly* 38(2), Apr. 1960: pp. 140-152.

217
*Potter, R.G., Jr.
"Some Relationships between the Short Range and Long Range Risks of Unwanted Pregnancy." *Milbank Memorial Fund Quarterly* 38(3), July 1960: pp. 255-263.

218
Potter, R.G., Jr.
"Additional Measures of Use-Effective-

ness of Contraception." *Milbank Memorial Fund Quarterly* 41(4, Part 1), Oct. 1963: pp. 400-418.

Develops life-table method of assessing effectiveness of contraceptive use to adjust for fact that the longer the period of observation the more selected the users are for low risk of failure.

219
Potter, R.G., Jr.
"Application of Life Table Techniques to Measurement of Contraceptive Effectiveness." *Demography* 3(2), 1966; pp. 297-304.

220
Potter, R.G., Jr.
"Parameters of the Menstrual Cycle: A Reply." *Population Studies* 20(2) Nov. 1966: pp. 223-232.

Reply to papers by James (see 210): discusses use of rhythm method and the quality of James' data and analysis.

221
Potter, R.G., Jr.
"The Multiple Decrement Life Table as an Approach to the Measurement of Use Effectiveness and Demographic Effectiveness of Contraception." In 1967 I.U.S.S.P. (*see* 21): pp. 869-883.

222
Potter, R.G., Jr. and Tietze, C.
"A Statistical Model of the Rhythm Method." In *Emerging Techniques of Population Research.* Proceedings of the 1962 Annual Conference of the Milbank Memorial Fund. New York: Milbank Memorial Fund, 1963: pp. 141-158.

223
Stoeckel, J. and Choudhury, M.A.
"Pakistan: Response Validity in a KAP Survey." *Studies in Family Planning* 1(47), Nov. 1969: pp. 5-9.

Merchants' records of sales of contraceptives give higher rates than survey response of customer, with underestimation especially high for those living in extended families and those not in sponsoring cooperative.

224
Tietze, C.
"Intra-Uterine Contraception: Recommended Procedures for Data Analysis." *Studies in Family Planning* (Supplement) 18, Apr. 1967: pp. 1-6.

225
Tietze, C. and Potter, R.G., Jr.
"Statistical Evaluation of the Rhythm Method." *American Journal of Obstetrics and Gynecology* 84(5), Sept. 1962: pp. 692-698.

226
***Westoff, C.F. et al.**
"Some Estimates of the Reliability of Survey Data of Family Planning." *Population Studies* 15(1), July 1961: pp. 52-69.

Important analysis of the reliability of reports on fetal deaths and contraceptive practice based on reinterviews after three years with the sample of the Princeton study (see 1534).

227
***Whelpton, P.K. and Kiser, C.V.**
"The Planning of Fertility." In Kiser and Whelpton, eds. (*see* 1512) Vol. 2: pp. 209-258.

Discusses the classification of couples by fertility planning success in the Indianapolis study.

II.B.3 Nuptiality

See also: 172, 630, 1268, 1295, 1627.

228
Bhate, V.
"Decline in Mortality and Change in Age at Marriage as Factors Affecting Incidence of Widowhood." *Artha Vijñāna* (Poona) 6(2), June 1964: pp. 92-105.

Estimation of interrelations between age-specific mortality rates and average age at marriage and the ratio of widows to ever-married women; illustration from Indian data.

229
Gilbert, J.P. and Hammel, E.A.
"Computer Simulation and Analysis of Problems in Kinship and Social Structure." *American Anthropologist* 68(1), Feb. 1966: pp. 71-93.

Computer program used to study kinship and marriage structure, with methodological discussion.

230
***Hajnal, J.**
"Age at Marriage and Proportions Marrying." *Population Studies* 7(2), Nov. 1953: pp. 111-136.

An important discussion of the post World War II increase in marriage rates in the Western world and of methods of measuring it.

231
Kunstadter, P. et al.
"Demographic Variability and Preferential Marriage Patterns." *American Journal of Physical Anthropology* 21(4), Dec. 1963: pp. 511-519.

Computer simulation model of marriage patterns based on specific demographic and marriage preference assumptions.

232
Mertens, W.
"Methodological Aspects of the Con-

struction of Nuptiality Tables." *Demography* 2, 1965: pp. 317-348.

233
Pollard, J.H.
"A Discrete-Time Two-Sex Age-Specific Stochastic Population Program Incorporating Marriage." *Demography* 6(2), May 1969: pp. 185-221.

Computer simulation model for projecting marriage probabilities and distributions.

234
Price, C.A. and Zubrzycki, J.
"Immigrant Marriage Patterns in Australia." *Population Studies* 16(2), Nov. 1962: pp. 123-133.

Develops two intermarriage indexes and discusses other social factors that explain marriage patterns.

235
Ryder, N.B.
"Measures of Recent Nuptiality in the Western World." In *International Population Conference.* New York, 1961. London: U.N.E.S.C.O., 1963: pp. 293-301.

Comparative nuptiality levels for countries with available data for preceding 40 years, with emphasis on methodological bases for comparative studies.

II.B.4 Others: fetal mortality, child spacing, etc
See also: 203, 226, 533, 1136, 1310, 1652.

236
Abernathy, J.R. et al.
"Estimates of Induced Abortion in Urban North Carolina." *Demography* 7(1), Feb. 1970: pp. 19-29.

Tests an interesting technique for estimating induced abortion from anonymous respondents in which the investigator does not know which of two questions has been answered.

237
de Bethune, A.J.
"Child Spacing: The Mathematical Probabilities." *Science* 142(3600), Dec. 1963: pp. 1629-1634.

238
Chase, H.C.
"The Current Status of Fetal Death Registration in the United States." *American Journal of Public Health and the Nation's Health* 56(10), Oct. 1966: pp. 1734-1744.
On the completeness and quality of U.S. registration system for fetal mortality.

239
*Dandekar, K.
"Intervals between Confinements." *Eugenics Quarterly* 6(3), Sept. 1959: pp. 180-186.

240
Dandekar, K.
"Analysis of Birth Intervals of a Set of Indian Women." *Eugenics Quarterly* 10(2), June 1963: pp. 73-78.
Comparative analyses for small samples of birth intervals and fecundability for Indian and French high-parity women.

241
Hammoud, E.I.
"Studies in Fetal and Infant Mortality. 1. A Methodological Approach to the Definition of Perinatal Mortality." *American Journal of Public Health and the Nation's Health* 55(7), July 1965: pp. 1012-1023.

Suggested approaches for separating biological and environmental factors in fetal and infant mortality.

242
Leridon, H.
"Some Comments on Article by K. Srinivasan: A Probability Model Applicable to the Study of Inter-Live Birth Intervals and Random Segments of the Same." *Population Studies* 23(1), Mar. 1969: pp. 101-104.
See comment on item 249.

243
Mantel, M. and Halperin, M.
"Analyses of Birth-Rank Data." *Biometrics* 19(2), June 1963: pp. 324-340.
Statistical tests (frequencies, variance, etc.) for birth rank order.

244
Mukherji, S.
"On the Fitting of a Mathematical Model to the Statistics of a First Birth." *Sankhyā* (Calcutta) (Series B) 27(3-4), Dec. 1965: pp. 265-270.
Probability models to estimate timing of birth based on previous survival experience.

245
Sheps, M.C.
"Pregnancy Wastage as a Factor in the Analysis of Fertility Data." *Demography* 1(1), 1964: pp. 111-118.

246
Sheps, M.C. and Perrin, E.B.
"The Distribution of Birth Intervals Under a Class of Stochastic Fertility Models." *Population Studies* 17(3), Mar. 1964: pp. 321-331.

247
Sheps, M.C. et al.
"Birth Intervals: Artifact and Reality."
In 1967 I.U.S.S.P. (*see* 21): pp. 857-868.
Computer simulation model used to demonstrate problems in use of incomplete series for estimating birth intervals paramaters.

248
Singh, S.N.
"On the Time of First Birth." *Sankhyā* (Calcutta) (Series B) 26(1-2), Nov. 1964: pp. 95-102.
Derivation of a probility distribution of time from marriage to first birth with application to 1956 Indian data.

249
Srinivasan, K.
"A Probability Model Applicable to the Study of Live Birth Intervals and Random Segments of the Same." *Population Studies* 21(1), July 1967: pp. 63-70.

250
Srinivasan, K.
"A Set of Analytical Models for the Study of Open Birth Intervals." *Demography* 5(1), 1968: pp. 34-44.

251
Szabady, E.
Some Problems of Studies in Family Planning. Budapest: Research Group for Population Studies, 1967; 27p.
Analyses of the problems of response and nonresponse in surveys about abortion and related matters where abortion is legal.

252
Taylor, W.F.
"On the Methodology of Measuring the

Probability of Fetal Death in a Prospective Study." *Human Biology* 36(2), May 1964: pp. 86-103.

II.C Social norms and values about family size
See also: 95, 444, 1050, 1196, 1501.

253
Bumpass, L.
"Stability and Change in Family Size Expectations over the First Two Years of Marriage." *Journal of Social Issues* 23(4), Oct. 1967: pp. 83-98.
A. U.S. longitudinal study.

254
Bumpass, L. and Westoff, C.F.
"The Prediction of Completed Fertility." *Demography* 6(4), Nov. 1969: pp. 445-454.
Based on the third reinterview of the Princeton fertility study sample, an important test of the predictive efficacy of desired family size at second parity in relation to contraceptive effectiveness, length of first two birth intervals, religion, and education; results indicate the usefulness of the preference measures at second parity.

255
Freedman, R. et al.
"Stability and Change in Expectations about Family Size: A Longitudinal Study." *Demography* 2, 1965: pp. 250-275.
Stability and change in expectations for additional births as related to age, parity, religion, status measures, desired family size, family interaction in Detroit sample.

256
Freedman, R. and Coombs, L.C.
"Expected Family Size and Family Growth Patterns: A Longitudinal Study." In Szabady et al., eds. (*see* 40): pp. 83-95.

Compares expectations at four successive interviews and considers some correlates of expectations in a longitudinal sample survey in Detroit.

257
Goldberg, D. and Coombs, C.H.
"Some Applications of Unfolding Theory to Fertility Analysis." In *Emerging Techniques in Population Research.* Proceedings of the 1962 Annual Conference of the Milbank Memorial Fund. New York: Milbank Memorial Fund, 1963: pp. 105-129.

Use of a psychometric method to measure the perceived distance between differing number of children desired in a sample survey.

258
Govindachari, A.
"Scale for Measuring Attitudes toward Small Family in a Rural Community." Institute of Rural Health and Family Planning. Ghandigram, Madurai District, Tamil Nadu, India. *Action Research Monographs* 3, 1966: pp. 31-47.

A scale on family-size attitudes combining Thurstone and Likert techniques tested on small samples of family planning acceptors and nonacceptors.

259
Knudsen, D.D. et al.
"Response Differences to Questions on Sexual Standards: An Interview-Questionnaire Comparison." *Public Opinion Quarterly* 31(2), Summer 1967: pp. 290-297.

Comparison of responses from small samples of premaritally pregnant women.

260
Myers, G.C. and Roberts, J.M.
"A Technique for Measuring Preferential Family Size and Composition." *Eugenics Quarterly* 15(3), Sept. 1968: pp. 164-172.

Preliminary report on a study using a small group of Puerto Rican women to test family size and sex preferences.

261
Pohlman, E.
"'Wanted' and 'Unwanted': Toward Less Ambiguous Definition." *Eugenics Quarterly* 12(1), Mar. 1965: pp. 19-27.

Problems of defining "unwanted" children.

262
Ryder, N.B. and Westoff, C.F.
"The Trend of Expected Parity in the United States: 1955, 1960, 1965." *Population Index* 33(2), Apr.-June 1967: pp. 153-168.

Trend series from survey samples used as basis for a critique of the usefulness of expected parity statements by respondents.

263
Ryder, N.B. and Westoff, C.F.
"Relationships among Intended, Expected, Desired and Ideal Family Size: United States, 1965." *Population Research,* Mar. 1969; 7p.

Based on the 1965 national fertility study, this analysis explores the relationships among four measures of attitudes toward family size, and their correlation to actual fertility, religion, race, and education.

264
Sastry, K.R.
"Instruments for Measuring Family Size Norm in a Rural Community." Institute of Rural Health and Family Planning.

Ghandigram, Madurai District, Tamil Nadu, India. *Action Research Monographs 3*, 1966: pp. 1-29.

A projective test for scoring attitudes toward a small family norm tested on small samples of family planning acceptors and nonacceptors.

265
Sengupta, A.
"Constructing a Scale for Measuring Attitude towards Family Planning: An Experiment with Thurstone." *Journal of Family Welfare* (Bombay) 13(2), Dec. 1966: pp. 45-60.

Report on 1964-65 experimental field study; discussion of concepts and terminology used in developing the scale.

266
Sheps, M.C.
"Effects of Family Size and Sex Ratio of Preferences Regarding the Sex of Children." *Population Studies* 17(1), July 1963: pp. 66-72.

A model for determining the number of children a couple desiring at least n children—b boys and g girls—must have on the average to achieve their goals.

267
Siegel, J.S. and Akers, D.S.
"Some Aspects of the Use of Birth Expectations Data for Sample Surveys for Population Projections." *Demography* 6(2), May 1969: pp. 101-115.

Ex-post-facto interpretation of expectation statements to test their validity for population forecasting.

268
Stycos, J.M.
"Haitian Attitudes toward Family Size." *Human Organization* 23(1), Spring 1964: pp. 42-47.

Unstructured interviewing technique in a small Haiti sample gives different results than poll-type questionnaires in other developing countries.

269
*Westoff, C.F. et al.
"Preferences in Size of Family and Eventual Fertility Twenty Years After." *American Journal of Sociology* 62(5), Mar. 1957: pp. 491-497.

Unique study of correlation between initial family size preferences and performance after 20 years, with controls for family planning; finds low correlations for individuals, although group as a whole predicted its ultimate fertility well.

II.D General methodological problems and models

See also: 7, 25, 64, 184, 364, 498, 606, 637, 638, 792, 801, 913, 1070, 1084, 1148, 1332, 1466, 1467, 1506, 1512, 1516, 1518, 1531, 1534.

270
Acsádi, G. et al.
Survey Techniques in Fertility and Family Planning Research: Experience in Hungary. Studies on Family Planning. Budapest: 1969; 152p.

Description of Hungarian fertility and family planning studies since 1958, samples of questionnaires, sampling procedures, estimates of error, survey of field experience, and bibliography of Hungarian publications on fertility and family planning, 1958-68.

271
Akers, D.S.
"Cohort Fertility versus Parity Progres-

sion as Methods of Projecting Births."
Demography 2, 1965; pp. 414-428.

272
*Bartlett, M.S.
Stochastic Population Models in Ecology and Epidemiology. London: Methuen; New York: John Wiley & Sons, 1960; 90p.

273
Basavarajappa, K.G.
"Effect of Declines in Mortality on the Birth Rate and Related Measures." *Population Studies* 16(3), Mar. 1963: pp. 237-256.
Effects of changes in mortality on birth rate, growth rate, and mean length of generation, when age-specific marital fertility rates and marriage patterns are held constant.

274
Beshers, J.M.
"Birth Projections with Cohort Models." *Demography* 2, 1965; pp. 593-599.
Model for cohort projections of fertility based on age, parity, birth control practice, and other variables.

275
Bodmer, W.F.
"Differential Fertility in Population Genetics Models." *Genetics* 51, Mar. 1965: pp. 411-424.

276
Bourgeois-Pichat, J.
"Some Unsolved Problems Raised by Human Reproduction." *Advances in Fertility Control* 2(4), Dec. 1967: pp. 45-48
Suggests need for basic interdisciplinary research on variations in fecundability and fetal mortality with coital frequency, the monthly cycle, and stages of family history.

277
Brass, W. and Coale, A.
"Methods of Analysis and Estimation." In Brass et al. (*see* 7): pp. 88-150.
Important exposition and illustration of methods of using incomplete or defective data for estimating fertility, nuptiality, and other important demographic parameters.

278
Campbell, A.
"Concepts and Techniques Used in Fertility Surveys." In *Emerging Techniques in Population Research* Proceedings of the 1962 Annual Conference of the Milbank Memorial Fund. New York: Milbank Memorial Fund, 1963: pp. 17-38.

279
Coale, A.J.
"Estimates of Various Demographic Measures through the Quasi-Stable Age Distribution." In *Emerging Techniques in Population Research* Proceedings of the 1962 Annual Conference of the Milbank Memorial Fund. New York: Milbank Memorial Fund, 1963: pp. 175-193.

280
Coale, A.J.
"Convergence of a Human Population to a Stable Form." *Journal of the American Statistical Association* 63 (322), June 1968: pp. 395-435.
Model for the sequence of births in a closed female population with constant fertility and mortality.

281
Coale, A.J. and Demeny, P.
Regional Model Life Tables and Stable Populations Princeton: Princeton University Press, 1966; 871p.

Important resource volume of nearly 5,000 stable population models with many parameters and with important methodological exposition.

282

Corsa, L.
"The Sample Survey in a National Population Program." *Public Opinion Quarterly* 28(3), 1964: pp. 383-388.

Discussion of the usefulness of national surveys in the development of family planning programs in developing countries, illustrated by Pakistan.

283

Demeny, P.
"Estimation of Vital Rates for Populations in the Process of Destabilization." *Demography* 2, 1965: pp. 516-530.

Examines the effect of declining mortality on quasi-stable population model biases.

284

Glick, P.C.
"Demographic Analysis of Family Data." In *Handbook of Marriage and the Family.* Edited by H.T. Christensen, Chicago: Rand McNally, 1964: pp. 300-334.

Broad review of the sources and methodology for analyzing fertility and other demographic variables in the context of family data, especially in the U.S.

285

Glick, P.C. and Heer, D.M.
"Joint Analysis of Personal and Family Characteristics." In *International Population Conference.* New York, 1961. London: U.N.E.S.C.O., 1963: pp. 217-228.

Advantages of considering jointly characteristics of the person and of the whole family in relation to other demographic facts.

286

Goodman, L.A.
"On the Age-Sex Composition of the Population That Would Result from Given Fertility and Mortality Conditions." *Demography* 4(2), 1967: pp. 423-441.

Formulas for ultimate sex ratios associated with specified patterns of vital rates.

287

Goodman, L.A.
"An Elementary Approach to the Population Projection Matrix, to the Population Re-productive Value, and to Related Topics in the Mathematical Theory of Population Growth." *Demography* 5(1), 1968: pp. 382-409.

288

Hackenberg, R.A.
"An Anthropological Study of Demographic Transition: The Papago Information System." *Milbank Memorial Fund Quarterly* 44(4, Part 1), Oct. 1966: pp. 470-494.

Model for information system that can be used for testing transition and other theories.

289

Hadden, J.K. and Borgatta, E.F.
"Family Growth in Metropolitan America: A Re-analysis." *Marriage and Family Living* 24(4), Nov. 1962: pp. 352-357.

Proper methods of factor analysis for data of Princeton fertility study.

290

Heer, D.M. and Smith, D.O.
"Mortality Level, Desired Family Size, and Population Increase." *Demography* 5(1), 1968: pp. 104-121.

Model of how mortality levels interacting with desired family size affect growth rates.

291
Henry, L.
"French Statistical Research in Natural Fertility." In Sheps and Ridley, eds. (*see* 73): pp. 333-350.

> *Review of the important work by French demographers on models for studying fecundability mainly from historical records.*

292
Hollingsworth, T.H.
Historical Demography. Ithaca, N. Y.: Cornell University Press, 1969; 448p.

> *Survey of data sources for historical demographic studies; evaluation of deductions that can be made from such data.*

293
Holmberg, I.V.
"Demographic Models." *Statistisk Tidskrift* (Stockholm) (3rd Series) 5(3), 1967: pp. 246-251.

> *Presents a micro model for simulating marital fertility.*

294
Holmberg, I.
Demographic Models: DM 4. Reports, 8. Goteborg, Sweden: Demographic Institute, University of Goteborg, 1968; 55p.

> *One of a series of reports on demographic models; deals with extreme levels of fertility and mortality.*

295
Hyrenius, H.
"New Technique for Studying Demographic-Economic-Social Interrelations." Conference on the Application of Science and Technology for Less Developed Areas. Goteborg, Sweden: Demographic Institute, University of Goteborg, 1965: pp. 1-24.

> *Discusses the usefulness and problems of building demographic models.*

296
Hyrenius, H. and Adolfsson, I.
A Fertility Simulation Model. Reports, 2. Demographic Institution, University of Goteborg. Goteborg, Sweden: Elanders Boktryckeri; Stockholm: Almqvist & Wilksell, 1964; 31p.

297
Hyrenius, H. et al.
Demographic Models: DM 2. Reports, 4. Demographic Institute, University of Goteborg. Goteborg, Sweden: Almqvist & Wiksell, 1966; 36p.

> *Report on demographic simulation model involving both fertility and mortality components.*

298
Hyrenius, H. et al.
Demographic Models: DM 3. Reports, 5. Demographic Institute, University of Goteborg. Goteborg, Sweden: Elanders Boktryckeri; Stockholm: Almqvist & Wiksell, 1967; 39p.

> *Theoretical aspects of a dynamic population model capable of handling demographic change analysis.*

299
International Union for the Scientific Study of Population.
International Population Conference. Ottawa, 21-26 Aug. 1963. Liege: 1964; 468p.
The following conference papers deal with obtaining vital statistics from limited data:
Ahmed, M. "Vital Rates of East Pakistan's Muslims: An Estimate from Stable Population Model": pp. 47-63.
Blacker, J.G.C. "The Use of Stable Population Models for the Construction

of Population Projections. Application of the African Population of Tanganyika": pp. 65-76.

Chandrasekaran, C. "Fertility Indices from Limited Data": pp. 91-105.

El-Badry, M.A. "Errors in Parity Data": pp. 121-129.

Das Gupta, A. "Estimation of Vital Rates for Developing Countries": pp. 131-150.

Khan, M.K.H. "Fertility Rates from Limited Data": pp. 151-157.

Krotki, K.J. "First Report on the Population Growth Estimation Experiment": pp. 159-173.

Lorimer, F. "Possibilities and Problems in the Estimation of Vital Rates in Africa": pp. 175-191.

Roberts, G.W. "Securing Demographic Data from Limited Historical Material": pp. 203-209.

Som, R.K. "On Adjustments for Non-Sampling Errors and Biases in the Estimation of Vital Rates": pp. 211-220.

Taeuber, I.B. "The Conundrum of the Chinese Birth rate": pp. 221-240.

300
International Union for the Scientific Study of Population. Committee on Comparative Studies of Fertility and Family Planning.
Variables for Comparative Fertility Studies: A Working Paper. Liege: 1967; 36p.
Suggested list of variables for comparative fertility studies together with notes, definitions, and some general suggestions about survey designs.

301
Kammeyer, K.
"Birth Order as a Research Variable." *Social Forces* 46(1), Sept. 1967: pp. 71-80.

Discusses the concept of birth order as it relates to many other phenemonon in potential research programs.

302
*Keyfitz, N.
"Differential Fertility in Ontario: Application of Factorial Design to Demographic Problem." *Population Studies* 6(2), Nov. 1952: pp. 123-134.
Replicates for English Protestants in Ontario the design developed for French Catholics in Quebec (see 303); demonstrates that distance from cities affects fertility independently of effect of income, education, and age.

303
*Keyfitz, N.
"A Factorial Arrangement of Comparisons of Family Size." *American Journal of Sociology* 58(5), Mar. 1953: pp. 470-480.
Example of the use of experimental design to study the interrelation of age at marriage, ethnicity, income level, education, and distance from city on fertility.

304
Keyfitz,N.
"Matrix Multiplication as a Technique of Population Analysis." *Milbank Memorial Fund Quarterly* 42(4 Part 1), Oct. 1964: pp. 68-84.
Report on exploratory computations by desk calculator and by electronic computer for summarizing fertility and survivorship patterns, as applied to the U.S. population.

305
Keyfitz, N.
"Changing Vital Rates and Age Distributions." *Population Studies* 22(2), July 1968: pp. 235-251.

Important anaylsis of the relation between various component demographic rates and the age structure; mathematical proofs and empirical illustrations include effects of varying mortality and fertility schedules, length of generation; provides a measure of aging effects of such changes.

306
Keyfitz, N.
Introduction to the Mathematics of Population. Series in Behavioral Science: Quantitative Methods. Reading, Mass.: Addison-Wesley, 1968; 450p.
Mathematical demography; many original contributions and reformulations of important models.

307
Keyfitz, N. and Murphy, E.M.
"Matrix and Multiple Decrement in Population Analysis." *Biometrics* 23(3), Sept. 1967: pp. 485-503.
Extension of one-sex population model to include migration, labor-force participation, and educational-marital status as well as parity.

308
Kusukawa, A.
"A Demographic Model of Fertility Related to Coitus for Populations not Practicing Family Limitation." *Kyushu Journal of Medical Science* (Fukuoka) 14, Dec. 1963: pp. 369-378.

309
Lauriat, P.
"Field Experience in Estimating Population Growth." *Demography* 4(1), 1967: pp. 228-243.
Problems encountered in various phases of field work and steps toward their solution in three nationwide population-estimation studies using fixed area samples in Pakistan, Thailand, and Turkey.

310
Liell, J. et al.
"A Research Design for a Comparative Study of Urbanism and Fertility: A Progress Report." *Nigerian Journal of Economic and Social Studies* (Ibadan) 7(1), Mar. 1965: pp. 63-69.
Research design for cross-cultural measurements of the impact of culture, urbanization, and industrialization on fertility.

311
Mauldin, W.P.
"Application of Survey Techniques to Fertility Studies." In Sheps and Ridley, eds. (*see* 73): pp. 93-118.

312
Namboodiri, N.K.
"On the Dependence of Age Structure on a Sequence of Mortality and Fertility Schedules: An Exposition of a Cyclical Model of Population Change." *Demography* 6(3), Aug. 1969: pp. 287-299.
Advances a method for consideration of the dependence of age structure and growth rate on a sequence of fertility and mortality schedules under the assumption of unchanging mortality and no migration, with fertility schedules repeating themselves in a cyclical fashion; the objective is to be "more realistic" than the assumptions of conventional stable population analysis.

313
*Orcutt, G.H. et al.
Microanlysis of Socioeconomic Systems: A Simulation Study. New York: Harper & Row, 1961; 425p.
Reports on a simulation study by computer of a micro-analytic model of the American economy, involving a simulated demographic model that includes reproduction.

314

Perrin, E.B. and Sheps, M.C.
"Human Reproduction: A Stochastic Process." *Biometrics* 20(1), Mar. 1964: pp. 28-45.

Model for reproduction as a stochastic process, the basis for important subsequent methodological work.

315

Population Council. Demographic Division.
Selected Questionnaires on Knowledge, Attitudes and Practice of Family Planning. New York: 1967; 2 vols.

Selected questionnaires from KAP studies, with relevant materials on interviewing, instructions, coding, etc. where feasible.

316

Population Council. Demographic Division.
A Manual for Surveys of Fertility and Family Planning: Knowledge, Attitudes, and Practice. New York: 1970; 405p.

317

Potter, R.G., Jr. et al.
"Improvement of Contraception during Course of Marriage." *Population Studies* 16(2), Nov. 1962: pp. 160-174.

Model for investigating how contraceptive effectiveness and desired family size are related over time as parity approaches desired level.

318

Potter, R.G., Jr., and Sakoda, J.M.
"A Computer Model of Family Building Based on Expected Values." *Demography* 3(2),1966: pp. 450-461.

Application of model to U.S. couples, considering family planning differentials related to contraceptive success, size of desired family, and child spacing.

319

Potter, R.G., Jr. and Sakoda, J.M.
"Family Planning and Fecundity." *Population Studies* 20(3), Mar. 1967: pp. 311-328.

Computer model to examine effects of varying levels of fecundity on child spacing, fetal mortality, and effective family planning.

320

Ridley, J.C. and Sheps, M.C.
"An Analytic Simulation Model of Human Re-production with Demographic and Biological Components." *Population Studies* 19(3), Mar. 1966: pp. 297-310.

Studies the determinants of human reproduction through an analytical simulation model.

321

Robinson, W.C. et al.
"Quasi-Stable Estimates of the Vital Rates of Pakistan." *Pakistan Development Review* (Karachi) 5(4), 1965: pp. 638-658.

Tests the methodology by comparing rates based on census data with those of a combined sample registration-survey procedure.

322

Ryder, N.B.
"The Process of Demographic Translation." *Demography* 1(1), 1964: pp. 74-82

Methodological discussion of the development of cohort rates from period data.

323

Ryder, N.B.
"The Measurement of Fertility Patterns." In Sheps and Ridley, eds. (*see* 73): pp. 287-306.

A summary of principles and problems in fertility measurement, moving from the simplest to the most complex approaches.

324
Ryder, N.B.
"The Emergence of a Modern Fertility Pattern: United States, 1917-66." In Behrman et al., eds. (*see* 51): pp. 99-123.
Measurements of both the quantity and the tempo of fertility; develops a procedure for assessing the relative importance of quantity and importance of nuptiality and marital parity for changes in the level of period fertility.

325
Sheps, M.C.
"On the Person-Years Concept in Epidemiology and Demography." *Milbank Memorial Fund Quarterly* 44(1), Jan. 1966: pp. 69-91.
Uses a mathematical model to show that conventional person-years concept may give misleading results in computing fertility or other vital rates.

326
Sheps, M.C.
"Applications of Probability Models to the Study of Patterns of Human Reproduction." In Sheps and Ridley, eds. (*see* 73): pp. 307-332.
A review of the approaches to the construction of such models.

327
Sheps, M.C. and Perrin, E.B.
"Changes in Birth Rates as a Function of Contraceptive Effectiveness: Some Applications of a Stochastic Model." *American Journal of Public Health* 53(7), July 1963: pp. 1031-1046.

328
Sheps, M.C. and Perrin, E.B.
"Further Results from a Human Fertility Model with a Variety of Pregnancy Outcomes." *Human Biology* 38(3) Sept. 1966: pp. 180-193.
Model of possible sequences of events during reproduction including fetal wastage.

329
Sheps, M.C. et al.
"Probability Models for Family Building: An Analytical Review." *Demography* 6(2), May 1969: pp. 161-183.
Review of the literature on stochastic models for the reproductive history of a cohort of couples, together with the classification of such models and proposals of more complex models to deal with greater variability in basic parameters.

330
Srivastava, M.L.
"The Relationship between the Birth Rate and the Death Rate in Stable Populations with the Same Fertility but Different Mortality Schedules." *Eugenics Quarterly* 13(3) Sept. 1966: pp. 231-239.

331
Srivastava, M.L.
"Effect of Rise in the Age of Marriage on the Fertility Rate." *Journal of Social Research* 10(2), Sept. 1967: pp. 63-79.
Develops a formula for the total fertility rate in a hypothetical population with no illegitimate births, employing two age-marriage duration specific fertility schedules.

332
Srivastava, M.L.
"The Relationships between Fertility and Mortality Characteristics in Stable Female Populations." *Eugenics Quarterly* 14(3), Sept. 1967: pp. 171-180.

333
Skyes, Z.M.
"On Discrete Stable Population Theo-

ry." *Biometrics* 25(2), June 1969: pp. 285-293.

334
Taeuber, C.
"Population Trends and Characteristics." In *Indicators of Social Change.* Edited by E.B. Sheldon and W.E. Moore. New York: Russell Sage Foundation, 1968: pp. 27-74.

Data and methodology available and needed for studying population trends in the U.S., including some considerations of fertility.

335
Thailand. National Statistical Office.
Final Report, Survey of Population Changes. Supplementary Survey on Knowledge, Attitude and Practice Concerning Official Registration of Births and Deaths. Bangkok: 1969; 84p.

A follow-up survey of cases unmatched in a program for comparing survey and registration data on births and deaths; survey probes reasons for discrepancies and failure to register.

336
Theiss, E. et al.
"Report and Discussion." In Szabady et al., eds. (*see* 39): pp. 112-132.

Summarizes recommendations for methodological refinements in fertility study.

337
Tietze, C.
"Pregnancy Rate and Birth Rates." *Population Studies* 16(1), July 1962: pp. 31-37.

Model of a hypothetical noncontracepting population applied to the evaluation of contraceptive effectiveness and resulting levels of pregnancy rates and crude birth rates; shows that high level of contraceptive effectiveness is needed to keep fertility low even if a large proportion of the population are contraceptors.

338
United Nations. Department of Economic and Social Affairs.
"Methods of Estimating Basic Demographic Measures from Incomplete Data." [Written by A. Coale and P. Demeny.] *Population Studies* 42. New York: 1967; 126p.

A major methodological work, presenting techniques for making estimates of fertility and other population parameters from imperfect data; many illustrations.

339
United Nations. Department of Economic and Social Affairs.
"The Concept of a Stable Population: Application to the Study of Populations of Countries with Incomplete Demographic Statistics." *Population Studies,* No. 39. ST/SOA. Ser. A/39. Sales No.: E.65. xiii 3. New York: 1968; 237p.

New techniques for the application of stable population models.

340
United Nations. Department of Economic and Social Affairs.
"Variables and Questionnaire for Comparative Fertility Surveys." *Population Studies,* No. 45. New York: 1970; 104p.

Model questionnaire and notes on its use for comparative study; prepared by a committee of the I.U.S.S.P.

341
Van de Walle, E.
"Characteristics of African Demographic Data." In *Brass et al.* (*see* 7): pp. 12-87.

An important discussion of the nature and limitations of the data sources in Africa, with special emphasis on the problems of getting age data, the functional relation of error to other parameters to be measured, and the problems of getting and using retrospective and recent fertility experience.

342
Vogt, J.
"Component Parts of the Number of Births." *Statsøkonomisk Tidsskrift* (Oslo) 78(4), Dec. 1964: pp. 287-307.

Changes in nuptiality and in numbers of childeren per marriage as components in fertility changes.

343
Wrigley, E.A., ed.
An Introduction to English Historical Demography from the Sixteenth to the Nineteenth Century. Cambridge Group for the History of Population and Social Structure, Publication No. 1. London: Weidenfeld & Nicolson, 1966; 283p.

An important exposition on historical demography by applying methods developed by Louis Henry to parish registers to reconstitute family histories and by analysis of early census records.

344
Wyon, J.B.
"Field Studies on Fertility of Human Populations." In *Human Fertility and Population Problems.* Edited by R.O. Greep. Cambridge, Mass.: Schenkman, 1963: pp. 79-99.

Outlines the ecological nature, purposes, methods, and sources of field studies.

III. DESCRIPTIVE AND HISTORICAL STUDIES: REGIONAL AND NATIONAL

III.A General

See also: 3, 182, 281, 667, 937.

345
Chandrasekhar, S., ed.
Asia's Population Problems with a Discussion of Population and Immigration in Australia. New York: Frederick A. Praeger, 1967; 311p.
> *Includes discussion of fertility and other population trends in six Asian countries.*

346
Cho, L.J.
"Estimated Refined Measures of Fertility for All Major Countries of the World." *Demography* 1(1), 1964: pp. 359-374.
> *Estimates fertility measures for 136 countries using regression equations developed by Bogue and Palmore. (see 142).*

347
***Connell, K.H.**
The Population of Ireland, 1750-1845. Oxford: Clarendon Press, 1950; 293p.
> *General treatment of a country with a unique demographic history reflecting both Catholicism and special economic problems.*

348
Cowgill, U.M.
"Recent Variations in the Season of Birth in Puerto Rico." *Proceedings of the National Academy of Sciences* 52(4), 1964: pp. 1149-1151.
> *Comparison of monthly birth rates of the U.S. and Puerto Rico for the period 1941-1961.*

349
***Davis, K.**
The Population of India and Pakistan. Princeton: Princeton University Press, 1951; 263p.
> *Early and still impressive general analysis of the population history and structure of a developing country, with considerable attention to fertility.*

350
Davis, K.
"The Place of Latin America in World Demographic History." *Milbank Memorial Fund Quarterly* 42(2, Part 2) Apr. 1964: pp. 19-47.
> *Places Latin American countries in world setting with respect to commonalities and differences in demographic measures, culture, and environment.*

351
Glass, D.V. and Grebenick, E.
"World Population, 1800-1950." In *The Cambridge Economic History of Europe.* Edited by H.J. Habakkuk and M. Poston. Cambridge, Eng.: Cambridge University Press, 1965; Part I, pp. 60-138.

352
Keyfitz, N. and Flieger, W.
World Population: An Analysis of Vital Data. Chicago: University of Chicago Press, 1968; 669p.

Major resource; official data on vital trends for many countries and periods, supplemented with estimates for many important parameters and projections of current vital rates as benchmarks for evaluating future trends.

353
Kwon, E.H. and Kim, T.R.
"The Population of Korea." *Journal of Population Studies* 7, 1968: pp. 113-181.

Demographic trends in fertility, mortality, nuptiality, and urbanization; population projections from various sources.

354
Miró, C.A.
"The Population of Latin America." *Demography* 1(1), 1964: pp. 15-41.

Excellent summary of broad demographic trends in Latin America, including summary of available data on fertility and fertility differentials.

355
Nevett, A.S.J.
Population: Explosion or Control? A Study with Special References to India. London: Geoffrey Chapman; Notre Dame, Ind.: Fides Publishers, 1964; 224p.

General discussion of population growth theories and population control from the Catholic viewpoint.

356
*Roberts, G.W.
The Population of Jamaica. Cambridge, Eng.: Cambridge University Press, 1957; 356p.

A major study of Jamaican population trends with significant analysis of fertility trends as related to changes in slave status, family forms, urbanization, and education.

357
Shorter, F.C. and Güvenc, B., eds.
Turkish Demography: Proceedings of a Conference. No. 7. Ankara: Institute of Population Studies, Hacettepe University, 1969; 310p.

Papers on fertility and family planning, with special reference to Turkey.

358
*Taeuber, I.B.
The Population of Japan. Princeton: Princeton University Press, 1958; 461p.

A monumental and definitive work on Japanese population trends, with considerable and sophisticated emphasis on fertility and related variables.

359
Taeuber, I.B.
"Population and Society." In *Handbook of Modern Sociology.* Edited by R.L. Faris. Chicago: Rand McNally, 1964: pp. 83-126.

A broad survey of population growth patterns, both historical and contemporary, with special emphasis on the U.S.

360
United Nations. Department of Economic and Social Affairs.
Population Bulletin No. 7 with Special Reference to Conditions and Trends of Fertility in the World. New York: 1965; 151p.

A historical landmark that presented for the first time frequency distributions for countries, regions, and the world of birth rates and gross reproduction rates; also presents gross relationships of development indicators to fertility measures.

III.B Fertility levels and norms before mature industrial development

III.B.1 Historical

See also: 48, 153, 292, 493, 509, 1054, 1070, 1148, 1296, 1394, 1561, 1562, 1565.

361
*Barclay, G.
Colonial Development and Population in Taiwan. Princeton: Princeton University Press, 1954; 274p.
    Well-documented analysis of stable reproductive patterns in a population subject to declining mortality under a carefully controlled colonial system designed to minimize change in family institutions.

362
Drake, M.
Population and Society in Norway 1735-1865. Cambridge, Eng.: Cambridge University Press, 1969; 255p.
    Based on early census data, parish register reports, and observations by Malthus, Sundt, and others, analyzes the interaction of fertility, nuptiality, family, and economic organization as it bears on relatively low birth rates in preindustrial Norway; advances the thesis that fertility responded to economic fluctuations through linkage to age at marriage, proportion married, and household-familial arrangements.

363
*Ford, C.S.
A Comparative Study of Human Reproduction. Yale University Publications in Anthropology, No. 32. New Haven: Yale University Press, 1945; 111p.
    Historically important review of the fragmentary evidence about childbearing, pregnancy, and contraception available in a sample of societies in the Yale cross-cultural files.

364
Glass, D.V.
"Notes on the Demography of London at the End of the Seventeenth Century." Daedalus 97(2), Spring 1968: pp. 581-592.
    Preliminary data from parish registers on nuptiality and family size; estimates of bias in records.

365
*Habakkuk, H.J.
"English Population in the Eighteenth Century." English History Review 6(2), Dec. 1953: pp. 117-133.

366
Helleiner, K.F.
"The Population of Europe from the Black Death to the Eve of the Vital Revolution." In The Economy of Expanding Europe in the Sixteenth and Seventeenth Centuries. Edited by E.E. Rich and C.H. Wilson. Cambridge, Eng.: Cambridge University Press, 1967: pp. 1-95.

367
Hofsten, E.
"Fertility for Birth Cohorts of Swedish

Women 1870/71." *Statistisk Tidskrift* (Stockholm) 4(4), 1966: pp. 295-309.

Cohort fertility by age, total fertility rates, and age at childbirth.

368
Kücheman, C.F. et al.
"A Demographic and Genetic Study of a Group of Oxfordshire Villages." *Human Biology* 39(3), Sept. 1967: pp. 251-276.

Data obtained from parish registers and census returns, 1578 to present, analyzed for population size, birth rate, age at marriage, family size, birth interval, infant mortality, marriage distance, and effective population size.

369
Laslett, P.
The World We Have Lost. London: Methuen, 1965; 208p.

Some aspects of English social and economic history since the Middle Ages, with reference to marriage, fertility, and other demographic factors, partly based on historical records and partly on speculative reconstructions.

370
Laslett, P.
"Size and Structure of the Household in England Over Three Centuries." *Population Studies* 23(2), July 1969: pp. 199-223.

371
*McKeown, T. and Brown, R.G.
"Medical Evidence Related to the English Population Changes in the Eighteenth Century." *Population Studies* 9(2), Nov. 1955: pp. 119-141.

Deals mainly with the causes of the decline of the death rate; also considers and rejects the possibilities that rising birth rates account for population growth in this period.

372
Pan, C.L.
"An Estimate of the Long-Term Crude Birth Rate of the Agricultural Population of China." *Demography* 3(1), 1966: pp. 204-208.

Estimates crude birth rates for Chinese provinces from crop yields and other demographic data.

373
Rich, E.E. and Wilson, C.H., eds.
The Economy of Expanding Europe in the Sixteenth and Seventeenth Centuries. Cambridge Economic History of Europe, vol. 4. Cambridge, Eng.: Cambridge University Press, 1967; 642p.

374
Roberts, G.W.
"The Present Fertility Position in Jamaica." In Szabady et al., eds. (*see* 40): pp. 259-275.

Analyzes differentials and trends in Jamaican fertility with special attention to family type variations and to explanations of the rising period rates in Jamaica, while cohort rates appear stable.

375
Thrupp, S.L.
"The Problem of Replacement Rates in Late Medieval English Population." *The Economic History Review* (2nd Series) 18(1), 1965: pp. 101-119.

376
Wojtun, B.
"Trends in Fertility in West Poland in the Nineteenth Century." *Susquehanna University Studies* 8(1), June 1967: pp. 69-78.

377

Wrigley, E.A.

"Family Limitation in Pre-Industrial England." *Economic History Review* (2nd Series) 19(1), Apr. 1966: pp. 82-109.

Extensive practice of family limitation in a seventeenth-century village inferred; family histories reconstituted to obtain data on nuptiality, marital age-specific fertility, birth intervals, and other important parameters.

III.B.2 Contemporary

See also: 8, 145, 159, 167, 185, 268, 321, 500, 542, 544, 550, 564, 734, 966, 1026, 1041, 1049, 1129, 1132, 1401, 1493, 1627.

378

Afzal, M.

"The Fertility of East Pakistan Married Women." In *Studies in the Demography of Pakistan.* Edited by W.C. Robinson. Karachi: Pakistan Institute of Development Economics, 1967: pp. 51-91.

Estimates age-specific fertility rates and mean age at marriage for rural and urban areas from census data on parity distributions by age and duration of marriage.

379

Aguirre, A.

"Colombia: The Family in Candelarie." *Studies in Family Planning* 11, Apr. 1966: pp. 1-5.

Descriptive study of the presumed social consequences of rapid population growth in a semirural village; infanticide practices, changes in sexual relations, contraception, impact of the Catholic church, role of physicians.

380

Aird, J.S.

"Estimates and Projections of the Population of Mainland China: 1953-1986." *U.S. Bureau of the Census International Population Reports.* Series P-91, 17. Washington: Government Printing Office, 1968; 73p.

A major effort to estimate and project the vital rates of mainland China on the basis of the 1953 census, fragmentary data, and speculations.

381

Anwar, A.A. and Bokhari, S.

A Methodological Study to Estimate the Birth Rate and the Death Rate of Rural Population of Lahore Tehsil. Board of Economic Inquiry (Pakistan Punjab). No. 128. Lahore: 1962; 84p.

Report of a three-phase interview survey; presents description of survey and computed demographic rates.

382

Baer, G.

Population and Society in the Arab East. New York: Frederick A. Praeger, 1964; 275p.

Chapter on demography, and one on the position of women and the family.

383

Bhatta, J.N.

An Estimate of Fertility Level of the Population of Djakarta by Polynomial Function. Departemen Angkatan Darat, No. 16. Djakarta: Dinas Geografi, Direktorat Topografi, 1966; 19p. [Summary in Indonesian.]

Report on application of the Brass method to data on child-woman ratios, children ever-born alive, and children still living as reported by ever-married women in Greater Djakarta.

384
Bonne, B.
"The Samaritans: A Demographic Study." *Human Biology* 3 (1), Feb. 1963: pp. 61-89.

> Demographic history and trends of an isolated religious sect in the Middle East; age-sex distribution, fertility and nuptiality patterns, and genetic implications of inbreeding patterns considered.

385
Cameroon. Ministry of Economic Affairs and Planning. Department of Statistics.
The Population of West Cameroon: Main Findings of the Demographic Survey of West Cameroon, 1964. Paris: Société d'Etudes pour le Developpement Economique et Social, 1966; 94p.

> Evaluates data on fertility and other demographic and social variables.

386
*Chandrasekhar, S.
China's Population: Census and Vital Statistics. Hong Kong: Hong Kong University Press, 1959; 69p.

> A report by an Indian demographer who had an early opportunity to visit mainland China.

387
Chidambaram, V.C.
"Fertility in Kerala." In 1967 I.U.S.S.P. (*see* 21): pp. 225-236.

> Uses incomplete data from various sources to estimate how much Kerala fertility differs from that for all of India and why.

388
Cho, L.J. and Hahm, M.J.
"Recent Change in Fertility Rates of the Korean Population." *Demography* 5(2), 1968: pp. 690-697.

> Estimates the significant decline in fertility between 1957-61 and 1962-66 after estimating the effect of declining portions married and the lack of any effect from changing age structures.

389
Cho, L.J. et al.
"Recent Fertility Trends in West Malaysia." *Demography* 5(2), 1968: pp. 732-744.

390
Coale, A.J. and Lorimer, E.
"Summary of Estimates of Fertility and Mortality." In Brass, et al. (*see* 7): pp. 151-182.

> Summaries of fertility and other measures for a considerable number of African countries and provinces for period since 1950, based on estimation by ingenious methods from incomplete data.

391
Cumper, G.E.
"Preliminary Analysis of Population Growth and Social Characteristics in Jamaica, 1943-60." *Social and Economic Studies* (Jamaica) 12(4), Dec. 1963: pp. 393-431.

392
*Das Gupta, A. et al.
"Couple Fertility, National Sample Survey No. 7." *Sankhyā* 16, 1955-56: pp. 230-434.

393
El-Badry, M.A.
"Trends in the Components of Population Growth in the Arab Countries in the Middle East; A Survey of Present Information." *Demography* 2, 1965: pp. 140-186.

Emphasizes regional variations in Egyptian fertility, trends, and possible explanations, with briefer treatment of general population trends in Lebanon, Jordan, and Syria.

394
Freedman, R.
"The Accelerating Fertility Decline in Taiwan." *Population Index* 31(4), Oct. 1965: pp. 430-435.
Analysis of change in age-specific birth rates, proportion married, and other fertility measures and their distributions in the 22 major administrative areas of Taiwan.

395
Freedman, R. and Muller, J.
"The Continuing Fertility Decline in Taiwan." *Population Index* 33(1), Jan.-Mar. 1967: pp. 3-17.
Describes and analyzes fertility decline from 1959-64, decomposing change into nuptiality trends, age-specific fertility trends, and regional variations in fertility and nuptiality.

396
Frothingham, N.
Population Concerns and Family Planning in Africa, South of the Sahara. New York: Pathfinder Fund, 1968; 133p.
Reviews demographic studies, statistical resources, and the development of family planning in Kenya.

397
Gaisie, S.K.
"Estimation of Vital Rates for Ghana." *Population Studies* 23(1), Mar. 1969: pp. 21-42.
Uses methods developed by Brass and Coale-Demeny.

398
Geisert, H.L.
The Control of World Population Growth.

Population Research Project. Washington: George Washington University, 1963; 50p.
General discussion of world population growth pressures; separate sections for many developing countries describing their demographic situations and family planning efforts.

399
Gille, H.
"National Seminar on Population Problems of Thailand: Conclusions of the Seminar." *Studies in Family Planning* 1(4), Aug. 1964: pp. 1-5.
Review of research and policy studies and recommended actions discussed at the seminar.

400
Gille, H.
"Twentieth Century Levels and Trends of Fertility in Developing Countries." In *Proceedings of the World Population Conference, 1965 (see 44):* pp. 85-91.
Draws on United Nations Bulletin No. 7 (see 360) and updates series for developing countries where available.

401
Gille, H. and Pardoka, R.H.
"A Family Life Study in East Java: Preliminary Findings." In Berelson et al., eds. *(see 53):* pp. 503-521.
Report on a pilot study in Indonesia.

402
Gosh, A.
Demographic Trends in West Bengal during 1901-1950. Census of India Monograph Series, No. 5, New Delhi: Office of the Registrar General, 1966; 40p.
Four papers dealing with trends in the birth rate (1911-51), differential fertility in Calcutta and Bombay, and the effect of urbanization on nuptiality.

403
Gupta, P.B.
"Estimation of All-India Birth and Death Rates, 1941-50." *Sankhyā* (Calcutta) (Series B) 20(1-2), June 1968: pp. 157-164.

Uses variants of differencing and reverse survival methods to estimate vital rates.

404
Hashmi, S.S.
The People of Karachi: Demographic Characteristics. Monographs in the Economics of Development, 13. Karachi: Pakistan Institute of Development Economics, 1965; 152p.

405
India. Cabinet Secretariat.
Fertility and Mortality Rates in Rural India. The National Sample Survey, No. 76, 14th Round: July 1958-June 1959. Delhi: Manager of Publications, 1963; 153p.

Age-specific fertility and mortality rates and demographic characteristics (age-sex composition, marital status); findings compared with earlier surveys.

406
Jamaica. Department of Statistics.
Population Census 1960. Some Notes on the Union Status, Marital Status and Number of Children of the Female Population of Jamaica. Kingston: 1963; 35p.

407
Jayewardene, C.H.S. and Selvaratnam, S.
"Fertility Level and Trends in Ceylon." In 1967 I.U.S.S.P. (*see* 21): pp. 237-244.

A brief statement of the major fertility trends developed in greater detail in the book-length treatment (see 1493).

408
Kim, Y.
"Some Demographic Measurements for Korea Based on the Quasi-Stable Population Theory." *Demography* 2, 1965: pp. 567-578.

Estimates of population trends in Korea and the effects of the Korean War, based on the quasi-stable population theory.

409
Kon, K.S.
The Fertility of Korean Women. 1960 Census Monograph Series. Seoul: Institute of Population Problems, 1966; 148p.

410
Mazur, D.P.
"Fertility among the Nationality Groups of Asia Adjacent to the ECAFE Region." In 1967 I.U.S.S.P. (*see* 21): pp. 245-255.

Analysis of the levels and correlates of fertility among 21 nationality groups in the U.S.S.R. that border on the countries of the E.C.A.F.E. region, presented as pertinent for understanding their E.C.A.F.E. neighbors where less data are available.

411
McArthur, N.
Island Populations of the Pacific. Canberra: Australian National University Press, 1967; 381p.

Includes data and analyses of fertility patterns in five Pacific island groups.

412
Miró, C.A.
"The Population of Twentieth Century Latin America." In *Population Dilemma*

in Latin America. Edited by J.M. Stycos and J. Arias, Washington: American Assembly, 1966: pp. 1-32.

413
Neville, R.J.W.
"Singapore: Recent Trends in the Sex and Age Composition of a Cosmopolitan Community." *Population Studies* 17(2), Nov. 1963: pp. 99-112.

Interrelation of sex and age distribution with population trends and policies in Singapore 1931-1957, with special reference to ethnic differentials.

414
Ridley, J.C.
"Recent Natality Trends in Underdeveloped Countries." In Sheps and Ridley, eds. (*see* 73): pp. 143-173.

415
Robinson, W.C. ed.
Studies in the Demography of Pakistan. Karachi: Pakistan Institute of Development Economics, 1967; 225p.

416
Romaniuk, L.
"The Demography of the Democratic Republic of the Congo." In Brass et al. (*see* 7): pp. 241-342.

Exhaustive analysis of fertility, nuptiality, and other demographic data in the period of the 1950s with perhaps the best combination of demographic data ever available for a native African population; important both substantively and methodologically.

417
Saw, S.H.
"Pattern of Fertility Decline in Malaya,

1956-1965." *Kajian Ekonomi Malaysis* (Kuala Lumpur) 3(1), June 1966: pp. 7-14.

418
Saw, S.H.
"A Note on the Fertility Levels in Malaya during 1947-1957." *Malayan Economic Review* (Singapore) 12(1), Apr. 1967: pp. 117-124.

Comparison of fertility and nuptiality indexes derived from the 1947 and 1957 censuses.

419
Shorter, F.C.
"Information on Fertility, Mortality and Population Growth in Turkey." In Shorter and Güvenc, eds. (*see* 357): pp. 19-41. [Also in *Population Index* 34(1), Jan.-Apr. 1968: pp. 3-21.]

National and regional trends for the early 1960s.

420
Smith, T.E. and Blacker, J.G.C.
Population Characteristics of the Commonwealth Countries of Tropical Africa. Commonwealth Papers, 9. London: University of London, Athlone Press, 1963; 72p.

Survey of fertility and other population trends in Africa.

421
Taeuber, I.B.
"Demographic Instabilities in Island Ecosystems." In *Man's Place in the Island Ecosystem.* Edited by F.R. Fosberg. Honolulu: Bishop Museum Press, 1963: pp. 226-251.

Reviews trends and projections for the principal islands or island groups of the Western Pacific.

422
United Nations. Department of Economic and Social Affairs.
"Guanabara Demographic Pilot Survey: A Joint Project of the United Nations and the Government of Brazil." *Population Studies* 35, New York: 1964; 77p.

> *Results of an experimental survey in a Brazilian state; data on nuptiality, migration, household size, sex ratios, age distributions, fertility, and mortality by age and social status.*

423
Van de Kaa, D.J.
"Fertility Patterns in New Guinea: An Appraisal of Present Knowledge." In 1967 I.U.S.S.P. (*see* 21): pp. 337-347.

> *Data for 13 groups for periods 1951-62 show varying results, with rates based on recent periods much higher than data for children ever born; some indications of changing patterns, although total fertility is high.*

424
Van de Walle, E.
"An Approach to the Study of Fertility in Nigeria." *Population Studies* 19(1), July 1965: pp. 5-16.

> *Calculates three sets of gross reproduction rates from child-adult ratios for provinces; description of methodology.*

425
Van de Walle, E. and Page, H.
"Some New Estimates of Fertility and Mortality in Africa." *Population Index* 35(1), Jan.-Mar. 1969: pp. 3-17.

426
Vásquez, J.L.
"Fertility Decline in Puerto Rico: Extent and Causes." *Demography* 5(2), 1968: pp. 855-865.

> *Analysis of the demographic components of the fertility decline 1940-67, with special reference to the more rapid decline in 1960-67 and on the effect of migration from 1950-60.*

427
Visaria, P.M.
"Mortality and Fertility in India, 1951-1961." *Milbank Memorial Fund Quarterly* 47(1, Part 1), Jan. 1969: pp. 91-116.

> *An important attempt to estimate vital rates for India (1941-51) and (1951-61) using Coale-Demeny estimation procedures.*

428
Zelnik, M. and Khan, M.R.
"An Estimate of the Birth Rate in East and West Pakistan." *Pakistan Development Review* 5(1), Spring 1965: pp. 64-93.

III.C Fertility trends and norms during the demographic transition through World War II for countries now industrially developed

See also: 10, 80, 152, 187, 188, 190, 324, 456, 458, 460, 586, 665, 1023, 1031, 1047, 1092, 1147, 1399, 1559, 1568, 1570, 1577.

429
Bash, W.H.
"Changing Birth Rates in Developing America: New York State, 1840-1875." *Milbank Memorial Fund Quarterly* 41(2), Apr. 1963: pp. 161-182.

An analysis that challenges the traditional demographic transition theory by showing that rural fertility rates fell as rapidly as urban fertility in New York State.

430
Coale, A.J. and Zelnik, M.
New Estimates of Fertility and Population in the United States: A Study of Annual White Births from 1855 to 1960 and of Completeness of Enumeration in the Censuses from 1880 to 1960. Princeton: Princeton University Press, 1963; 186p.

An important set of estimates of fertility trends in the U.S. and methodology for making the estimates.

431
*Gille, H.
"The Demographic History of the Northern European Countries in the Eighteenth Century." *Population Studies* 3(1), June 1949: pp. 3-65.

432
Good, D.
"Some Aspects of Fertility Change in Hungary." *Population Index* 30(2), Apr. 1964: pp. 137-171.

Reviews data (1787-1962) on birth and death rates, rural and urban fertility patterns, migration, and state population policy.

433
*Habakkuk, H.J.
"Family Structure and Economic Change in Nineteenth-Century Europe." *Journal of Economic History* 15(1), Winter 1955: pp. 1-12.

434
*Habakkuk, H.J.
"The Economic History of Modern Britain." *Journal of Economic History* 18(4), Dec. 1958: pp. 486-501.

435
*Krause, J.T.
"Changes in English Fertility and Mortality, 1781-1850." *English History Review* 11(1), Aug. 1958: pp. 52-70.

Concludes from national materials that rising fertility was the main cause of population growth in England 1781-1850, probably resulting from higher marriage rates and higher illegitimacy rates.

436
Matthiessen, P.C.
"The Fertility for Birth Cohorts of Danish Women." In Szabady et al., eds. (*see* 40): pp. 209-218.

437
Mazur, D.P.
"Reconstruction of Fertility Trends for the Female Population of the U.S.S.R." *Population Studies* 21(1), July 1967: pp. 33-52.

Examination of Soviet cohort fertility rates over a 40-year period; comparisons with U.S. experience.

438
Myers, P.F.
"Demographic Trends in Eastern Europe." In *Economic Developments in Countries of Eastern Europe.* Subcommittee on Foreign Economic Policy of the Joint Economic Committee, Congress of the United States. Washington: Government Printing Office, 1970: pp. 68-148.

Description of demographic change in six countries of Eastern Europe; impact of World War II on population growth and composition, postwar fertility and nuptiality patterns, incidence of abortion, and age-specific population projections to 1990.

439
*Van den Brink, T.
"Birth Rate Trends and Changes in Marital Fertility in the Netherlands after 1937." *Population Studies* 4(3), Dec. 1950: pp. 314-332.

440
Wrigley, E.A.
Industrial Growth and Population Change. Cambridge, Eng.: Cambridge University Press, 1961; 193p.

> *A detailed study of regional demographic (including fertility) trends in the coal fields of Northwest Europe, 1850-1914, including comparisons with other urban and rural regions in Prussia and France; stresses the considerable regional variations in fertility, nuptiality, sex ratios, and net reproduction as making national averages or gross rural-urban comparisons misleading.*

441
Yasukawa, M.
"Estimates of Annual Births and of the General Fertility Rates in Japan, 1890-1920." *Keio Economic Studies* (Tokyo) 1, 1963: pp. 53-88.

442
Basavarajappa, K.G.
"Recent Trends and Patterns of Non-Maori Fertility in New Zealand." *Journal of Biosocial Science* 1, 1969: pp. 101-108.

443
Bednarski, B.
"Some Demographic Aspects of Family Unit Evolution." In *Proceedings of the Third Conference of the Region for Europe, Near East and Africa of the International Planned Parenthood Foundation.* International Congress Series, 71. The Hague: Excerpta Medica 1963: pp. 17-23.

> *Discussion of some of the important factors in the postwar demographic history of Europe.*

444
Blake, J.
"Ideal Family Size among White Americans: A Quarter of a Century's Evidence." *Demography* 3(1), 1966: pp. 154-173.

> *Uses data from Gallup surveys and the Growth of American Families studies to investigate trends in various measures of ideal and expected family size, emphasizing a rise in the average and concentration in two-to-four child range.*

III.D Postwar fertility trends and norms in mature industrialized countries

See also: 31, 140, 151, 187, 188, 190, 262, 313, 323, 430, 438, 546, 548, 692, 703, 1029, 1050, 1577.

445
Blake, J.
"Family Size in the 1960's—A Baffling Fad?" *Eugenics Quarterly* 14(1), Mar. 1967: pp. 60-74.

> *Disputes the view that postwar fertility trends are a result of "fads" or that they cannot be explained; interpretation based on series of data on desired family size.*

446

Brackett, J.W.

"Demographic Trends and Population Policy in the Soviet Union." In *Dimensions of Soviet Economic Power*. Joint Economic Committee, Congress of the United States, 87th Congress, 2nd Session, 91126. Washington: Government Printing Office, 1962: pp. 487-589.

Detailed statistical analysis of growth trends and component changes of the Soviet population from the period of the revolution: age-sex structure, ethnic differentials, trends in fertility including rural-urban and regional differentials, future trends, comparison with U.S. growth; recent developments in Marxist-Leninist population theory and Soviet population policy.

447

Brackett, J.W. and De Pauw, J.W.

"Population Policy and Demographic Trends in the Soviet Union." In *New Directions in the Soviet Economy*. Parts 3 and 4. Studies prepared for the Subcommittee on Foreign Economic Policy of the Joint Economic Committee, Congress of the United States, 89th Congress, 2nd Session. Washington: Government Printing Office, 1966: pp. 593-705.

448

Erskine, H.

"The Polls: More on the Population Explosion and Birth Control." *Public Opinion Quarterly* 31(2), Summer 1967: pp. 303-313.

Reproduces questions asked and tabulates replies given in three nationwide interview surveys in the U.S. in 1965, 1966, and 1967.

449

Glass, D.V.

"Fertility Trends in Europe since the Second World War." In Behrman, et al., eds. (*see* 51): pp. 25-74. [Also in *Population Studies* 22(1), Mar. 1968: pp. 103-146.]

Comprehensive review of European trends and patterns in fertility, nuptiality, family planning, and other pertinent data where available; very useful collection of data from a wide variety of sources.

450

Goldberg, D.

"Some Observations on Recent Changes in American Fertility Based on Sample Survey Data." *Eugenics Quarterly* 14(4), Dec. 1967: pp. 255-264.

Discussion of the possibilities for reconciling apparent discrepancies between cohort and period fertility rates for the period 1955-67.

451

Kuroda, T.

"An Analysis of the Change of Fertility in Postwar Japan." In *Archives of the Population Association of Japan* No. 4. Tokyo: 1963: pp. 24-40. [English edition.]

452

McArthur, N.

"Australia Birth Rate in Perspective." *Economic Record* (Melbourne) 43(101), Mar. 1967: pp. 57-64.

Report on cohort analysis of marital fertility.

453

Mitra, S.

"Child-Bearing Pattern of American Women." *Eugenics Quarterly* 13, June 1966: pp. 133-140.

Study of U.S. fertility using 1960 census data on childlessness and number of children born to cohorts of once-married women by color and such demographic variables as age and marriage duration.

454
*Ramholt, P.
"Nuptiality, Fertility, and Reproduction in Norway." *Population Studies* 7(1), July 1953: pp. 46-61.
   Cohort fertility and nuptiality analyses covering about 1920-50.

455
Rosenberg, H.
"Seasonal Variations of Births, United States, 1933-63." *Vital and Health Statistics* 6, May 1966; 59p.

456
Ryder, N.B.
"Fertility in Developed Countries during the Twentieth Century." In *Proceedings of the World Population Conference, 1965* (*see* 44): pp. 105-109.

457
Somogy, S.
"Variations in the Italian Population in the Decade 1951-1961." *Review of the Economic Conditions in Italy* (Rome) 16(4), July 1962: pp. 291-300.

458
Srb, V.
"The Population of Czechoslovakia in 1918-1968." In *Czechoslovak Population Problems.* Prague: Czechoslovak State Population Committee, 1968: pp 3-15.

459
Sweetser, F.L. and Piepponen, P.
"Postwar Fertility Trends and Their Consequences in Finland and the United States." *Journal of Social History* 1(2), Winter 1967: pp. 101-118.

   Cohort analysis of postwar fertility trends related to changes in the age distribution and the sociopolitical climate.

460
*United Nations. Department of Economic and Social Affairs.
Recent Trends in Fertility in Industrialized Countries. ST/SOA/Ser. A/27. New York: 1958; 182p.

461
Whelpton, P.K.
"Why Did the United States Crude Birth Rate Decline during 1957-1962?" *Population Index* 29(2), Apr. 1963: pp. 120-125.
   The role of changes in timing of births and age distributions.

462
Whelpton, P.K. et al.
"Trends and Determinants of Family Size in the U.S." *American Journal of Public Health and the Nation's Health* 54(11), Nov. 1964: pp. 1834-1840.

III.E The use of contraception and induced abortion

See also: 95, 363, 438, 670, 681, 932, 1021, 1204, 1208, 1218, 1231, 1304, 1343, 1344, 1525.

463
Allingham, J.D. et al.
"The End of Rapid Increase in the Use of Oral Anovulants: Some Problems in

the Interpretation of Time Series of Oral Use among Married Women." *Demography* 7(1), Feb. 1970: pp. 31-41.

On the basis of a metropolitan Toronto area sample, rate of use of oral contraception decreases when duration or marriage and other variables are taken into account.

464
Blacker, C.P.
"Voluntary Sterilization: Transitions throughout the World." *Eugenics Review* 54(3), Oct. 1962: pp. 143-162.

Current practice and legal regulation in Japan, Sweden, Denmark, United Kingdom, U.S., and Puerto Rico.

465
Coale, A.J.
"Voluntary Control of Fertility." *Proceedings of the American Philosophical Society* 111(3), 1967: pp. 164-169.

Brief history of the conditions under which voluntary fertility control appears; speculations about extension to populations where it is not yet general.

466
Erskine, H.G.
"The Polls: The Population Explosion, Birth Control, and Sex Education." *Public Opinion Quarterly* 30(3), Fall 1966: pp. 490-501.

Reproduces results of a variety of polls from the 1930s through the early 1960s on a variety of questions related to contraception and sex education; in general shows trend to more favorable attitudes toward use of contraception, government intervention, and provision of information and services, with increasing approval by Catholics and lower status groups especially in the more recent period.

467
Finch, B.E. and Green, H.
Contraception through the Ages. Springfield, Ill.: Charles C Thomas, 1963; 174p.

Traces the history of the development of contraceptive methods from ancient times; considers cultural and legal aspects.

468
Freundt, L.
"Surveys of Induced and Spontaneous Abortions in the Copenhagen Area." *Acta Psychiatrica Scandinavica* (Copenhagen) (Supplement) 40, 1964: pp. 180-235.

469
Hardin, G.
"The History and Future of Birth Control." *Perspectives in Biology and Medicine* 10(1). Autumn 1966: pp. 1-18.

Historical view of contraception policies and need for abortion as a supplement to contraceptive practices.

470
Himes, N.E.
Medical History of Contraception. New York: Gamut Press, 1964; 521p.

Reissue of the major history of the use of contraception for the period before 1936.

471
Hopkins, K.
"Contraception in the Roman Empire." *Comparative Studies in Society and History* (The Hague) 8(1), Oct. 1965: pp. 124-151.

References in literature and circumstantial evidence on practice of contraception and its consequence.

472
Saxton, G.A., Jr. et al.
"The Place of Intra-uterine Contracep-

tive Devices in East Africa." *East African Medical Journal* (Nairobi) 42, Nov. 1965: pp. 646-660.

473
Suyin, H.
"Family Planning in China Today." *Eastern Horizon* (Hong Kong) 4(11), Nov. 1965: pp. 5-8.

474
Tien, H.Y.
"Sterilization, Oral Contraception, and Population Control in China." *Population Studies* 18(3), Mar. 1965: pp. 215-235.

Discussion of the promotion of sterilization and traditional contraceptive methods and the need for modern oral contraceptives in mainland China.

475
Tietze, C.
"History of Contraceptive Methods." *Journal of Sex Research* 1(2), July 1965: pp. 69-85.

Short summary, with excellent bibliography, of all major methods of contraception—history, advantages, and weaknesses.

476
Valoaras, V.G. et al.
"Control of Family Size in Greece." *Population Studies* 18(3), Mar. 1965: pp. 265-278.

Survey of clients coming to general health facilities indicating a combination of poor contraception and considerable illegal abortion used to explain low birth rates and need for legitimate sources of better information and services.

III.F Descriptive studies of other intermediate variables: fetal mortality, nuptiality, birth spacing, etc.

See also: 199, 200, 228, 230, 235, 363, 364, 368, 384, 418, 422, 438, 508, 529, 1021, 1268, 1292, 1295, 1299, 1312, 1340, 1358, 1636.

477
Agrawal, B.L.
"Some Birth Interval and Order of Live Birth Data in Sample Registration." *Sample Registration Bulletin, Provincial Statistics* (New Delhi) no. 29, May 1969: pp. 3-4.

Summary of data on births by order and age of mother in a large sample involving 12 Indian states for the period 1965-67.

478
Amundsen, D.W. and Diers, C.J.
"The Age of Menarche in Classical Greece and Rome." *Human Biology* 41(1), Feb. 1969: pp. 125-132.

479
Basavarajappa, K.G.
"Pre-Marital Pregnancies and Ex-Nuptial Births in Australia, 1911-66." *Australian and New Zealand Journal of Sociology* 4(2), Oct. 1968: pp. 126-145.

480
Benjamin, B.
"Changes in Marriage Incidence in

Western Society in the Last Thirty Years." *Journal of the Institute of Actuaries* 89(II, 382) 1963: pp. 125-134.

481
Bhate, V.
"Rate of Incidence of Widowhood." *Artha Vijñāna* (Poona) 4(3), Sept. 1962: pp. 198-209. [Hindi summary.]

482
Bierman, J.M. et al.
"Analysis of the Outcome of All Pregnancies in a Community: Kauai Pregnancy Study." *American Journal of Obstetrics and Gynecology* 91, Jan. 1965: pp. 37-45.

An unusually intensive canvass to determine all pregnancies in an area and to follow up until all live-born were two years of age; yields an estimate of about 240 per 1,000 for fetal mortality and other estimates for infant mortality and for perinatal handicaps to the age of two.

483
*Dandekar, K.
"Widow Remarriage in Six Rural Communities in India." In *International Population Conference* New York, 1961. London: U.N.E.S.C.O. 1963: pp. 191-207.

484
Drake, M.
"Marriage and Population Growth in Ireland, 1750-1845." *Economic History Review* (2nd Series) 16(2), Dec. 1963: pp. 301-313.

485
Goubert, P.
"Legitimate Fecundity and Infant Mortality in France during the Eighteenth Century: A Comparison." *Daedalus* 97(2), Spring 1968: pp. 593-603.

486
Hopkins, M.K.
"The Age of Roman Girls at Marriage." *Population Studies* 18(3), Mar. 1965: pp. 309-327.

487
*Hyrenius, H.
"Fertility and Reproduction in a Swedish Population Group without Family Limitation." *Population Studies* 12(2), Nov. 1958: pp. 121-130.

488
Jeanneret, O. and MacMahon, B.
"Secular Changes in Rates of Multiple Births in the United States." *American Journal of Human Genetics* 14(4), Dec. 1962: pp. 410-425.

Examines trends, maternal age, parity, racial and regional variations.

489
Matthiessen, P.C.
"Infant and Perinatal Mortality in Denmark." Analytical Studies. *Vital and Health Statistics* (Series 3) 3(9), Nov. 1967; 67p.

Analysis of level and trends of perinatal and infant mortality in Denmark, with emphasis on the period 1951-62.

490
Mehlan, K.H. and Falkenthal, S.
"Birth Intervals and Their Effect on the Fertility and Health of Women." In Szabady et al., eds. (*see* 39): pp. 27-39.

Describes trends in number of children and birth intervals in Germany 1901-60, with inference about relation to mother's health.

491
Muller-Dietz, H.
"Abortion in the Soviet Union and in the East European States." *Review of Soviet Medical Sciences* (Munich) 1(2), 1964: pp. 28-35.

492
Roth, D.B.
"The Frequency of Spontaneous Abortion." *International Journal of Fertility* 8(1), Jan.-Mar. 1963: pp. 431-434.

On basis of scanty American data, indicates probability of higher rate of spontaneous abortion for the general population and lower rate for consecutive aborters than previously assumed.

493
*Stone, L.
"Marriage among the English Nobility in the 16th and 17th Centuries." *Comparative Studies in Society and History* (The Hague) 3(2), Jan. 1961: pp. 182-206.

IV. STUDIES RELATING STRATIFICATION VARIABLES TO FERTILITY AND FERTILITY NORMS

IV.A Economic strata

See also: 256, 648, 710, 918, 1035, 1051, 1438, 1528.

494
*Becker, G.S.
"An Economic Analysis of Fertility." In *Demographic and Economic Change in Developed Countries*. Princeton: Princeton University Press, 1960: pp. 209-240.
Argues that "quality" as well as quantity of children is relevant in analysis of possible positive relation of fertility and income in mature industrial society.

495
Blake, J.
"Income and Reproductive Motivation." *Population Studies* 21(3), Nov. 1967: pp. 185-206.
Examines results from 13 U.S. studies, 1936-66, to argue that there is no positive association between income and family size preferences; suggests findings invalidate theory of consumer demand for children; considers intervening effect of Catholicism.

496
Cho, L.J.
"Income and Differentials in Current

Fertility." *Demography* 5(1), 1968: pp. 198-211.
On the basis of 1960 U.S. census data, studies relation between fertility measures and income, taking into account race, urban-rural residence and wife's labor-force participation.

497
Davtyan, L.M.
"The Influence of Socio-Economic Factors on Natality (as Exemplified in the Armenian Soviet Socialist Republic.)" In *Proceedings of the World Population Conference, 1965 (see 44):* pp. 73-77.
Survey data cited indicate negative correlations between income, education, wife's participation in labor force, and adequacy of housing; author interprets how the socialist conditions may alter the measuring or character of these relationships.

498
Duncan, O.D.
"Residential Areas and Differential Fertility." *Eugenics Quarterly* 11(2), June 1964: pp. 82-89.
Both median rent for census tract and individual rental data had an effect on fertility in Indianapolis in 1941, independent of other individual characteristics.

499
Freedman, D.S.
"The Relation of Economic Status to Fertility." *American Economic Review* 53(3), June 1963: pp. 414-426.

Supports the hypothesis that fertility is affected less by actual income than by the relation between actual income and income expected in a family's occupational and educational reference group.

500
Gupta, P.B. and Malaker, C.R.
"Fertility Differentials with Level of Living and Adjustment of Fertility, Birth and Death Rates." *Sankhyā* (Calcutta) (Series B) 25(1-2), Nov. 1963: pp. 26-48.

Relation between levels of living and fertility levels in a national Indian study; methodological contributions to the estimation of fertility rates from a retrospective survey.

501
Orshansky, M.
"Counting the Poor: Another Look at the Poverty Profile." *Social Security Bulletin* Jan. 1965: pp. 3-29.

Relation of family size to poverty, incidental to a larger discussion of measurement and distribution of poverty.

502
Orshansky, M.
"Who's Who among the Poor: A Demographic View of Poverty." *Social Security Bulletin* July 1965: pp. 3-32.

Detailed profile of the demographic and socioeconomic characteristics of the poor in the U.S.

503
*Sinha, J.N.
"Differential Fertility and Family Limitation in an Urban Community of Uttar Pradesh." *Population Studies* 11(2), Nov. 1957: pp. 157-169.

Distinctively negative correlation between income or caste level and fertility, resulting in part from differential use of contraception.

504
*Stys, W.
"The Influence of Economic Conditions on the Fertility of Peasant Women." *Population Studies* 11(2), Nov. 1957: pp. 136-148.

Positive relation between economic status and fertility in a peasant population as a result of marriage postponement for poorer economic groups.

505
Wunderlich, G.S.
Educational Attainment of Mother and Family Income: White Legitimate Births, United States—1963. Vital Health and Statistics. Washington: Government Printing Office, 1968; 46p.

506
Zelnik, M.
"Socioeconomic and Seasonal Variations in Births: A Replication." *Milbank Memorial Fund Quarterly* 47(2), Apr. 1969: pp. 159-165.

During 1961-65 there was no significant differential in seasonal pattern of births for low- and high-status births in Baltimore; high-status groups did not have a rectilinear pattern over the seasons as postulated in an earlier study by Pasamanick and others (see 512).

IV.B Occupation
See also: 362, 515, 534, 591, 968, 1022, 1025, 1035, 1353, 1494, 1529.

507
Blau, P.M. and Duncan, O.D.
The American Occupational Structure.
New York: John Wiley & Sons, 1967;
520p.
> *A landmark systematic analysis of U.S. occupational stratification system; includes sections on differential fertility and nuptiality.*

508
*Glass, D.V. and Grebenik, E.
"The Trend and Pattern of Fertility in
Great Britain." In *Papers of the Royal
Commission on Population* London:
H.M.S.O., 1954; 2 Vols.
> *A Major cohort analysis of fertility and nuptiality trends in relation to broad socio-occupational strata; important methodological sections.*

509
Loschky, D.J. and Krier, D.F.
"Income and Family Size in Three Eighteenth-Century Lancashire Parishes: A
Reconstitution Study," *Journal of Economic History* 29(3), Sept. 1969: pp.
429-448.
> *Occupational class as a proxy for income is related to age at marriage, average number of births, and age differences between spouses; applies findings to demographic transition theory.*

510
Mitra, S.
"Occupation and Fertility in the United
States." *Eugenics Quarterly* 13(2), June
1966: pp. 141-146.
> *Analysis of occupational differentials in fertility based on comparisons of 1950 and 1960 U.S. census.*

511
Nazaret, F.V.
"Differential Fertility by Occupational

Groups in the Philippines." *Philippine
Statistician* (Manila) 11(1), Mar. 1962:
pp. 516-522.

512
*Pasamanick, B. et al.
"Socio-Economic and Seasonal Variations in the Birth Rates." *Milbank Memorial Fund Quarterly* 38(3), July 1960:
pp. 248-254.

513
Windle, C. and Sabagh, G.
"Social Status and Family Size of Iranian Industrial Employees." *Milbank Memorial Fund Quarterly* 41(4, Part 1), Oct.
1963: pp. 436-443.
> *A study of more than 18,000 employees of an oil company finds a U-shaped relation between job rank and fertility for both Moslems and Christians, but higher Moslem rates at every rank, apparently because of differences in age at marriage.*

IV.C Education and literacy

See also: 134, 136, 138, 263, 356, 497,
505, 538, 988, 1016, 1022, 1025, 1031,
1039, 1045, 1063, 1228, 1498, 1501, 1616.

514
Bajema, C.J.
"Relation of Fertility to Educational
Attainment in a Kalamazoo Public
School Population: A Follow-up
Study." *Eugenics Quarterly* 13(4), Dec.
1966: pp. 306-315.
> *Analyzes the interrelation of educational attainment and I.Q. scores with fertility by follow-up of an age cohort tested in the sixth grade.*

515
Bajema, C.J.
"Relation of Fertility to Occupational Status, IQ, Educational Attainment, and Size of Family of Origin: A Follow-up Study of a Male Kalamazoo Public School Population." *Eugenics Quarterly* 15(3), Sept. 1968: pp. 198-203.

516
Blake, J.
"Reproductive Ideals and Educational Attainment among White Americans, 1943-1960." *Population Studies* 21(2), Sept. 1967: pp. 159-174.

Using historical series of poll and survey data, examines educational differentials in actual and desired (ideal) family size, with controls for age, religion, and rural-urban residence; reaches policy conclusion that significant decline in fertility requires change in values for all major educational strata.

517
Bouvier, L.F. and Macisco, J.J., Jr.
"Education of Husband and Wife and Fertility in Puerto Rico, 1960." *Social and Economic Studies* (Jamaica) 17(1), Mar. 1968: pp. 49-59.

Uses 1960 census data to consider the relation of education of husband and wife to fertility.

518
Breznik, D.
"Sterility of First Marriages." In Szabady et al., eds. (*see* 39): pp. 19-26.

The effects of region, education, and demographic factors on sterility, based on data in the 1953 Yugoslav census.

519
Dice, L.R. et al.
"Relation of Fertility to Education in Ann Arbor, Michigan, 1951-1954." *Eu-

genics Quarterly* 11(2), Mar. 1964: pp. 30-45.

On basis of small sample, correlation of education and fertility has no significant genetic effect.

520
***Duncan, O.D. and Hodge, R.W.**
"Cohort Analysis of Differential Natality." In *International Population Conference.* New York, 1961. London: U.N.E.S.C.O., 1963: pp. 59-68.

Uses census data to trace fertility history of cohorts classified by age and education.

521
El-Badry, M.A.
"A Study of Differential Fertility in Bombay." *Demography* 4(2), 1967: pp. 626-640.

Birth registration data used to relate standardized average parity rates to overcrowding, religion, illiteracy, and migration status for 67 areal divisions of Bombay.

522
Godley, E.H.
"Fertility and Educational Attainment, Puerto Rico, 1962." *Vital and Health Statistics* (Series 21) 12, Sept. 1967; 20p.

Birth registration data used to analyze the relation of educational attainment and nuptiality variables to fertility.

523
Liu, A.
"Education as a Factor in Limiting Population Growth." *Advances in Fertility Control* (Amsterdam) 3(3), Sept. 1968: pp. 38-43.

524
Mitra, S.
"Education and Fertility in the United

States." *Eugenics Quarterly* 13(3), Sept. 1966: pp. 214-222.

525
Olusanya, P.O.
"The Educational Factor in Human Fertility: A Case Study of the Residents of a Suburban Area in Ibadan, Western Nigeria." *Nigerian Journal of Economic and Social Studies* (Ibadan) 9(3), Nov. 1967: pp. 351-374.
A KAP survey for small samples of women in a migrant and suburban community.

526
Schuman, H. et al.
"Some Social Psychological Effects and Non-effects of Literacy in a New Nation." *Economic Development and Cultural Change* 16(1), 1967: pp. 1-14.
A study of East Pakistan (now Bangladesh) finds literacy positively associated with favorable view of family planning but only if it is combined with industrial experience.

527
Sutton, G.F. and Wunderlich, G.S.
"Estimating Marital Fertility Rates by Educational Attainment Using a Survey of New Mothers." *Demography* 4(1), 1967: pp. 135-142.

528
Westoff, C.F. and Potvin, R.H.
College Women and Fertility Values. Princeton: Princeton University Press, 1967; 237p.
Large survey of women from Catholic and non-Catholic colleges. Studies the effect of different types of higher education on family size values, the socioeconomic, religious, ethnic, and parental family characteristics relevant to family size and family planning attitudes; derives theory about how fertility values are learned in early adolescence.

529
Whelpton, P.K.
"Trends and Differentials in the Spacing of Births." *Demography* 1(1), 1964: pp. 83-93.
Analysis of changes in birth spacing over the time and the relation of recent birth interval changes to religion and education in the U. S.

IV.D Other specific measures: prestige, caste, etc.
See also: 503, 507, 509, 970, 1504, 1531.

530
*Hollingsworth, T.H.
"A Demographic Study of the British Ducal Families." *Population Studies* 11(1), July 1957: pp. 4-26.
Fertility history of this elite group from preindustrial period to the present.

531
Hollingsworth, T.H
"The Demography of the British Peerage." *Population Studies* (Supplement) 18(2), Nov. 1964; 108p.
Cohort analysis of trends in nuptiality, fertility, and mortality of British nobility, 1550-1949.

532
Hollingsworth, T.H.
"The Demographic Background of the Peerage, 1603-1938." *Eugenics Review* 57(2), June 1965: pp. 56-66.
Summary of Hollingsworth's 1964 study (see 531), with some additional information.

533
Potter, R.G., Jr. et al.
"A Fertility Differential in Eleven Punjab Villages." *Milbank Memorial Fund Quarterly* 43(2, Part 1), Apr. 1965: pp. 185-201.
Analysis of differential fertility related to caste in a carefully maintained control-group experiment to study fertility histories with and without a family planning program; finds persistent caste differences antedating the study.

534
Saxena, G.B.
"Differential Fertility in Rural Hindu Community: A Sample Survey of the Rural Uttar Pradesh, India." *Eugenics Quarterly* 12(3), Sept. 1965: pp. 137-145.
Study to assess effect of caste and occupation on fertility; reports no use of contraception in any of the groups; high birth rate related to early marriage and long span of fertility; caste inversely related to fertility, but occupation of little independent importance.

IV.E Social mobility between strata
See also: 39, 507, 538, 1196, 1512, 1534.

535
*Berent, J.
"Fertility and Social Mobility." *Population Studies* 5(3), Mar. 1952: pp. 244-260.
Negative relation between upward social mobility and fertility in postwar British data.

536
*Blacker, J.G.G.
"Social Ambitions of the Bourgeoisie in

18th Century France and Their Relation to Family Limitation." *Population Studies* 11(1), July 1957: pp. 46-63.
Relates the family limitation practices of the French bourgeoisie to their desire for social mobility for the family.

537
*Hutchinson, B.
"Fertility, Social Mobility, and Urban Migration in Brazil." *Population Studies* 14(3), Mar. 1961: pp. 182-189.
Finds that fertility is negatively related both to status and upward mobility, and these relations are not affected by rural or urban background.

538
Perrucci, C.C.
"Social Origins, Mobility Patterns and Fertility." *American Sociological Review* 32(4), Aug. 1967: pp. 615-625.
Family size and child spacing related to mobility patterns and educational levels for sample of engineering graduates.

539
Tien, H.Y.
Social Mobility and Controlled Fertility: Family Origins and Structure of the Australian Academic Elite. New Haven: College and University Press, 1965; 224p.
Relation of family size and birth spacing to intergenerational mobility in a small sample of Australian professors.

IV.F Combinations of several of the preceding status criteria, or generalized status measures, or

parallel treatments of different status criteria

See also: 1, 56, 64, 130, 132, 255, 302, 303, 349, 358, 422, 449, 499, 528, 599, 633, 868, 922, 971, 975, 978, 980, 1016, 1018, 1019, 1032, 1076, 1087, 1093, 1096, 1097, 1098, 1099, 1101, 1102, 1106, 1140, 1142, 1184, 1186, 1199, 1209, 1220, 1222, 1223, 1228, 1296, 1362, 1473, 1493, 1502, 1503, 1504, 1506, 1508, 1509, 1510, 1511, 1512, 1516, 1518, 1519, 1520, 1521, 1522, 1527, 1531, 1532, 1533, 1534, 1535, 1537, 1538.

540
Abu-Lughod, J.
"The Emergence of Differential Fertility in Urban Egypt." *Milbank Memorial Fund Quarterly* 43(2, Part 1), Apr. 1965: pp. 235-253.

Compares 1947 and 1960 fertility data for Cairo, finding persistent negative correlations with education and occupation.

541
Anand, K.
"Opinion and Attitude towards Family Planning in Chandigarh." *Journal of Family Welfare* (Bombay) 10(4), June 1964: pp. 60-65.

Results of survey of 100 married women relating ideal and actual family size to income, literacy, occupation, and residence.

542
Carleton, R.O.
"Fertility Trends and Differentials in Latin America." *Milbank Memorial Fund Quarterly* 43(4, Part 2), Oct. 1965: pp. 15-35.

543
*Chandrasekaran, C. and George, M.V.
"Mechanisms Underlying the Differences in Fertility Patterns of Bengalese Women from Three Socio-Economic Groups." *Milbank Memorial Fund Quarterly* 40, Jan. 1962: pp. 59-89.

Beginnings of fertility decline in Bengal may be present in urban practices resembling those of the West at a similar stage.

544
Chinnatamby, S.
"Fertility Trends in Ceylonese Women." *Journal of Reproduction and Fertility* 3(3), June 1962: pp. 342-355.

From records of 5,223 female clients of family planning clinics; relationship of fertility to age at puberty, age at marriage, income, educational level, and urban-rural residence.

545
Cowgill, U.M.
"The Season of Birth in Man." *Man* 1(2), June 1966: pp. 232-239.

Critical study of data from Europe and South America on socioeconomic factors related to seasonality in births.

546
Dobbelaere, K.
"Ideal Number of Children in Marriage in Belgium and the U.S.A." *Journal of Marriage and the Family* 29(2), 1967: pp. 360-367.

Comparisons of Belgian and U.S. surveys of relation between ideal family size and income, occupation, education, and mobility.

547
El-Badry, M.A. and Rizk, H.
"Regional Fertility Differences among Socio-Economic Groups in the United Arab Republic." In *Proceedings of the World Population Conference, 1965* (*see* 44): pp. 137-141.

Survey and census data for 1957 and 1960 used to relate educational and occupational strata for fertility within rural-urban strata; finds interaction between social and urban variables, with farmers having lowest rural rates and professional or administrative workers lowest urban rates.

548
Freedman, R. and Bumpass, L.
"Fertility Expectations in the United States: 1962-64." *Population Index* 32(2), Apr. 1966: pp. 181-197.
Last of a series of five trend reports with data on period and cohort fertility rates and expectations, differentials by religion, education, occupation, income, race, farm background. Earlier reports were all published in Population Index:
Axelrod, M. et al. "Fertility Expectations of the United States Population: A Time Series" 29(1), Jan. 1963: pp. 25-31.
Freedman, R. et al. "Current Fertility Expectations of Married Couples in the United States" 29(4), Oct. 1963: pp. 366-391.
Freedman, R. et al. "Fertility Expectations of Married Couples in the United States: 1963" 30(2), Apr. 1964: pp. 171-175.
Freedman, R. et al. "Current Fertility Expectations of Married Couples in the United States: 1963" 31(1), Jan. 1965: pp. 3-20.

549
Fuchs, Z. and Marshall, D.G.
Fertility Trends in Wisconsin, 1900-1964. Madison, Wisc.: Department of Rural Sociology, College of Agriculture, University of Wisconsin, 1966; 67p.
Fertility differentials by socioeconomic status, race, age, marital status, and labor-force status of women.

550
Gendell, M.
"Fertility and Development in Brazil." *Demography* 4(1), 1967: pp. 143-157.
Fertility trends and changes in differential fertility during the period of Brazilian development.

551
*Goldberg, D.
"The Fertility of Two-Generation Urbanites." *Population Studies* 12(3), Mar. 1959: pp. 214-222.
Shows that the relation of status measures to fertility depends on rural background in Detroit, Michigan.

552
*Goldberg, D.
"Another Look at the Indianapolis Fertility Data." *Milbank Memorial Fund Quarterly* 38(1), Jan. 1960: pp. 23-36.
Correlations of status measures to fertility become more positive when only couples without any farm background are considered.

553
Goldberg, D.
"Fertility and Fertility Differentials: Some Observations on Recent Changes in the United States." In Sheps and Ridley, eds. (*see* 73): pp. 119-142. [Also in *Eugenics Quarterly* 14(4), Dec. 1967: pp. 255-264.]
An interpretative review of U.S. studies; suggests hypotheses to explain time trends and cross-sectional differentials.

554
*Hawley, A.H.
"Rural Fertility in Central Luzon." *American Sociological Review* 20(1), Feb. 1955: pp. 21-27.

Finds positive relation between fertility and size of land holding, although relation to educational and occupational status is negative.

555
Hicks, W.W.
"A 'Reproduction Function' for Young Women in Mexico." *Social and Economic Studies* (Jamaica) 15(2), June 1966: pp. 121-125.

Estimates effects of various socioeconomic variables on fertility by ecological data for 32 Mexican states, 1960.

556
Higgins, E.
"Some Fertility Attitudes among White Women in Johannesburg." *Population Studies* 16(1), July 1962: pp. 70-78.

Analysis of ideal family size by ethnic, religious group, and socioeconomic status measures for urban whites in 1957-58 in South Africa.

557
Hutchinson, B.
"Colour, Social Status and Fertility in Brazil." *America Latina* (Rio de Janeiro) 8(4), Oct.-Dec. 1965: pp. 3-25.

Differential fertility, nuptiality, and fetal mortality studied in relation to color, social status, and life-cycle variables based on a Brazil survey, 1962-63.

558
*Kiser, C.V. and Whelpton, P.K.
"Fertility Planning and Fertility Rates by Socio-Economic Status." In Kiser and Whelpton, eds. (*see* 1512) Vol. 2: pp. 359-416.

An important demonstration that fertility differentials are related to differential contraceptive practice in the Indianapolis study.

559
*Kitagawa, E.M.
"Differential Fertility in Chicago, 1920-1940." *American Journal of Sociology* 58(5), Mar. 1953: pp. 481-492.

Analyzes the trends of nuptial and total fertility for five socioeconomic groups and demonstrates convergence toward a positive relation of nuptial fertility and socioeconomic status with rising fertility even before 1940; shows the importance of nuptiality as an intervening variable.

560
Kono, S.
"Social and Economic Factors Affecting Fertility in Japan." In *Annual Reports of the Institute of Population Problems,* 11. Tokyo: Institute of Population Problems, 1966: pp. 39-42, 86.

561
Kunz, P.B.
"The Relation of Income and Fertility." *Journal of Marriage and the Family* 27(4), Nov. 1965: pp. 509-513.

Tests the relation between income and fertility within education-occupation categories, on the basis of the 1960 census.

562
Lee, H.Y. et al.
Differential Fertility Survey of a Korean Middle Town, Ichon Eup. Seoul: Population Studies Center, Seoul National University, 1965; 183p.

563
Liu, P.K,C.
"Differential Fertility in Taiwan." In 1967 I.U.S.S.P. (*see* 21): pp. 363-370.

Reports on 1966 differentials in fertility as related to extended family type, education of wife and husband's occupation, wife's labor-force status, and the type of area; based on samples from Taiwan's population register.

564

Macisco, J.J., Jr.

"Fertility in Puerto Rico: An Ecological Study." *Sociological Analysis* 26(3), Fall 1965: pp. 157-164.

1960 U.S. census data used to develop correlations between fertility and socioeconomic areal measures.

565

Matras, J.

"The Social Strategy of Family Formation: Some Variations in Time and Space." *Demography* 2, 1965: pp. 349-362.

One of a series of studies by Matras that analyzes the relation of socioeconomic measures to age at marriage and fertility levels and makes inferences about levels of contraceptive practice and the social strategy of family formation. (See following articles and see also 1021.)

566

Matras, J.

"Social Strategies of Family Formation: Some Comparative Data for Scandinavia, The British Isles, and North America." *International Social Science Journal* 17(2), 1965: pp. 1-16.

567

Matras, J.

"Social Strategies of Family Formation: Data for British Female Cohorts Born 1831-1906." *Population Studies* 19(2), Nov. 1965: pp. 167-181.

568

Mitra, S.

"Income, Socioeconomic Status, and Fertility in the United States." *Eugenics Quarterly* 13(3), Sept. 1966: pp. 223-230.

569

*Moore, W.P.

"Attitudes of Mexican Factory Workers toward Fertility Control." In *Approaches to Problems of High Fertility in Agrarian Societies.* New York: Milbank Memorial Fund, 1952: pp. 74-101.

Higher education and literacy linked to low-fertility values but much of this relation is a function of age differences; income directly related to family size for this sample of factory workers.

570

Morris, J.K.

"Changing Patterns of Fertility: A Study in Depth." *Population Bulletin* 20(5), Sept. 1964: pp. 118-139.

A summary of U.S. 1950-60 fertility differentials with reference to education, income, religion, wife's work status, urbanization, and religion; not in depth.

571

Okediji, F.O.

"Some Social Psychological Aspects of Fertility among Married Women in an African City." *Nigerian Journal of Economic and Social Studies* (Ibadan) 9(1), Mar. 1967: pp. 67-79.

Study of relationship of education, occupation, and income to ideal family size, actual family size, and attitudes toward use of contraceptives.

572

Okediji, F.O.

"Some Social Psychological Aspects of Fertility among Married Women in an African City: Rejoinder." *Nigerian Journal of Economic and Social Studies* (Ibadan) 10(1), Mar. 1968: pp. 125-133.

Rejoinder to Olusanya's review (see 573).

573
Olusanya, P.O.
"Some Social Psychological Aspects of Fertility among Married Women in an African City : Comments." *Nigerian Journal of Economic and Social Studies* (Ibadan) 10(1), Mar. 1968: pp. 117-123.
Critical review of Okediji's 1967 article (see 571).

574
Powers, M.G.
"Socioeconomic Status and the Fertility of Married Womem." *Sociology and Social Research* 50(4), July 1966: pp. 472-482.
Uses the 1-in-1,000 sample of the 1960 U.S. census to relate a multiple-item index of socioeconomic status and a measure of status consistency to fertility of married women 35-44 years of age.

575
Rele, J.R.
"Fertility Differentials in India: Evidence from a Rural Background." *Milbank Memorial Fund Quarterly* 41(2), Apr. 1963: pp. 183-199.
Analysis of rural Uttar Pradesh fertility differentials in 1956 with reference to caste, occupation, and literacy.

576
Rizk, H.
"Social and Psychological Factors Affecting Fertility in the United Arab Republic." *Marriage and Family Living* 25(1), Feb. 1963: pp. 69-73.
Brief report on a social survey relating education, occupation, and urbanization to fertility and family planning.

577
Scott, J.W.
"Sources of Social Changes in Community Family, and Fertility in a Puerto Rican Town." *American Journal of Sociology* 72(5), Mar. 1967: pp. 520-530.
Sample data (206 interviews) on fertility attitudes and performance in relation to socioeconomic characteristics of married women in a mountain town.

578
Stockwell, E.G.
"Use of Socioeconomic Status as a Demographic Variable." *Public Health Reports* 81(11), Nov. 1966: pp. 961-966.
Analyzes the relation between several socioeconomic measures and fertility (as well as migration and mortality) for 169 towns in the state of Connecticut.

579
Stoeckel, J. and Choudhury, M.A.
"Differential Fertility in a Rural Area of East Pakistan." *Milbank Memorial Fund Quarterly* 47(2), Apr. 1969: pp. 189-198.
Total and age-specific marital fertility rates by occupation, education, land holding, religion, family-structure type, and age.

580
Stycos, J.M.
"Social Class and Preferred Family Size in Peru." *American Journal of Sociology* 70(6), May 1965: pp. 651-658.
Comparisons of relationships of social status to actual and desired fertility and to knowledge and attitudes about family planning based on sample surveys in Lima and in a Peruvian mountain town.

581
Tabah, L.
"A Study of Fertility in Santiago, Chile." *Marriage and Family Living* 25(1), Feb. 1963: pp. 20-26.

A 1959 survey in Santiago on the relation of economic status, education, and labor-force status of wife to fertility, fertility norms, contraception and abortion, premarital pregnancies, and age at marriage.

582

Takeshita, J.Y.

"Population Control in Japan: A Miracle or Secular Trend." *Marriage and Family Living* 25(1), Feb. 1963: pp. 44-52.

Intensive survey in Osaka in 1956 indicates that postwar legislation in Japan served chiefly to facilitate diffusion of fertility norms and controls already begun under industrial-urban transformation; material on socioeconomic status, rural background, and wife's work experience.

583

Verster, J.

"The Trend and Pattern of Fertility in Soweto: An Urban Bantu Community." *African Studies* (Johannesburg) 24(3-4), 1965: pp. 131-198.

Detailed survey findings of fertility levels and differentials related to occupation, education, tribe, rural-urban, age at first birth; analysis of age structure and age-specific activity rates.

584

*Whelpton, P.K. and Kiser, C.V.

"Differential Fertility among 41,498 Native-White Couples in Indianapolis." In Kiser and Whelpton, eds. (*see* 1512) Vol. 1: pp. 1-60.

Analysis of differential fertility based on large-scale survey from which sample for the Indianapolis study was selected.

585

Zarate, A.O.

"Differential Fertility in Monterrey, Mexico: Prelude to Transition?" *Milbank Memorial Fund Quarterly* 45(2, Part 1), Apr. 1967: pp. 213-228.

Sample survey data on fertility differentials by education, occupation, income, wife's work status, and age at marriage.

V. STUDIES RELATING FAMILY STRUCTURE TO FERTILITY AND FERTILITY NORMS

V.A Types of family structure and their relation to other institutions

V.A.1 The roles of women (especially as workers)

See also: 56, 64, 132, 134, 136, 138, 358, 449, 497, 548, 549, 563, 570, 581, 585, 608, 615, 620, 678, 692, 1097, 1440, 1493, 1506, 1508, 1511, 1512, 1527, 1529, 1534, 1537.

586
Banks, J.A. and Banks, O.
Feminism and Family Planning in Victorian England. Liverpool: University Press, 1964; 142p. [Also in *Studies in Sociology* Series New York: Schocken Books, 1964; 142p.]
Economic forces and male decisions more important than feminist movement in fertility decline in Victorian England.

587
*Blake, J.
Family Structure in Jamaica: The Social *Context of Reproduction.* New York: Free Press, 1961; 262p.
Intensive analysis of how form of Jamaican sexual and marital relationships affects fertility, nuptiality patterns, illegitimacy, and stability of sexual unions.

588
Collver, O.A.
"Women's Work Participation and Fertility in Metropolitan Areas." *Demography* 5(1), 1968: pp. 55-60.
A multivariate analysis for 65 metropolitan areas in the U.S. (1960-61) of the relation between labor-force participation of women and fertility rates, taking into account marital status, race, and educational levels.

589
Federici, N.
"The Influence of Women's Employment on Fertility." In Szabady et al., eds. (*see* 40): pp. 77-82.
Regression analysis of regional Italian age-specific female activity and fertility rates for various sectors of the economy.

590
*Jaffe, A.J. and Azumi, K.
"The Birth Rate and Cottage Industries in Underdeveloped Countries." *Economic Development and Cultural Change* 9(1, Part 1), Oct. 1960: pp. 52-63.

Evidence that fertility is lower when women work in nonfamilial enterprises but not when work is in home or cottage industries.

591
Klinger, A.
"Trends of Differential Fertility by Social Strata in Hungary." In *International Population Conference.* New York, 1961. London: U.N.E.S.C.O., 1963: pp. 87-96.
Differential fertility by broad occupational strata and by wife's labor-force status and occupation.

592
Myers, G.C.
"Labor Force Participation of Suburban Mothers." *Journal of Marriage and the Family* 26(3), Aug. 1964: pp. 306-311.
Labor-force participation of mothers of Seattle, Washington, high school students in relation to family size and other variables.

593
Namboodiri, N.K.
"The Wife's Work Experience and Child Spacing." *The Milbank Memorial Fund Quarterly* 42(3), July 1964: pp. 67-77.
Based on multivariate analysis of data from 1955 Growth of American Families national sample survey.

594
Pfeil, E.
"An Empirical Study on the Employment of Married Women in Western Germany." In *International Population Conference.* New York, 1961. London: U.N.E.S.C.O., 1963: pp. 235-242.
How different female employment situations and attitudes relate to familial attitudes and behavior.

595
Poffenberger, T.
"Motivational Aspects of Resistance to Family Planning in an Indian Village." *Demography* 5(2), 1968: pp. 757-766.
Based on intensive village studies, a generalized (nonquantitative) summary of how the following factors make high fertility and a lack of interest in family planning a rational response: subordinate role of very young wife in husband's family, preference for sons for economic and ritual reasons, dependence of old parents on children, and high rate of mortality of children.

596
***Pratt, L. and Whelpton, P.K.**
"Extra-Familial Participation of Wives in Relation to Interest and Liking for Children, Fertility Planning, and Actual and Desired Family Size." In Kiser and Whelpton, eds. (*see* 1512) Vol. 5: pp. 1245-1280.
Shows that activity of wives outside the home in either work or club situation is related to effective family planning and smaller families.

597
***Ridley, J.C.**
"Number of Children Expected in Relation to Non-Familial Activities of the Wife." *Milbank Memorial Fund Quarterly* 37(3), July 1959: pp. 277-296.
Finds the history of the wife's labor-force participation affects fertility and family planning even after allowance is made for fecundity impairment.

598
Ridley, J.C.
"Demographic Change and the Roles and Status of Women." *Annals of the American Academy of Political and Social Science* 375, Jan. 1968: pp. 16-25.

Brief summary of changing roles of women during industrialization and the demographic transition in the West; cross-sectional analysis of contemporary situation with implications for developing countries.

Measures how social and economic factors affect the relationship between female labor-force participation and fertility by their effect on the compatibility of roles of mother and worker.

599
Stycos, J.M.
"Female Employment and Fertility in Lima, Peru." *Milbank Memorial Fund Quarterly* 43(1), Jan. 1965: pp. 42-54.

Three urban studies in Peru show no direct causal relation between female employment and lower fertility.

600
Stycos, J.M. and Weller, R.H.
"Female Working Roles and Fertility." *Demography* 4(1), 1967: pp. 210-217.

Based on 1963 survey in Turkey, examines relation of female labor-force participation to fertility behavior and attitudes, controlling for residential, educational, and exposure risk factors.

601
Weller, R.H.
"The Employment of Wives, Dominance, and Fertility." *Journal of Marriage and the Family* 30(3), Aug. 1968: pp. 437-442.

Puerto Rican survey data used to test relationship between female labor-force status, female influence in decision making, and fertility.

602
Weller, R.H.
"The Employment of Wives, Role Incompatibility and Fertility: A Study among Lower and Middle Class Residents of San Juan, Puerto Rico." *Milbank Memorial Fund Quarterly* 46(4), Oct. 1968: pp. 507-526.

V.A.2 Other aspects of family organization, including its place in the division of labor
See also: 81, 129, 358, 361, 362, 374, 382, 433, 515, 551, 562, 579, 587, 600, 648, 696, 1104, 1125, 1134, 1229, 1498, 1504, 1505, 1508, 1510, 1511, 1512, 1516, 1526, 1527, 1531, 1534, 1538.

603
*Berent, J.
"The Relationship between Family Sizes of Two Successive Generations." *Milbank Memorial Fund Quarterly* 31(1), Jan. 1953: pp. 39-50.

A small but significant positive relation is found for family size in two successive British generations even within social class.

604
Beresford, J.C. and Rivlin, A.M.
"Characteristics of "Other" Families." *Demography* 1(1), 1964: pp. 242-246.

Composition and growth of "other" families 1950-60 and the higher cumulative fertility of female heads of household compared to husband-wife families.

605
Burch, T.K.
"The Size and Structure of Families." *American Sociological Review* 32(3), June 1967: pp. 347-363.

International comparison of family size; relates total family size to size of nuclear family.

606
Burch, T.K.
"Some Demographic Determinants of Average Household Size: An Analytic Approach." *Demography* 7(1), Feb. 1970: pp. 61-69.
Important simulation model of how differing fertility and mortality levels affect household size depending on type of family system (stem, joint-extended, nuclear); shows that with high fertility and low mortality extended family systems imply household sizes far larger than actually found, thus implying pressures for fission and fertility control.

607
Caldwell, J.C.
"The Erosion of the Family: A Study of the Fate of the Family in Ghana." *Population Studies* 20(1), July 1966: pp. 5-26.
Reports on interviews with a sample of retired persons over 60 to analyze interaction of family size and mortality of children on assistance to parents.

608
Camilleri, C.
"Modernity and the Family in Tunisia." *Journal of Marriage and the Family* 29(3), Aug. 1967: pp. 590-595.
Results from six surveys of young people for the period 1960-66 on attitudes toward family size, family organization, and the role of women.

609
Coale, A.J. et al.
Aspects of the Analysis of Family Structure. Princeton: Princeton University Press, 1965; 248p.
Five authors discuss theories about the connection between vital rates, norms about family composition, and actual family composition.

610
Collver, A.
"The Family Cycle in India and the United States." *American Sociological Review* 28(1), Feb. 1963: pp. 86-96.
Comparison of family life cycle stages of marriage, reproduction, death, etc., in India and the U.S.

611
Davis-Blake, J.
"Parental Control, Delayed Marriage, and Population Policy". In *Proceedings of the World Population Conference, 1965* (*see* 44): pp. 132-136.
Under different sociocultural conditions parents may have motives for encouraging either early or late marriages; therefore, parental influence need not necessarily lead to early or universal marriage.

612
*Dorjahn, V.R.
"Fertility, Polygyny and Their Interrelations in Temne Society." *American Anthropologist* 60(5), Oct. 1958: pp. 838-860.

613
Dubey, D.C.
"Family Life Cycle Hypothesis and Its Importance in Explaining Fertility Behavior in India." *Journal of Family Welfare* (Bombay) 14(2), Dec. 1967: pp. 42-52.
Attempts to use a dynamic and functional view of the family to explain fertility control behavior.

614
Duncan, O.D. et al.
"Marital Fertility and Size of Family of Orientation." *Demography* 2, 1965: pp. 508-515.

Analysis of U.S. marriage cohorts based on several sample surveys of relation between fertility and size of family orientation.

615
Geiger, J.K.
The Family in Soviet Russia. Cambridge, Mass.: Harvard University Press, 1968; 381p.

Examines changes in the Russian family, including aspects of family policy, fertility control, and abortion.

616
Goode, W.J.
World Revolution and Family Patterns. New York: Free Press; London: Collier-Macmillian, 1963; 432p.

Examines changes in family structure in Arabia, China, Japan, India, Sub-Saharan Africa and the West; considers such aspects as polygamy, age at marriage, courtship practices, divorce, kin networks, legal sanctions of marriage, fertility, and birth control.

617
Goode, W.J.
"The Theory of Measurement of Social Change." In *Indicators of Social Change.* Edited by E.B. Sheldon and W.E. Moore. New York: Russell Sage Foundation, 1968: pp. 295-348.

A general review of the concepts and data appropriate for studying social change in the family, with some reference to fertility, mainly for the U.S.

618
*Greenfield, S.M.
"Industrialization and the Family in Sociological Theory." *American Journal of Sociology* 67(3), Nov. 1961: pp. 312-322.

Rejects the view that the nuclear family is a necessary condition for or consequence of industrialization.

619
Heer, D.M.
"The Childbearing Functions of the Soviet Family." In *The Role and Status of Women in Soviet Union.* Edited by D.R. Brown. New York: Bureau of Publications, Teachers College, Columbia University, 1968: pp. 125-129.

620
*Hill, R.
The Sociology of Marriage and Family Behavior, 1945-1956. U.N.E.S.C.O. Trend Report. Oxford: Basil Blackwell, 1958; 98p.

Summary of research before 1958 and annotated bibliography.

621
*Muhsam, H.V.
"The Fertility of Polygamous Marriages." *Population Studies* 10(1), July 1956: pp. 3-16.

622
Namboodiri, N.K.
"Another Look at Structural-Functional Analysis: An Exercise in Axiomatic Theory Construction." *Sociological Bulletin* (Bombay) 15(1), Mar. 1966: pp. 75-89.

Relates long-term secular decline in Western fertility and the postwar reversal to a long-term increase of disjunctiveness in husband-wife roles and recent reversal of this trend.

623
Olusanya, P.O.
"Nigeria: Cultural Barriers to Family Planning among the Yorubas." *Studies in Family Planning* 1(37), Jan. 1969: pp. 13-16.

Traditional values stressing male dominance and support for numerous progeny persist despite erosion of some traditional relationships and use of birth control.

624

Pakrasi, K. and Malaker, C.
"The Relationship between Family Type and Fertility." *Milbank Memorial Fund Quarterly* 45(4), Oct. 1967: pp. 451-460.

Relates average number of children to family type (single or joint) by Hindu groups in West Bengal, controlling for duration of marriage and occupational class.

625

Pool, D.I.
"Conjugal Patterns in Ghana." *Canadian Review of Sociology and Anthropology* 5(4), 1969: pp. 241-253.

Relates marriage type to fertility, age, place of residence, tribe; reasons for marriage termination.

626

Prag, A.
"Some Demographic Aspects of Kibbutz Life in Israel." *Jewish Journal of Sociology* 4(1), June 1962: pp. 39-46.

A mainly descriptive comparison of the fertility and other demographic characteristics of kibbutz population with the rest of the Israeli population.

627

*Roberts, G.W. and Braithwaite, L.
"Fertility Differentials by Family Type in Trinidad." *Annals of the New York Academy of Sciences* 84(17), Dec. 1960: pp. 963-980.

628

*Talmon-Garber, Y.
"Social Structure and Family Size." *Human Relations* 12(2), 1959: pp. 121-146.

Deals with norms for family size in different types of collective communities in Israel.

629

Uhlenberg, P.R.
"A Study of Cohort Life Cycles: Cohorts of Native Born Massachusetts Women, 1830-1920." *Population Studies* 23(3), Nov. 1969: pp. 407-420.

A cohort reconstruction from Massachusetts data of life-cycle types and their frequency for birth, 1830-1920; shows distributions as well as averages for six family life-cycle types, taking into account probabilities for mortality, marriage, childbearing, and widowhood.

630

Van de Walle, E.
"Marriage in African Censuses and Inquiries." In Brass et al. (*see* 7): pp. 183-238.

Sources of data and methods of estimation; estimates of levels and form of marriage status, with especially interesting discussion of the levels and correlates of polygyny.

631

Wilkinson, T.O.
"Family Structure and Industrialization in Japan." *American Sociological Review* 27(5), Oct. 1962: pp. 678-682.

Strong family controls in Japan permitted retention of traditional values while making necessary adjustments to industrialization without disorganization and individualization reported elsewhere in transition.

V.B Intrafamilial organizational variables

V.B.1 Communication and dominance patterns

See also: 587, 595, 601, 620, 1185, 1508, 1511, 1512, 1523, 1526.

632
Michel, A.
"Interaction and Family Planning in the French Urban Family." *Demography* 4(2), 1967: pp. 615-625.
Relative importance of socioeconomic status and familial communication to success in family planning, based on sample survey.

633
*Stycos, J.M.
Family and Fertility in Puerto Rico: A Study of the Lower Income Group. New York: Columbia University Press, 1955; 332p.
Intensive case-study analysis of the way intrafamilial relations affect attitudes to sexuality, family planning, and fertility in Puerto Rico.

634
Yaukey, D. et al.
"Couple Concurrence and Empathy on Birth Control Motivation in Dacca, East Pakistan." *American Sociological Review* 32(5), Oct. 1967: pp. 716-726.
Communication patterns concerning ideal family size among couples; comparison with Indian and Puerto Rican study findings.

V.B.2 Sex-preference for children
See also: 266, 595, 620, 1221, 1493, 1508, 1511, 1512, 1526.

635
*Clare, J.E. and Kiser, C.V.
"Preference for Children of a Given Sex in Relation to Fertility." In Kiser and Whelpton, eds. (*see* 1512) Vol. 3: pp. 621-674.

636
*Freedman, D.S. et al.
"Size of Family and Preference for Children of Each Sex." *American Journal of Sociology* 66(2), Sept. 1960: pp. 141-146.
Based on data in the 1955 Growth of American Families study, finds that preference for a child of each sex rather than for a male or female child was dominant in U.S. in 1955.

637
Heer, D.M. and Smith, D.O.
"Mortality Level and Desired Family Size." In 1967 I.U.S.S.P. (*see* 21): pp. 26-36.
Uses a computer simulation model to show that even with perfect contraception the amount of fertility reduction depends on the assurance that a son will be alive to support the father at age 65.

638
Heer, D.M. and Smith, D.O.
"Mortality Level, Desired Family Size and Population Increase: Further Variations on a Basic Model." *Demography* 6(2), May 1969: pp. 141-149.
Further development of earlier model (see 637 showing that varying fecundity and other assumptions still lead to the conclusion that high life expectancy is required to lower fertility if one son must survive until the father is 65; compares this assumption with condition that two children must survive regardless of their sex.

639
May, D.A. and Heer, D.M.
"Son Survivorship Motivation and Family Size in India: A Computer Simulation." *Population Studies* 22(2), July 1968: pp. 199-210.

Computer simulation used to study the effect of son survivorship motivation on family size.

640
Patel, T.
"Some Reflections on the Attitudes of Married Couples towards Family Planning in Ahmedabad." *Sociological Bulletin* (Bombay) 12(2), Sept. 1963: pp. 1-13.
Survey results indicating that strong desire for sons is a powerful deterrent to use of family planning methods.

641
Pohlman, E.
"Some Effects of Being Able to Control Sex of Offspring" *Eugenics Quarterly* 14(4), 1967: pp. 274-281.
Brief survey of research on sex preferences is the basis for speculation on the possible psychological and demographic effects of being able to control sex of children.

V.B.3 Other aspects of intrafamilial interaction, size of family of origin

See also: 255, 620, 633, 1187, 1511, 1512.

642
Deyrup, F.J.
"Family Dominance as a Factor in Population Growth of Developing Countries." *Social Research* 29(2), Summer 1962: pp. 177-189.
Theoretical discussion of how traditional family structure maintains high fertility and proposals for policies to change this relationship indirectly.

643
Misra, B.D.
"A Comparison of Husbands' and Wives' Attitudes toward Family Planning." *Journal of Family Welfare* (Bombay) 12(4), June 1966: pp. 9-23.
Based on a sample of 118 Negro couples in Chicago.

VI. STUDIES OF THE EFFECTS OF NONFAMILIAL INSTITUTIONS WITH EXPLICIT PROGRAMS TO AFFECT FERTILITY, THE INTERMEDIATE VARIABLES, OR THE NORMS ABOUT THEM

VI.A General population policy: discussions of the merits of different strategies of changing birth rates by providing birth control, by changing institutions, by changing social norms, etc.

See also: 1, 17, 31, 87, 88, 97, 104, 355, 432, 446, 447, 465, 516, 611, 642, 716, 803, 922, 938, 1062, 1064 1076, 1193, 1273, 1284, 1328, 1344, 1425, 1546, 1552, 1553, 1560, 1564, 1566, 1567, 1571.

644
Agarwala, S.N.
"Social Dynamics of Family Planning." *Indian Conference of Social Work, Thirteenth Session.* 24-28 Dec. 1964. Delhi: Demographic Research Centre, Institute of Economic Growth, 1965; pp. 1-9.

Discussion of need for social scientists to take a leading role in India to change social behavior and help establish new patterns of family planning.

645
Back, K.W. and Winsborough, H.H.
"Population Policy: Opinions and Actions of Governments." *Public Opinion Quarterly* 32(4), Winter 1968-69: pp. 634-645.

Responses of United Nations survey of governmental population policies are related to socioeconomic conditions and action programs.

646
Beaney, W.M.
"The Griswold Case and the Expanding Right to Privacy." *Wisconsin Law Review* 1966: pp. 979-996.

Discussion of issues in the Griswold v. Connecticut case concerning the constitutionality of a state law forbidding prescription or use of contraceptives.

647
Berelson, B.
"National Family Planning Programs:

Where We Stand." In Behrman et al., eds. (*see* 51): pp. 341-387. [Also in *Studies in Family Planning* 1(39) (Supplement) Mar. 1969.]

An important review of the progress, problems, and correlates of family planning programs as of 1967; includes unique tabulations of some of the conditions under which governmental action in this field emerge.

648
Blake, J.
"Demographic Science and the Redirection of Population Policy." In Sheps and Ridley, eds. (*see* 73): pp. 41-69.

Evidence from a variety of sources for the thesis that motivation for having children arises from the role of familial institutions in society and that policies to change fertility should make this a central concern.

649
Blake, J.
"Population Policy for Americans: Is the Government Being Misled?" *Science* 164(3879), May 1969: pp. 522-529.

Public-opinion poll results argue that policies to supply contraception to the poor are misguided because they will be ineffective in that sector and fail to make the changes in desired number of children only possible by social structural changes, e.g., role of women.

650
Bogue, D.J.
"The Demographic Breakthrough: From Projection to Control." *Population Index* 30(4), Oct. 1964: pp. 449-454.

Unusually optimistic assessment of the actual prospect and progress of programs to limit fertility; possibility of reducing world birth rate to 25 in a decade and of universal success in current efforts.

651
Bogue, D.J.
"The End of the Population Explosion." *Public Interest* 7, Spring 1967: pp. 11-20.

Optimistic evaluation of current factors acting to control population growth.

652
Brayer, F.T., ed.
World Population and U.S. Government Policy and Programs. Washington: Georgetown University Press, 1968; 116p.

653
Castellano, V.
Population Growth, Economic Development and the Dangers of National Policies of Birth Control. Rome: Istituto di Statistica della Facoltà di Scienze Statistiche, Demografiche ed Attuariali, 1963; 22p.

654
Coale, A.J.
"Should the United States Start a Campaign for Fewer Births?" *Population Index* 34(3), Oct.-Dec. 1968: pp. 467-474.

Discusses the advisability of an explicit anti-natalist policy in the U.S.; critical of the view that reducing population growth is an effective method of solving social and ecological problems.

655
Council of Europe. Social Committee.
Family Policy. Laws and Regulations Designed to Compensate for Family Commitments. Strasbourg: 1967; 96p.

656
Davis, K.
"Population Policy: Will Current Programs Succeed?" *Science* 158, Nov. 1967: pp. 730-739.

Important critique of family planning programs as inadequate to reduce birth rates sharply to zero population growth rate levels because they fail to change social structure to facilitate low fertility.

657
Day, L.H. and Day, A.T.
Too Many Americans. Boston: Houghton Mifflin, 1964; 298p.
> General discussion of factors in the growth of American population, religious and secular attitudes toward fertility, and pronatalist arguments against achievement of stable population.

658
Dickens, B.
Abortion and the Law. London: Macgibbon and Kee, 1966; 219p.
> Traces the history, effectiveness, and enforcement of English abortion law.

659
Dow, T.E.
"Family Planning: Theoretical Considerations and African Models." *Journal of Marriage and the Family* 31(2), May 1969: pp. 252-256.

660
Dowse, R.E. and Peel, J.
"The Politics of Birth-Control." *Political Studies* 13(2), June 1965: pp. 179-197.
> History of the birth control movement in England with emphasis on the interaction of a voluntary social movement and public policy.

661
*Eldridge, H.T.
Population Policies: A Survey of Recent Developments. Prepared under the Auspices of the Committee on Investigation of Population Policies. Washington: International Union for the Scientific Study of Population, 1954; 154p.
> Early review of programs designed to affect fertility levels either directly or indirectly.

662
Gardner, R.N.
Population Growth: A World Problem. Statement of U.S. Policy. Department of State Publication 7485. International Organization and Conference Series 36. Washington: Government Printing Office, 1963; 16p.

663
Gardner, R.N.
"Toward a World Population Program." *International Organization* 22, Winter 1968: pp. 332-361.

664
Ghana, Republic of.
Population Planning for National Progress and Prosperity. Ghana Population Policy. Accra-Tema: Ghana Publishing Corporation, 1969; 23p. [Abstracted in *Studies in Family Planning* 1(44), Aug. 1969: 1-7.]
> One of the most comprehensive and coherent official statements on population policy, with references both to family planning and to changes in social and economic situations that will foster smaller families.

665
Glass, D.V.
"Fertility and Birth Control in Developed Societies and Some Questions of Policy for Less Developed Societies." *Malayan Economic Review* (Singapore) 8(1), Apr. 1963: pp. 29-39.
> Reviews processes of fertility decline in the West, suggesting importance of inducing basic social change in developing areas today.

666
Glass, D.
"Fertility, Birth Control, and Policy Questions." *Family Planning News* 4(8), Aug. 1963: pp. 144-150.

Reviews history of fertility decline in the West and suggests policy orientations for developing countries involving emphasis on education, general development, and concentration on groups that will have early motivation to accept and, thus, serve as models.

667
*Great Britain. Royal Commission on Population.
Report. Parliament Command Papers, 7695. London: H.M.S.O., 1949; 259p.
Important government report summarizing results of many special investigations; concern with low rather than high fertility.

668
Harkavy, O. et al.
"Family Planning and Public Policy: Who Is Misleading Whom?" *Science* 165(3891), 25 July 1969: pp. 367-373.
Critical response to item 649.

669
*Harrod, R.F.
"Memoranda Presented to the Royal Commission." In *Papers of the Royal Commission on Population,* vol. 5. London: H.M.S.O., 1950; pp. 77-120.
A program for increasing fertility by endowments for children; illustrates the concern with low fertility in the period just before and after World War II.

670
Heer, D.M.
"Abortion, Contraception, and Population Policy in the Soviet Union." *Demography* 2, 1965; pp. 531-539.
Discusses the policy implications and the effects of the relegalization of induced abortion in 1955.

671
Jain, S.C. and Sinding, S.W.
North Carolina Abortion Law 1967. A

Study in Legislative Process. No. 20 Chapel Hill: Carolina Population Center, University of North Carolina, 1968; 74p.
Traces the political developments leading to the enactment of abortion legislation.

672
Kantner, J.F.
"American Attitudes on Population Policy: Recent Trends." *Studies in Family Planning* 1(30), May 1968: pp. 1-7.
Comparison of results from 1965 and 1967 Gallup polls concerning the relative importance of the population problem, government family planning policies, and abortion law reform; educational, income and religious differentials presented.

673
Kantner, J.F. and Berelson, B.
"American Attitudes on Population Policy." *Studies in Family Planning* 1(9), Jan. 1966: pp. 5-8.
Results of Gallup opinion poll concerning awareness of the population problem, attitudes toward the role of government, and general availability of birth control information; differentials by age, sex, and religion.

674
Kirk, D.
"Prospects for Reducing Natality in the Underdeveloped World." *Annals of the American Academy of Science* 369, Jan. 1967: pp. 48-60.

675
Kirk, D. and Nortman, D.
"Population Policies in Developing Countries" *Economic Development and Cultural Change* 15(2, Part 1), Jan. 1967: pp. 129-142.

Regional survey of problems of rapid population growth as handicaps to social and economic development and of government policies on family planning, including those of international bodies, the U.S., and other developed countries.

676
Krotki, K.J.
"The Feasibility of an Effective Population Policy for Pakistan." *Pakistan Development Review* (Karachi) 4(2), Summer 1964: pp. 283-313.

677
Lal, A.
"Fertility Management and Concern with Over-Population in Mainland China." *Eugenics Quarterly* 11(3), Sept. 1964: pp. 170-174.

678
Mahadevan, M.S.
"The Conflicting Effects of Family Planning Measures and Maternity Benefit Measures." *Journal of Family Welfare* (Bombay) 10(4) June 1964: pp. 40-50.
Argues for changes to eliminate opposing effects of maternity benefits and the family planning program in India.

679
Mars, J.
"A Population Stop Policy for Developing Countries." *Nigerian Journal of Economic and Social Studies* (Ibadan) 5(2), July 1963: pp. 145-185.
Advocates a terminable "population stop policy" for lower rates of growth until desired objectives are fulfilled.

680
Mehta, J.K.
"Population, Time-Lag and Depreciation." *Indian Journal of Economics* (Allahabad) 45(177), Oct. 1964: pp. 113-123.

Discusses the need for fertility control efforts to be concentrated in areas where there is a surplus of labor.

681
Muramatsu, M.
"Policy Measures and Social Changes for Fertility Decline in Japan." In *Proceedings of the World Population Conference, 1965 (see* 44): pp. 96-99.
Analyzes the postwar situation, indicating that abortion probably only facilitated the rapid fertility decline that would have occurred sooner or later anyway, given all favorable predisposing factors.

682
National Institutes of Health.
"The Behavioral Sciences and Family Planning Programs: Report on a Conference." *Studies in Family Planning* 1(23), Oct. 1967: pp. 1-12.
Two papers and a summary of discussion.

683
Notestein, F.W.
"The Population Crisis: Reasons for Hope." *Foreign Affairs* 46(1), Oct. 1967: pp. 167-180.
Political, attitudinal, and technical developments that permit a cautiously optimistic view of the population problem.

684
Ohlin, G.
Population Control and Economic Development. Development Centre Studies Series. Paris: Development Center of the Organization of Economic Cooperation and Development, 1967; 138p.
Summary view of the interrelation of population growth and development; sections on population policy, fertility attitudes, and contraceptive effectiveness.

685
Petersen, W.
The Politics of Population. Garden City, N.Y.: Doubleday, 1964; 350p.
> Role of population policy in social welfare, urban planning, and international migration.

686
Podyachikh, P.
"Population and Progress." *Current Digest of the Soviet Press* 18(9), Mar. 1966: pp. 10-11.
> Soviet Union's position on demographic aspects of development.

687
Population Reference Bureau.
"United Nations: Population Opinion Survey." *Population Bulletin* 20(6), Oct. 1964: pp. 141-171.
> Brief excerpts from the responses of 49 governments to opinion survey concerning general population growth, general socioeconomic development, and family planning.

688
Population Reference Bureau.
"Needed: A Population Policy for the World." *Population Bulletin* 21(2), May 1965: pp. 17-47.
> Notes and comments on recent developments in policy—especially toward fertility controls—on the part of agencies of the U.S. and the U.N.

689
*St. John-Stevas, N.
Birth Control and Public Policy. Santa Barbara, Calif.: Center for the Study of Democratic Institutions, 1960; 83p.

690
Samuel, T.J.
"Population Control in Japan: Lessons for India." *Eugenics Review* 58(1), Mar. 1966: pp. 15-22.
> Socioeconomic and psychological factors affecting fertility, the influence of tradition, and the role of government in population control.

691
Segal, A. and Earnhardt, K.C.
Politics and Population in the Caribbean. Rio Piedras, Puerto Rico: University of Puerto Rico, 1969; 158p.
> Population policy and public and private family planning programs in nine Caribbean countries.

692
Srb, V.
"Population Development and Population Policy in Czechoslovakia." *Population Studies* 16(2), Nov. 1962: pp. 147-159.
> Population change and official policy since World War II, with discussion of the role of legal abortion, the employment of women, and survey reports on family planning and desired family size.

693
Stycos, J.M.
"Population Growth and the Alliance for Progress." *Eugenics Quarterly* 9(4), Dec. 1962: pp. 231-236.
> Adverse consequences of uncontrolled population growth and policy suggestions.

694
Stycos, J.M.
"Obstacles to Programs of Population Control: Facts and Fancies." *Marriage and Family Living* 25(1), Feb. 1963: pp. 5-13.
> Analysis of the possible explanations of the failure of governments to introduce, or to implement successfully, population-control programs.

695
Stycos, J.M.
"Opposition to Family Planning in La-

tin America: Conservative Nationalism." *Demography* 5(2), 1968; pp. 846-854.

Cites the work of three Latin American writers who oppose family planning programs as well as population-limitation ideas as being imperialistic in origin, subversive of traditional moral and religious values, calculated to weaken Latin American countries, and unnecessary because of the low densities and vast resources attributed to the area.

696
Sussman, M.B., ed.
Journal of Marriage and the Family. 29(1), Feb. 1967: pp. 5-205.

Nine articles on governmental programs and the family in the U.S.

697
Tien, H.Y.
"Induced Abortion and Population Control in Mainland China." *Marriage and Family Living* 25(1), Feb. 1963: pp. 35-43.

Traces opposition to induced abortion; concludes that it is unlikely abortion can be an important means of population control.

698
United States Presidential Committee on Population and Family Planning.
Population and Family Planning: The Transition from Concern to Action. Washington: Government Printing Office, 1968; 48p.

Report on the domestic and international needs for family planning programs and population policy.

699
Wadia, S.A.B.
"Some Thoughts on the Educational Programme for Family Planning." *Journal of Family Welfare* (Bombay) 11(3), Mar. 1965: pp. 13-18.

Proposals for educational programs and activities to make changes in traditional aspects of society.

700
Weinberg, R.D.
Laws Governing Family Planning. Legal Almanac Series, 18. Dobbs Ferry, N.Y.: Oceana, 1968; 118p.

Survey of current American laws pertaining to family planning, contraception, abortion, and artificial insemination; texts of recent statutes and statements by related organizations.

701
Wood, H.C., Jr.
Sex without Babies: A Comprehensive Review of Voluntary Sterilization as a Method of Birth Control. Philadelphia: Whitmore, 1967; 229p.

A case for voluntary sterilization: legal, medical, and religious aspects.

VI.B Programs specifically concerned with affecting the practice of birth control

VI.B.1 Policies, plans, or proposals for specific birth-control programs or critical analysis of programs
See also: 52, 469, 647, 650, 691, 900, 922, 1388, 1392.

702
Aromin, B.B.
"Consideration for a Philippine Population Policy." *Philippine Statistician* (Manila) 12(4), Dec. 1963: pp. 122-144.

Discussion of the need for and the requirements of a national family planning program.

703

Brackett, J.W. and Huyck, E.
"The Objectives of Government Policies on Fertility Control in Eastern Europe." *Population Studies* 16(2), Nov. 1962: pp. 134-146.

Reviews state policies (1949-61) toward population size and contraception, especially abortion.

704

Chandrasekhar, S.
"How India is Tackling Her Population Problem." *Foreign Affairs* 47(1), Oct. 1968: pp. 138-150.

A general description by India's minister of family planning and health.

705

Demeny, P.
"The Economics of Government Payments to Limit Population: A Comment." *Economic Development and Cultural Change* 9(4, Part 1), July 1961: pp. 641-644.

A comment on the cost criteria used by Enke (see 707).

706

El-Hefnawi, F.
"The Place of Sterilization in Egypt." *International Journal of Fertility* 11(4), Oct.-Dec. 1966: pp. 381-388.

Review of Egyptian demographic trends; proposes policy of tubal ligation for women who have had six or more live births.

707

Enke, S.
"The Economics of Government Payments to Limit Population." *Economic Development and Cultural Change* 8(4, Part 1), July, 1960: pp. 339-348.

Presents plan for economic incentive payments to reduce fertility; application of plan to India (further discussion of scheme in item 1392).

708

Enke, S.
"A Rejoinder to Comments on the Superior Effectiveness of Vasectomy-Bonus Schemes." *Economic Development and Cultural Change* 9(4, Part 1), July 1961: pp. 645-647.

A rejoinder to Demeny (see 705).

709

Enke, S.
"Some Misconceptions of Krueger and Sjaastad Regarding the Vasectomy-Bonus Plan to Reduce Births in Overpopulated and Poor Countries." *Economic Development and Cultural Change* 10(4), July 1962: pp. 427-431.

A rejoinder to Krueger and Sjaastad (see 721).

710

Enke, S.
"Fewer Births—More Welfare." In *Contributions to the Analysis of Urban Problems: A Selection of Papers from the RAND Workshop on Urban Programs.* 18 Dec. 1967-12 Jan. 1968. Edited by A.H. Pascal, Santa Monica, Calif.: RAND Corporation, 1968: pp. 103-121.

Relation of family size to poverty, need for family planning services to the poor, and how to provide it.

711

Freeberne, M.
"Birth Control in China." *Population Studies* 18(1), July 1964: pp. 5-16

Study of mainland China's fluctuating birth control campaigns based on official documents and periodicals.

712

Freedman, R.

"Family Planning Programs Today: Major Themes of the Conference." In Berelson et al., eds. (*see* 53): pp. 811-825.

Summary and interpretation of the major issues raised by a large conference on national family planning programs.

713

Glass, D.V.

"Family Planning Programmes and Action in Western Europe." In Szabady et al., eds. (*see* 40): pp. 105-125. [Also in *Population Studies* 19(3), Mar. 1966: pp. 221-238.]

Outline of changes in programs in the period 1945-65 and of possible factors involved.

714

Guttmacher, A.F., ed.

The Case for Legalized Abortion Now. Berkeley: Diablo Press, 1967; 154p.

Papers by various professionals dealing with the need for legal reform of U.S. abortion laws.

715

Harkavy, O. et al.

"Implementing DHEW Policy on Family Planning and Population: A Consultant's Report." In *Family Planning and Population Research, 1970.* Hearings before the Subcommittee on Health of the Committee on Labor and Public Welfare, United States Senate. Washington: Government Printing Office, 1970; Appendix A: pp. 333-377.

Historically important review of U.S. policies on family planning with specific recommendations for far-reaching changes.

716

Hauser, P.M.

"Family Planning and Population Pro-

grams: A Book Review Article." *Demography* 4(1), 1967: pp. 397-414.

Critical survey of assumptions, methods, and conclusions of the work cited in item 53.

717

India. Chamber of Commerce.

New Approach to Family Planning: Proceedings of the Industrial Conference on Family Planning Held in Calcutta in January 1966. Calcutta: 1966; 132p.

718

Jaffe, F.S.

"Family Planning, Public Policy and Intervention Strategy." *Journal of Social Issues* 23(4) July 1967: pp. 145-163.

Summarizes changes in U.S. public policy and evaluates adequacy of existing family planning services.

719

Jaffe, F.S. and Polgar,S.

"Family Planning and Public Policy: Is the 'Culture of Poverty' the New Cop-Out?" *Journal of Marriage and the Family* 30(2), May 1968: pp. 228-235.

Critical examination of the underlying rationale of the current approach to providing family planning services to the poor in the U.S.; suggests alternative viewpoint.

720

Kenya. Ministry of Economic Planning and Development.

Family Planning in Kenya. No. 4. Nairobi: 1966; 45p.

Report to the Kenya government by an advisory mission concerning the scope of a government family planning program.

721

Krueger, A.O. and Sjaastad, L.A.

"Some Limitations of Enke's Economics of Population." *Economic Development and Cultural Change* 10(4), July 1962: pp. 423-426.

A comment on the welfare criteria used by Enke (see 707).

722
Lader, L.
Abortion. Indianapolis: Bobbs-Merrill, 1966; 212p.

Abortion policy and practice in the U.S. and suggested legal reform.

723
Orleans, L.A.
"A New Birth Control Campaign?" *China Quarterly* 12, Oct.-Dec. 1962: pp. 207-210.

Notes on reports and pronouncements on official policy in mainland China.

724
Pakistan. Family Planning Division.
Proposals of the Family Planning Division for Family Planning Sector During the Fourth Five Year Plan (1970-75). Islamabad: 1968; 140p.

725
Ridker, R.G.
"Synopsis of a Proposal for a Family Planning Bond." *Studies in Family Planning* 1(43), June 1969: pp. 11-16.

Detailed plans for an incentive system of retirement bonds to couples who limit their fertility.

726
Ridker, R.G.
"Desired Family Size and the Efficacy of Current Family Planning Programmes." *Population Studies* 23(2), July 1969: pp. 279-284.

Critical assessment of the ability of family planning programs,—notably the Indian program—to reach target reduction of the birth rate without resorting to incentives and coercion.

727
Robinson, W.C.
"Family Planning in Pakistan's Third Five Year Plan." *Pakistan Development Review* (Karachi) 6(2), Summer 1966: pp. 255-281.

Critical review of population policy and plans.

728
Simon, J.L.
"The Value of Avoided Births to Underdeveloped Countries." *Population Studies* 23(1), Mar. 1969: pp. 61-68.

Questions public versus private cost elements and discount rate used by Enke (see 707); applies incentive scheme to Indian population growth estimates.

729
Singapore. Parliament.
White Paper on Family Planning Cmd. 22 of 1965. Singapore: 1965; 28p.

Historical setting, organization, and budget goals of a five-year plan.

730
Social Action (POONA).
"Family Planning in India." [A group of articles.] *Social Action* (Poona) Aug. 1962: pp. 361-411.

Demographic problems and programs of family planning.

731
*Stycos, J.M.
"A Critique of the Traditional Planned Parenthood Approach in Underdeveloped Areas." In *Research in Family*

Planning. Edited by C.V. Kiser. Princeton: Princeton University Press, 1962: pp. 447-501.

A critique of middle-class feminist biases in the planned parenthood movement.

732
Taylor, H.C., Jr.
"A Family Planning Program Related to Maternity Service" *American Journal of Obstetrics and Gynecology* 95, July 1966: pp. 726-731.

Argues for a prepartum and postpartum family planning service; presents delivery rates by place for various cities and nations of the world.

733
Taylor, H.C., Jr. and Berelson, B.
"Maternity Care and Family Planning as a World Program." *American Journal of Obstetrics and Gynecology* 100(7), Apr. 1968: pp. 885-893.

Possible effectiveness and feasibility of postpartum family planning services.

734
Thakur, H.N.
"The Demographic Quest for Family Planning in Nepal." *Journal of Family Welfare* (Bombay) 11(1), Sept. 1964: pp. 20-28.

Proposes a family planning program and better data for Nepal where the demographic situation is estimated to be difficult.

735
Tien, H.Y.
"Birth Control in Mainland China: Ideology and Politics." *Milbank Memorial Fund Quarterly* 41(3), July 1963: pp. 269-290.

Traces official attitudes and actions related to birth control in mainland China 1949-62.

736
United Nations. Programme of Technical Assistance.
Report on the Family Planning Programme in India by a United Nations Advisory Mission. New York: 1966; 123p.

737
United States. Department of Health, Education, and Welfare.
Report on Family Planning: Activities of the U.S. Department of Health, Education, and Welfare in Family Planning, Fertility, Sterility, and Population Dynamics. Washington: Government Printing Office, 1966; 35p.

Initial policy statement and subsequent developments.

738
Visaria, P.
"Population Assumptions and Policy." *Economic Weekly* 16(33), Aug. 1964: pp. 1339-1344.

Analysis of the Indian population policies and suggested changes, based on review of unexpected demographic trends indicated by 1961 census.

VI.B.2 Organization and implementation: including aspects of administration; personnel, budgets, educational activities, incentives, methods, etc.

VI.B.2.a Description of what is done
See also: 82, 127, 358, 396, 398, 699, 894, 896, 904, 922, 1153, 1387, 1508.

739

The private and public programs in various countries and regions as of 1965 are described in Berelson et al., eds. (*see* 53), in the following papers:

Adil, E. "Pakistan": pp. 123-134.

Asavasena, W. et al. "Thailand": pp. 95-104.

Caldwell, J.C. "Africa": pp. 163-181.

Cha, Y.K. "South Korea": pp. 21-30.

Chun, D. "Hong Kong": pp. 71-84.

Corsa, L., Jr. "The United States": pp. 259-275.

Curt, J.N. "Puerto Rico": pp. 227-233.

Daly, A. "Tunisia": pp. 151-161.

Delgado Garcia, R. "Latin America": pp. 249-257.

Glass, D.V. "Western Europe": pp. 183-206.

Hsu, T.C. and Chow, L.P. "Taiwan, Republic of China": pp. 55-70.

Husein, H.M. "United Arab Republic": pp. 143-150.

Kim, T.I. and Kim, S.W. "Mass Use of Intra-Uterine Contraceptive Devices in Korea": pp. 425-432.

Kinch, A. "Ceylon": pp. 105-110.

Lim, M. "Malaysia and Singapore": pp. 85-94.

Mahlan, K.H. "The Socialist Countries of Europe": pp. 207-226.

Metiner, T. "Turkey": pp. 135-141.

Muramatsu, M. "Japan": pp. 7-19.

Raina, B.L. "India": pp. 111-121.

Romero, M. "Chile": pp. 235-247.

Taeuber, I. and Orleans, L.A. "Mainland China": pp. 31-54.

740

Broad summaries of actual and proposed family planning programs and background data for countries and areas appeared in the following articles in *Demography* 5(2), 1968:

Adil, E. "Measurement of Family Planning Progress in Pakistan": pp. 659-665.

Agarwala, S.N. "How Are We Doing in Family Planning in India?": pp. 710-713.

Brown, G.F. "Moroccan Family Planning Program: Progress and Problems": pp. 627-631.

Chandrasekaran, C. "How India is Tackling Her Population Problem": pp. 642-649.

Fisek, N.H. and Shorter, F.C. "Fertility Control in Turkey": pp. 578-589.

Harewood, J. "Recent Population Trends and Family Planning Activity in the Caribbean Area": pp. 874-893.

Jaffe, F.S. and Guttmacher, A.F. "Family Planning Programs in the United States": pp. 910-923.

London, G.D. "Family Planning Programs of the Office of Economic Opportunity: Scope, Operation, and Impact": pp. 924-930.

Mendoza-Hoyos, H. "The Colombian Program for Public Education, Personnel Training and Evaluation": pp. 827-835.

Povey, W.G. and Brown, G.F. "Tunisia's Experience in Family Planning": pp. 620-626.

Rodrigues, W. "Progress and Problems of Family Planning in Brazil": pp. 800-810.

Ross, J.A. and Finnigan, O.D., III "Within Family Planning—Korea": pp. 679-689.

Sardari, A.M. and Keyhan, R. "The Prospect of Family Planning in Iran": pp. 780-784.

Toppozada, H.K. "Progress and Problems of Family Planning in the United Arab Republic": pp. 590-597.

Wright, N.H. "Recent Fertility Change in Ceylon and Prospects for the National Family Planning Program": pp. 745-756.

741
American Public Health Association. Program Area Committee on Population and Public Health.
"Public Health Programs in Family Planning." [A group of 15 papers.] *American Journal of Public Health and the Nation's Health* 56(1, Part 2), Jan. 1966; 93p.
Organizational aspects and results of family planning services in the U.S.

742
Apte, M.L.
"Industrial Units and Family Planning." *Journal of Family Welfare* (Bombay) 12(4), June 1966: pp. 38-41.
Description and preliminary results of a voluntary family planning clinic initiated by a private industry in Bombay.

743
Bain, I.
"The Development of Family Planning in Canada." *Canadian Journal of Public Health* 55(8), Aug. 1964: pp. 334-340.
The history of activities in seven centers since 1929 and motivation behind the movement.

744
Balfour, M.
"Population and Family Planning Programs in U.S. Schools of Public Health." *Studies in Family Planning* 29, Apr. 1968: pp. 12-16.
Description of population training programs in major U.S. schools of public health.

745
Ball, D.W.
"An Abortion Clinic Ethnography." *Social Problems* 14, Winter 1967: pp. 293-301.
Social, psychological, economic, and medical characteristics of a relatively costly abortion clinic on the California-Mexico border.

746
Bean, L.L. and Bhatti, A.D.
"Three Years of Pakistan's National Family Planning Program." *The Pakistan Development Review* 9(1), Spring 1969: pp. 35-57.
Organization and progress, including an estimate of the proportion of eligible couples using program services at the end of three years.

747
Begum, A.I.
"Training of Thana Family Planning Officers of Bakergang District, East Pakistan." In *Seminar on Research in Family Planning.* 2nd, Karachi, Oct. 1966. Karachi: National Research Institute of Family Planning, 1966: pp. 18-30.
Description of the training of family planning officers and their knowledge and attitudes toward family planning and the villagers they serve.

748
Bogue, D.J., ed.
The Rural South Fertility Experiments, Report Number 1. Community and Family Study Center Publications in Family Planning, 5. No. 30. Chicago: Community and Family Study Center, University of Chicago, 1966; 26p.
Description and first evaluation of results of family planning clinics in southern U.S.

749
Bogue, D.J., ed.
Mass Communication and Motivation for

Family Planning. Chicago: Community and Family Study Center, University of Chicago, 1967; 551p.

Papers from the summer workshop at the University of Chicago.

750
Corsa, L., Jr.
"Family Planning in Pakistan." *American Journal of Public Health and the Nation's Health* 55(3), Mar. 1965: pp. 400-403.

Description of organization and progress of the Pakistan program during the first half of its program for 1960-65.

751
Eliot, J.W. et al.
"Family Planning Activities of Official Health and Welfare Agencies, United States, 1966." *American Journal of Public Health and the Nation's Health* 58(4), Apr. 1968: pp. 700-712.

1966 findings of a national survey of agencies providing the services.

752
*Florence, L.S.
Progress Report on Birth Control. London: William Heinemann, 1956; 256p.

An early, detailed, frank report on the functioning of a family planning clinic.

753
Garnier, J.C.
"Morocco: Training and Utilization of Family Planning Field Workers." *Studies in Family Planning* 1(47), Nov. 1969: pp. 1-5.

Description of the training program with recommendations for restructuring the course.

754
Gustafson, H.C. et al.
"Educational Efforts in the Implementa-tion of Rural Family Planning Programs in East Pakistan." *Demography* 4(1), 1967: pp. 81-89.

755
Hatcher, R.A. and Tiller, M.J.
"Acceleration of a Public Health Department Family Planning Program: Referral from Well Baby Clinics in Muscogee County, Georgia." *American Journal of Public Health* 59(7), July 1969: pp. 1217-1225.

756
Howell, K.
IPPF World Survey. Factors Affecting the Work of the Family Planning Associations. Part 1. London: International Planned Parenthood Federation, 1966; 102p.

Manual includes sections on finance, staff, training, publicity, type of patients, and methods available at clinics.

757
Mahajan, B.M.
"Vasectomy versus IUCD." *Artha Vijñāna* (Poona) 8(2), June 1966: pp. 149-160.

Comparison of costs and personnel needs of contraceptive methods.

758
Muramatsu, M. and Harper, P.A.
Population Dynamics: International Action and Training Programs. Baltimore: Johns Hopkins Press, 1965; 248p.

Conference papers include descriptions of national family planning programs and discussions of personnel training.

759
O'Conner, R.W. et al.
"United States: Information Flow and

Service-oriented Feedback in Family Planning Programs." *Studies in Family Planning* 46, Oct. 1969: pp. 6-10.

Description of computer-centered information system used in Georgia.

760
Peng, J.Y. et al.
"A Pilot Programme for Family Planning in Thailand: Review of one Year of Operation in Potharam, 1964-65." Parts 1 and 2. *Medical Gynaecology and Sociology* 2(7), 1967: pp. 5-8; and 2(8), 1967: pp. 7-15.

Organization of a family planning program in a rural district, and results of a baseline survey of fertility and fertility control.

761
Population Council.
"International Postpartum Family Planning Program: Report on the First Year." *Studies in Family Planning* 1(22), Aug. 1967: pp. 1-23.

762
Roberts, G.W.
"Some Problems of Fertility Control in Developing Societies." *Advances in Fertility Control* 3(3), Sept. 1968: pp. 33-37.

Description of the development and organization of the family planning programs in the West Indies.

763
Ross, J.A. et al.
"Korea and Taiwan: Review of Progress in 1968." *Studies in Family Planning* 1(41), Apr. 1969: pp. 1-11.

764
Samuel, T.J.
"The Development of India's Policy of Population Control." *Milbank Memorial Fund Quarterly* 44(1, Part 1), Jan. 1966: pp. 49-67.

Historical development and factors retarding implementation of India's family planning program.

765
United Nations. Economic Commission for Asia and the Far East.
Administrative Aspects of Family Planning Programmes: Report of a Working Group. Asian Population Studies Series, 1. New York: 1966; 64p.

Report on deliberations of meeting at Bangkok, March 1966, organized by the United Nations Development Program in cooperation with The Population Council; individual reports on 10 member countries and proposals for cooperative arrangements.

766
Wilder, F. and Tyagi, D.K.
"India's New Departures in Mass Motivation for Fertility Control." *Demography* 5(2), 1968: pp. 773-779.

The Indian program's attempt to convey a fairly simple message by repetition in many mass media and public information contexts.

767
Zalduondo, C.
"A Family Planning Program Using Volunteers as Health Educators." *American Journal of Public Health and the Nation's Health* 54(2), Feb. 1964: pp. 301-307.

Description of Puerto Rico's private Family Planning Association and its special use of local community leaders.

VI.B.2.b Suggestions and estimates of what should be done
See also: 58, 749, 753, 1140, 1150, 1220, 1387.

768
Discussions of the various aspects of organization, personnel, budget issues

are described in Berelson et al., eds. (*see* 53), in the following papers:

Baumgartner, L. "Family Planning Around the World": pp. 277-294.

Cummings, G.T.M. and Vaillant, H.W. "The Training of the Nurse-Midwife for a National Program in Barbados Combining the IUD and Cervical Cytology": pp. 451-454.

Fisek, N.H. "Problems in Starting a Program": pp. 297-304.

Freymann, M.W. "Organizational Structure in Family Planning Programs": pp. 321-334.

Hsu, S.C. "Personnel Problems in Family Planning Programs": pp. 335-343.

Kantner, J.F. "The Place of Conventional Methods in Family Planning Programs": pp. 403-409.

Keeny, S.M. "Budget and Timetable": pp. 363-372.

Ross, J.A. "Cost of Family Planning Program": pp. 759-778.

Taylor, H.C., Jr. "A Family Planning Program Related to Maternity Service": pp. 433-441.

Wayland, S.R. "Family Planning and the School Curriculum": pp. 353-362.

Yang, J.M. "Planning and Program": pp. 305-320.

769
Berelson, B.
"Communication, Communication Research, and Family Planning." In *Emerging Techniques in Population Research*. Proceedings of the 1962 Annual Conference of the Milbank Memorial Fund. New York: Milbank Memorial Fund, 1963: pp. 159-171.

770
*Bogue, D.J.
"Some Tentative Recommendations for a 'Sociologically Correct' Family Planning Communication and Motivation Program in India." In *Research in Family Planning*. Edited by C.V. Kiser. Princeton: Princeton University Press, 1962: pp. 503-538.

771
Bogue, D.J. and Heiskanen, V.S.
How to Improve Written Communication for Birth Control. No. 2. Chicago: Community and Family Study Center, University of Chicago, 1963; 90p.

772
Carolina Population Center.
Final Report: International Workshop on Communication Aspects of Family Planning Programs. Monograph 3. Chapel Hill: 1969; 128p.

A report of a workshop designed to provide intensive training for information specialists serving health ministries and family planning agencies of countries in the Near East, South Asia, and East Asia.

773
Center for Family Planning Program Development. Technical Assistance Division of Planned Parenthood-World Population.
Need for Subsidized Family Planning Services: United States, Each State and County, 1968. Washington: Government Printing Office, 1969; 255p.

Data for U.S. counties on medical and welfare resources and need for government family planning services.

774
Chilman, C.S.
"Poverty and Family Planning in the United States: Some Social and Psychological Aspects and Implications for

Programs and Policy." *Welfare in Review* 5, Apr. 1967: pp. 3-15.

Reviews social and psychological research on family planning and poverty; suggests program and policy orientations.

775

Dandekar, K.

"Possible Targets and Their Attainment in the Field of Family Planning in India during 1966-76." *Artha Vijñāna* (Poona) 8(3), Sept. 1966: pp. 239-249.

Estimates the size of the work program required to reduce the birth rate by one third, based on assumption that childbearing would cease after three living children.

776

Jaffe, F.S.

"Family Planning and the Medical Assistance Program." *Medical Care* 6(1), Jan.-Feb. 1968: pp. 69-77.

Assesses the potential role of Medicaid in family planning services, legislative, and administrative aspects.

777

Jaffe, F.S.

"A Strategy for Implementing Family Planning Services in the United States." *American Journal of Public Health and the Nation's Health* 58(4), Apr. 1968: pp. 713-725.

Resource allocation, priorities, and distribution of responsibilities among various agencies.

778

Jaffe, F.S. et al.

"Planning for Community-Wide Family Planning Services." *American Journal of Public Health* 59(8), Aug. 1969: pp. 1339-1354.

Model for organizational and resource allocative aspects of a community family planning program based on a functioning metropolitan program in the U.S.

779

Kanagaratnam, K. and Balfour, M.

"Administrative Aspects of Family Planning Programmes in Asia: Report on a Workshop." *Studies in Family Planning* 14, Sept. 1966: pp. 1-8.

Summary of a conference dealing with administrative aspects of Asian family planning programs.

780

Perkin, G.W.

"Pregnancy Prevention in 'High Risk' Women: A Strategy for New National Family Planning Programs." *Studies in Family Planning* 1(44), Aug. 1969: pp. 19-24.

781

Polgar, S. and Jaffe, F.S.

"Evaluation and Recordkeeping for U.S. Family Planning Services." *Public Health Reports* 83(8), Aug. 1968: pp. 639-651.

Reviews and recommends changes in present systems of evaluation and record keeping.

782

Simon, J.L.

"The Role of Bonuses and Persuasive Propaganda in the Reduction of Birth Rates." *Economic Development and Cultural Change* 16(3), Apr. 1968: pp. 404-411.

Suggests a complementary role for incentive payments and educational programs in the family planning programs.

783

Simon, J.L.

"Some 'Marketing Correct' Recommendations for Family Planning Campaigns." *Demography* 5(10), 1968: pp. 504-507.

Takes issue with some recommendations that have been made for communication and motivation programs and suggests some ways in which family planning marketing may be improved.

784
United Nations. Economic Commission for Asia and the Far East.
"ECAFE: Working Group on Communications Aspects of Family Planning Programs." *Studies in Family Planning* 1(31), May 1968: pp. 1-8.
Brief review of family planning communication efforts in the E.C.A.F.E. region countries; organizational and media message system models.

785
United Nations. World Health Organization Advisory Mission.
"Pakistan: Report on the Family Planning Program by the UN/WHO Advisory Mission." *Studies in Family Planning* 1(40), Apr. 1969: pp. 4-10.
Evaluation of the administrative aspects of the program with summary of recommendations for further expansion.

786
United States Congress. Senate Committee on Labor and Public Welfare. Subcommittee on Employment, Manpower, and Poverty.
Family Planning Program. Hearing before the Subcommittee on Employment, Manpower, and Poverty of the Committee. Washington: Government Printing Office, 1966; 135p.
Congressional hearings on bill to provide financial assistance to public and private agencies for family planning programs.

787
Wilber, G.
"Fertility and the Need for Family Planning among Rural Poor in the United States." *Demography* 5(2), 1968: pp. 894-909.

788
Wishik, S.M.
"Designs for Family Planning Programs and Research in Developing Countries." *American Journal of Public Health and the Nation's Health* 57(1), Jan. 1967: pp. 15-21.
Notes on typical difficulties (illiteracy, identifications of individuals, inaccurate vital statistics, special health conditions, channels of communication) and on adaptations to cultural and environmental circumstances in Pakistan.

VI.B.3 Evaluative studies (these often overlap with research on general studies of factors affecting fertility)

VI.B.3a Models or methodologies for evaluation
See also: 191, 192, 206, 214, 219, 889, 910, 1403.

789
Back, K.W.
"A Model of Family Planning Experiments: The Lessons of the Puerto Rican and Jamaican Studies." *Marriage and Family Living* 25(1), Feb. 1963: pp. 14-19.
Theoretical framework developed to examine fertility change at the individual level in the context of a family planning program.

790
Bean, L.L. and Seltzer, W.
"Couple Years of Protection and Births

Prevented: A Methodological Examination." *Demography* 5(2), 1968: pp. 947-959.

A detailed critique of the Pakistan system for converting statistics on couples receiving certain services to estimates of couple years of protection and then converting that to births averted; clearly demonstrates that the methodology is imperfect and probably overestimates program success.

791
Bogue, D.J.
"Family Planning Research: An Outline of the Field." In Berelson et al., eds. (*see* 53): pp. 721-735.

Comprehensive program for evaluating family planning progress.

792
Bogue, D.J.
Inventory, Explanation, and Evaluation by Interview of Family Planning Motives—Attitudes—Knowledge—Behavior.
Chicago: Community and Family Study Center, University of Chicago, 1965; 192p.

A very detailed plan for sample surveys to estimate changing levels of fertility, family planning attitudes, and behavior, with illustrative data for a small Negro sample in Chicago; specimens for questionnaire, code, and tabulation.

793
Brackett, J.W. and Akers, D.S.
Projections of the Population of Pakistan, by Age and Sex, 1965. A Measure of the Potential Impact of a Family Planning Program. Washington: Bureau of the Census, 1965; 63p.

794
Chandrasekaran, C. and Freymann, M.W.
"Evaluating Community Family Planning Programs." In Sheps and Ridley, eds. (*see* 73): pp. 266-286.

Proposes an index of fertility change after reviewing general evaluation needs of family planning programs.

795
Coulter, E.J. and Greenberg, B.G.
"Methods of Evaluating Family Planning Programs with Special Reference to North Carolina." In *Proceedings of the Social Statistics Section, 1967.* Washington: American Statistical Association, 1968: pp. 190-205.

796
Freedman, R.
"Sample Surveys for Family Planning Research in Taiwan." *Public Opinion Quarterly* 28(3), 1964: pp. 373-382.

Practical and scientific utility of sample surveys related to a family planning program.

797
*Freymann, M.W. and Lionberger, H.F.
"A Model for Family Planning Action-Research." In *Research in Family Planning.* Edited by C.V. Kiser. Princeton: Princeton University Press, 1962: pp. 443-461.

An early program for action-oriented research.

798
Green, L.W. and Jan, Y.A.
"Family Planning and Attitude Surveys in Pakistan." *Pakistan Development Review* (Karachi) 4(2), Summer 1964: pp. 332-355.

Critical discussion of survey results with suggestions for improving studies and programs.

799
Gupta, P.B.
"A Method of Estimating the Reduction

in Birth Rate by Sterilization of Married Couples." *Sankhyā* (Calcutta) (Series B) 27(3-4), Dec. 1965: pp. 225-250.

800
Haider, S.J. and Millar, R.A.
"Conducting Family Planning Research in Rural East Pakistan: Some Experience with the Standardized Interview." In *Seminar on Research in Family Planning.* 2nd, Karchi, Oct. 66. Karachi: National Research Institute of Family Planning, 1966: pp. 151-161.

801
Masnick, G. S. and Potter, R.G., Jr.
"Contraceptive Acceptance and Pregnancy: A Matrix Approach to the Analysis of Competing Risks." *Population Studies* 23(2), July 1969: pp. 267-277.

802
Mauldin, W.P.
"Births Averted by Family Planning Programs." In Shorter and Güvenc, eds. (*see* 357): pp. 281-297. [Also in *Studies in Family Planning* 1(33), Aug. 1968: pp. 1-7.]
Discussion of techniques to measure the effect of a family planning program on fertility.

803
Namboodiri, N.K.
"On the Problem of Measuring the Impact of F.P. Action Programmes." *Journal of Family Welfare* (Bombay) 11(1), Sept. 1964: pp. 29-35.

804
***Ogburn, W.F.**
"A Design for Some Experiments in the Limitation of Population Growth in India." *Economic Development and Cultural Change* 1(5), Feb. 1953: pp. 376-389.

Early suggestion for the use of experimental designs to study population limitation.

805
Potter, R.G., Jr.
"Estimating Births Averted in a Family Planning Program." In Behrman et al., eds. (*see* 51): pp. 413-434.
Presents a model and tests it with Taiwan data; further developed in item 1508.

806
Ross, J.A. and Bang, S.
"The AID Computer Programme, Used to Predict Adoption of Family Planning in Koyang." *Population Studies* 20(1), July 1966: pp. 61-75.
Computer program to predict acceptance of alternative family planning programs using presurvey measurements.

807
Ross, J.A. et al.
A Handbook for Service Statistics in Family Planning Programs. New York: Population Council, 1968; 151p.
Summarizes the alternative methods of keeping and analyzing the statistics about the service and organization aspects of a family planning program; an important summary and source.

808
Sheps, M.C.
"Contributions of Natality Models to Program Planning and Evaluation." *Demography,* 3(2), 1966: pp. 445-461.

809
Sheps, M.C.
"Uses of Stochastic Models in the Evaluation of Population Policies. 1. Theory and Approaches to Data Analysis." In *Proceedings of the Fifth Berkeley Symposium on Mathematical Statistics and*

Probability. Vol. 4, Biology and Health. Berkeley: University of California Press, 1968: pp. 115-136.

Summarizes work done on mathematical models of reproduction and their application to fertility control efforts.

810
Stephan, F.F.
"Demonstrations, Experiments, and Pilot Projects: A Review of Recent Designs." In Berelson et al., eds. (*see* 53): pp. 711-720.

Reviews possible experimental designs for programs.

811
Stycos, J.M.
"Survey Research and Population Control in Latin America." *Public Opinion Quarterly* 28, Fall 1964: pp. 367-372.

Outlines the purposes of attitude, use, and knowledge surveys in Latin America; gives examples with special reference to policy implications.

812
Tabbarah, R.B.
"Birth Control and Population Policy." *Population Studies* 18(2), Nov. 1964: pp. 187-196.

An index of acceptability of contraception based on desired number of children is suggested for evaluating acceptance of family planning in population programs.

813
Takeshita, J.Y.
"Lessons Learned from Family Planning Studies in Taiwan and Korea." In Berelson et al., eds. (*see* 53): pp. 691-710.

Discusses possible implications of evaluation studies and experiments for programs.

814
Takeshita, J.Y. and Freedman, R.
"Measuring Acceptances in a Family Planning Program: The Decomposition of Rates by Eligibility Criteria." *Demography* 4(1), 1967: pp. 158-171.

Illustrates advantage of separating acceptance rates into eligibility rates and acceptance for the eligible in relevant subgroups of population, with illustrations from Taiwan.

815
Tietze, C. and Lewit, S.
"Statistical Evaluation of Contraceptive Methods: Use-Effectiveness and Extended Use-Effectiveness." *Demography* 5(2), 1968: pp. 931-940.

816
United Nations. Economic Commission for Asia and the Far East.
"Report of the Expert Group on Assessment of Acceptance and Use-Effectiveness of Family Planning Methods." *Asian Population Studies Series* 4, Oct. 1969; 69p.

Conference report on evaluation of acceptance, use-effectiveness, and program effects on fertility rates.

817
Wolfers, D.
"An Evaluation Criterion for a National Family Planning Program." *American Journal of Public Health and the Nation's Health* 58(8), Aug. 1968: pp. 1447-1451.

Presents projections of monthly number of births over a five-year period for the several ethnic groups of Singapore as a basis for evaluating what happens.

818
Yaukey, D.
"Some Designs for Rural Action Studies

on Family Planning." *Journal of Pakistan Academy for Village Development* (Comilla) 3, July 1962: pp. 48-55.

VI.B.3.b Studies of the administrative aspects of the program
See also: 773, 1152.

819
Beasley, J.D. et al.
"The Orleans Parish Family Planning Demonstration Program." *Milbank Memorial Fund Quarterly* 47(3, Part 1), July 1969: pp. 225-253.
> *Reports on the first year of an important, carefully planned and monitored program to reach all of the indigent women at childbearing risk in the Orleans parish through a health-based family planning program; organization, method on contact, and rather high rate of acceptance in first year of program discussed.*

820
Hartman, P.
"Information and Educational Programs." In Berelson et al., eds. (*see* 53): pp. 345-351.
> *Assessment of efficacy of various communication media in Korea.*

821
Kantner, J. and Stycos, J.M.
"A Non-Clinical Approach to Contraception." In *Research in Family Planning*. Edited by C.V. Kiser. Princeton: Princeton University Press, 1962: pp. 573-590.
> *A survey of leadership motivation and contraceptive use in the family planning program in Puerto Rico.*

822
Mathen, K.K. and Sen, M.
"The Singur Population Study as an Action Research Model for Family Planning." *Journal of Family Welfare* (Bombay) 10(4), June 1964: pp. 4-15.
> *Discussion of the Singur family planning experiment in terms of stages desirable for an action research program.*

823
Mitchell, R.E.
"Hong Kong: An Evaluation of Field Workers and Decision Making in Family Planning Programs." *Studies in Family Planning* 1(30), May 1968: pp. 7-22.

824
Murty, D.V.R.
"Evaluation of Family Planning Programme in India." In 1967 I.U.S.S.P. (*see* 21): pp. 468-475.

825
Raina, B.L. et al.
A Study in Family Planning Communication-Meerut District. Monograph Series, 3. New Delhi: Central Family Planning Institute, 1967; 82p. [Also in *Studies in Family Planning* 1(21), June 1967: pp. 1-5.]
> *Experimental intensive information program, with before and after surveys to measure knowledge; also describes the contemporaneous sale of commercial contraceptives and the acceptance of the IUD and sterilization.*

826
Ross, J.A.
"Cost Analysis of the Taichung Experiment." *Studies in Family Planning* 1(10), Feb. 1966: pp. 6-15.
> *Comparison of efficiency of different program methods used in separate sectors of a Taiwanese town.*

VI.B.3.c Studies of the attitudes and related characteristics of the population toward birth control or the program

See also: 582, 640, 961, 1160, 1161, 1219, 1240, 1513, 1526.

827
Gomez, M.J.
"Medellin: A Case of Strong Resistance to Brith Control." *Demography* 5(2), 1968: pp. 811-826.

Unusual case history of the interplay in a Colombian city between the opinions of the public, various elites, government officials, and church leaders, and the use of survey data on the practices and opinions of each of these sectors.

828
Hawley, A.H. and Prachuabmoh, V.
"Family Growth and Family Planning in a Rural District of Thailand." In Berelson et al., eds. (*see* 53): pp. 523-544.

Baseline survey for a family planning experiment with preliminary data on correlates of fertility and family planning.

829
Morsa, J.
"The Tunisia Survey: A Preliminary Analysis." In Berelson et al., eds. (*see* 53): pp. 581-593.

Benchwork survey for a family planning program, providing data on social and demographic correlates of fertility and family planning.

830
Nag, M.
"Attitudes toward Vasectomy in West Bengal." *Population Review* (Madras) 10(1), Jan. 1966: pp. 61-64.

A 1960 survey of reasons for almost universal opposition to sterilization among rural women, interpreted to result from misinformation that could be removed by the proper program.

831
Opler, M.E.
"Cultural Context and Population Control Programs in Village India." In *Fact and Theory in Social Science.* Edited by E.W. Count and G. T. Bowles. Syracuse, N.Y.: Syracuse University Press, 1964: pp. 201-221.

832
Poffenberger, T.
"Urban Indian Attitudinal Response and Behavior Related to Family Planning: Possible Implications for the Mass Communication Program." *Journal of Family Welfare* (Bombay) 14(4), June 1968: pp. 31-38.

A survey of levels and correlates of general attitudes and information about family planning used as basis for recommendations.

833
Raman, M.V.
"A Study of Current Attitudes toward Family Planning." *Journal of Family Welfare* (Bombay) 9(4), June 1963: pp. 18-29.

Evaluating various Indian surveys on attitudes toward family size and toward birth control; desire for male heir and joint family makes the male the primary program target.

834
Roberts, B.J. et al.
"Family Planning Survey in Dacca, East Pakistan." *Demography* 2, 1965: pp. 74-96.

Report of a benchmark survey prior to a program for testing the relative effectiveness of three alternative education approaches.

835
Ross, J.A. and Smith, D.P.
"Korea: Trends in Four National KAP Surveys, 1964-67." *Studies in Family Planning* 1(43), June 1969: pp. 6-11.

135

836

Saw, S.H.

"Family Planning Knowledge, Attitudes, and Practice in Malaya." *Demography* 5(2), 1968: pp. 702-709.

Brief summary of materials drawn from the Report on the West Malaysian Family Survey (see 1516).

837

Stycos, J.M.

"Politics and Population Control in Latin America." *World Politics* 20(1), Oct 1967: pp. 66-82.

Newspaper items and interviews with university professors used to discuss the view of intellectuals in Brazil and Colombia toward family planning and U.S. aid.

838

Verma, S.S. et al.

"A Base-line Survey of Attitude, Knowledge and Practice of Family Planning on the Eastern Railway." *Journal of Family Welfare* (Bombay) 12(4), June 1966: pp. 56-60.

Report on program initiated by the Eastern Railway, India, in 1962.

VI.B.3.d Studies of the characteristics of the clients, including changes in their fertility or birth-control practices and attitudes, or success of specific contraceptive methods used

See also: 587, 742, 748, 750, 752, 761, 819, 890, 914, 1225, 1325, 1462.

839

Agarwala, S.N.

Fertility Control through Contraception: A Study of Family Planning Clinics of Metropolitan Delhi. New Delhi: Directorate of Health Services, Ministry of Health, Government of India, 1960; 85p.

840

Agarwala, S.N.

"A Follow-up Study of Intrauterine Contraceptive Devices: An Indian Experience." *Eugenics Quarterly* 15(1), Mar. 1968: pp. 41-50.

One of the first systematic follow-up reports on the IUD in India, based on clients of an urban clinic in Delhi.

841

Balakrishnan, T.R. and Mathai, R.J.

"Evaluation of a Family Planning Publicity Program in India." In 1967 I.U.S.S.P. (*see* 21): pp. 413-423.

A mass publicity program for the IUD is shown to have increased the numbers practicing family planning by increasing the knowledge about it rather than by increasing IUD practice among the knowledgeable.

842

Basu, R.N.

"Experience with a Poorly Effective Oral Contraceptive in an Indian Village." *Demography* 1(1), 1964: pp. 106-110.

Repercussions of using a contraceptive with a 50-percent failure rate.

843

Begum, A.I.

"IUD Clinic Follow Up Study." In *Seminar on Research in Family Planning.* 2nd, Karachi, Oct. 1966. Karachi: National Research Institute of Family Planning, 1966: pp. 61-75.

IUD use differentials by age, family size, income, source of information, length of use.

844

Bhatia, B. et al.

"A Study in Family Planning Communication—Direct Mailing." *Demography* 3(2), 1966: pp. 343-351. [Based on Central Family Planning Institute Monograph 1. Delhi: June 1966.]

Report on field tests of information and attitudes about family planning in five villages one month after direct mailing of family planning literature.

845

Bogue, D.J.

"United States: The Chicago Fertility Control Studies." *Studies in Family Planning* 1(15), Oct. 1966: pp. 1-8.

Description of the study design and action results of an experiment in family planning mass communication; presents data on changes in clinic attendance and commercial distribution of contraceptives and their suggested relation to the decline in fertility.

846

Chandrasekaran, C. and Kuder, K.

Family Planning through Clinics. Report of a Survey of Family Planning Clinics in Greater Bombay. Demographic Training and Research Centre. Research Monograph 2. Bombay: Allied Publishers, 1965; 272p.

Pioneering study of who comes to clinics, under what influences, and with what effect on later reproductive behavior; based on both analysis of clinic records and sample survey of clients.

847

Chow, L.P. et al.

"Evaluation of Intrauterine Contraceptive Devices Program by Follow-up Interview." *Journal of the Formosan Medical Association* (Taipei) 64, July 1965: pp. 345-357.

848

Chow, L.P. et al.

"Correlates of IUD Termination in a Mass Family Planning Program: The First Taiwan IUD Follow-up Survey." *Milbank Memorial Fund Quarterly* 46(2, Part 1), Apr. 1968: pp. 215-235.

One of the first reports for a significant probability sample on IUD termination rates, their correlates, and the postinsertion contraceptive history of program acceptors.

849

Cobb, J. et al.

"Oral Contraceptive Program Synchronized with Moon Phase." *Fertility and Sterility* 17(4), July-Aug. 1966: pp. 559-567.

Description of experiment to regulate oral pill use by phases of the moon.

850

Collver, A. et al.

"Factors Influencing the Use of Maternal Health Services." *Social Science and Medicine* 1, 1967: pp. 293-308.

Socioeconomic, racial, religious, and demographic correlates of use of prenatal, postpartum, and family planning services for a sample of Detroit area obstetric patients.

851

Dingle, J.T. and Tietze, C.

"Comparative Study of Three Contraceptive Methods: Vaginal Foam Tablets, Jelly Alone, and Diaphragm with Jelly or Cream." *American Journal of Obstetrics and Gynecology* 85(8), Apr. 1963: pp. 1012-1022.

Assesses acceptability and effectiveness of three contraceptive methods in three-year planned parenthood program for low-income women in Cleveland, Ohio.

852

Dubey, D.C.

Adoption of a New Contraceptive in Ur-

ban India. Monograph Series, 6. New Delhi: Central Family Planning Institute, 1969; 132p.

Study of IUD acceptors in clinics serving civil servants in the Delhi area; demographic characteristics, sources of information, patterns of communication, decision-making process, religiosity, consumption patterns.

853
Dubey, D.C. and Choldin, H.M.
"Communication and Diffusion of the IUCD: A Case Study in Urban India." *Demography* 4(2), 1967: pp. 601-614.

Communication sources and adoption stages in the diffusion of the IUCD in New Delhi housing colonies.

854
Edmands, E.M.
"A Study of Contraceptive Practices in a Selected Group of Urban, Negro Mothers in Baltimore." *American Journal of Public Health and the Nation's Health* 58(2), Feb. 1968: pp. 263-273.

Contraceptive and fertility knowledge and practices of small sample of mothers coming to a child-health clinic.

855
Fawcett, J.T. et al.
"Thailand: An Analysis of Time and Distance Factors at an IUD Clinic in Bangkok." *Studies in Family Planning* 1(19), May 1967: pp. 8-12.

856
Frank, R. and Tietze, C.
"Acceptance of an Oral Contraceptive Program in a Large Metropolitan Area." *American Journal of Obstetrics and Gynecology* 93, Sept. 1965: pp. 122-127.

Early field study (1960-63) showing high acceptability and long continuous use of an oral contraceptive in a young, largely Negro population in Chicago, with life-table continuation rates of over 70 percent at 30 months.

857
Freedman, R. and Sun, T.H.
"Taiwan: Fertility Trends in a Crucial Period of Transition." *Studies in Family Planning* 1(44), Aug. 1969: pp. 15-19.

Recent trends in program acceptors' characteristics, age structure, and age-specific fertility and nuptiality as they potentially affect the birth rate.

858
Green, L.W. and Krotki, K.J.
"Proximity and Other Geographical Factors in Family Planning Clinic Utilization in Pakistan." *Pakistan Development Review* (Karachi) 6(1), Spring 1966: pp. 80-104.

Residential distribution and proximity analysis of family planning clients.

859
Hall, M.F.
"Field Effectiveness of the Oral and Intrauterine Methods of Contraception: The Baltimore Public Program, 1964-66." *Milbank Memorial Fund Quarterly* 47(1, Part 1), Jan. 1969: pp. 55-71.

Comparison of oral and device users as to sociodemographic characteristics and age-adjusted probabilities of continuing contraception.

860
Hall, M.F. and Reinke, W.A.
"Factors Influencing Contraception Continuation Rates: The Oral and the Intrauterine Methods." *Demography* 6(3), Aug. 1969: pp. 335-346.

For a Baltimore sample the IUD has higher continuation rates than the pill in a public program; relates characteristics of age, duration of use, and race to termination rates by a new multivariate method (multisort analysis).

861
Hsu, T.C. et al.
"Preliminary Report on the Medical Follow-up Study of the New Inter-Uterine Contraceptive Device." *Journal of the Formosan Medical Association* (Taipei) 63, Sept. 1964: pp. 427-436.

862
Hyrenius, H. and Ahs, U.
The Swedish-Ceylon Family Planning Pilot Project. Reports, 6. Goteborg, Sweden: Demographic Institute, University of Goteborg, 1968; 34p.
Report on fertility and nuptiality changes and contraceptive use in two different programs in Ceylon involving different ethnic groups.

863
Demographic Research Centre, India. Kerala. (Trivandrum).
Published and unpublished articles on knowledge, attitudes, and practice toward family planning; demographic and socioeconomic correlates, knowledge and attitudes toward sterilization. (For an annotated listing of the reports see 117.)

864
India. Uttar Pradesh.
Acceptance of Family Planning Methods as a Function of the Nature and Intensity of Contact. Lucknow: Planning Research and Action Institute, 1961; 67p.
Sample survey results used to study the number of visits by family planning workers prior to acceptance of method and the relative value of contacting both husband and wife; demographic and socioeconomic correlates of acceptance.

865
Jarret, W.H.
"Family Size and Fertility Patterns of Participants in Family Planning Clinics." *Sociological Analysis* 25(3), Summer 1964: pp. 113-120.
The relation of education and occupation to fertility for couples seeking information from a Catholic clinic.

866
Jones, G.W. and Mauldin, W.P.
"Use of Oral Contraceptives: With Special Reference to Developing Countries." *Studies in Family Planning* 1(24), Dec. 1967: pp. 1-13.

867
Kanagaratnam, K. and Khoo, K.C.
"Singapore: The Use of Oral Contraceptives in the National Program." *Studies in Family Planning* 1(48), Dec. 1969: pp. 1-9.
Analysis of the level and correlates of termination rates for use of oral contraception in the large-scale Singapore program.

868
Khan, M.
"Population Control: A Two-Year Rural Action Experience." *Demography* 1, 1964: pp. 126-129.
Brief description of characteristics of the population, organization, and results of the action program; comparisons of clients with nonclients.

869
Khan, A.M. and Choldin, H.M.
"New 'Family Planners' in Rural East Pakistan." *Demography* 2, 1965: pp. 1-7.
Compares the characteristics of family planning acceptors in villages with and without a development program.

870
Korea. Ministry of Health and Social Affairs.
National Intrauterine Contraception Report. [Korean and English text.] Seoul: Planned Parenthood Federation of Korea, 1967; 86p.

A report on factors affecting acceptance of IUD and termination of use in the important Korean family planning program.

871
Koya, Y.
"A Family Planning Program in a Large Population Group." *Milbank Memorial Fund Quarterly* 40(3), July 1962: pp. 319-327.

Discusses the Japanese National Railway's family planning program for its employees, which was followed by sharp birth-rate declines.

872
Koya, Y.
"Lessons from Contraceptive Failure." *Population Studies* 16(1), July 1962: pp. 4-11.

Inferences about family planning programs drawn from analyses of 4,300 case records in health clinics; demographic facts and data on adoption of and success with contraception failure.

873
Kurup, R.S.
"Sterilization Operations in Kerala State, India." In 1967 I.U.S.S.P. (*see* 21): pp. 440-448.

Examines demographic and socioeconomic aspects.

874
Lafitte, F.
"The Users of Birth Control Clinics." *Population Studies* 16(1), July 1962: pp. 12-30.

Report on the characteristics of clients of the Family Planning Association in Great Britain as of 1960.

875
Mauldin, W.P. et al.
"Retention of IUDs: An International Comparison." *Studies in Family Planning* 1(18), Apr. 1967: pp. 1-12.

876
McDaniel, E.B.
"Trial of a Long-Acting, Injectable Contraceptive as a Substitute for the IUCD and the Pill in a Remote Region in Thailand." *Demography* 5(2), 1968: pp. 699-701.

Reports initial success in acceptability, retention, and effectiveness of a new method in a remote area.

877
Poffenberger, S.B. and Sheth, D.L.
"Reaction of Urban Employees to Vasectomy Operations." *Journal of Family Welfare* 10(2), Dec. 1963: pp. 1-17.

878
Polgar, S.
"United States: The PPFA Mobile Service Project in New York City." *Studies in Family Planning* 1(15), Oct. 1966: pp. 9-15.

Report on the effectiveness of communication efforts in a low-income neighborhood to initiate family planning services.

879
Roberts, B.J. et al.
"A Post-Operative Study of Ligatees in Dacca, East Pakistan." *Journal of the Pakistan Academy for Rural Development* (Comilla) 4(3), Jan. 1964: pp. 1-21.

Survey of patients of a maternity center in Pakistan.

880
Satterthwaite, A.P.
"Oral Contraceptives." In Berelson et al., eds. (*see* 53): pp. 411-424.
Reports on tests in Puerto Rico, 1957-64, with special reference to high termination rates.

881
Satterthwaite, A.P.
"Experience with Oral and Intrauterine Contraception in Rural Puerto Rico." In Sheps and Ridley, eds. (*see* 73): pp. 474-480.
Early field experience with IUD and oral contraception in Puerto Rico.

882
Schuman, H.
Economic Development and Individual Change: A Social-Psychological Study of the Comilla Experiment in Pakistan. Occasional Papers in International Affairs, 15. Cambridge, Mass.: Center for International Affairs, Harvard University, 1967; 59p.
Birth-control attitudes and motivation related to standard of living and social and educational status, as small part of a larger study.

883
Stoeckel, J.
"Social and Demographic Correlates of Contraceptive Adoption in a Rural Area of East Pakistan." *Demography* 5(1), 1968: pp. 45-54.
Study of social and demographic situations of women purchasing contraceptives in villages, 1962-66.

884
Stoeckel, J. and Choudhury, M.A.
"East Pakistan: Fertility and Family Planning in Comilla." *Studies in Family Planning* 1(39), Mar. 1969: pp. 14-16.

Reconstructed fertility histories used to analyze the impact of "organizer" and commercial-distribution approaches of family planning on fertility rates.

885
Tietze, C.
"Fertility after Discontinuation of Intrauterine and Oral Contraception." *International Journal of Fertility* 13(4), Oct.-Dec. 1968: pp. 385-389.
Estimates conception rates after voluntary discontinuance of IUD contraception by age at removal and duration of use.

886
Timur, S. and Fincancioglu, N.
"Demographic and Socio-Economic Characteristics of Turkish IUD Acceptors." In Shorter and Güvenc, eds. (*see* 357): pp. 175-217.

887
Viel, B.
"Results of a Family Planning Program in the Western Area of the City of Santiago." *American Journal of Public Health* 59(10), Oct. 1969: pp. 1898-1909.
Finds that postpartum and postabortion IUD insertion program has led to a large increase in contraceptive use, as well as lowering the abortion and birth rates.

VI.B.3.e Studies of the effect of the program on contraceptive practice or fertility of the larger population of which the directly served clients are only one part, or studies comparing clients and nonclients
See also: 426, 533, 746, 805, 868, 1156, 1238, 1530, 1646.

888

Beasley, J.D. and Parish, V.W.

"Family Planning and the Reduction of Fertility and Illegitimacy: A Preliminary Report on Rural Southern Program." *Social Biology* 16(3), Sept. 1969: pp. 167-178.

Comparison of one parish with a family planning program and four without, showing that "experimental" parish had a larger reduction than "controls" in medically indigent births, both for total and illegitimate births.

889

Chang, M.C. and Chow, L.P.

"A Study by Matching of the Demographic Impact of an IUD Program." *Milbank Memorial Fund Quarterly* 47(2), Apr. 1969: pp. 135-157.

Compares postinsertion fertility of a sample of IUD acceptors in Taiwan with a carefully controlled group matched in age, parity, education, and interval since last birth at time of IUD insertion; while fertility fell substantially for both groups, it fell by widest margin for IUD acceptors; an important model.

890

Chow, L.P.

"A Study on the Demographic Impact of an IUD Programme." *Population Studies* 22(3), Nov. 1968: pp. 347-359.

Attempts to assess the impact of the island-wide program on the reduction of the birth rate; data on fertility and contraceptive use levels, termination rates by cause, and estimates of births prevented.

891

Dandekar, K.

Communication in Family Planning: Report on an Experiment. Gokhale Institute Studies, 49. Bombay: Asia Publishing House, 1967; 109p.

Statistical report on a four-stage field test of the efficacy of the work of a family planning clinic attached to a small hospital.

892

Dandekar, K. and Bhate, V.

"Family Planning in the City of Poona." *Journal of Institute of Economic Research* (Dharwar) 3(1), Jan. 1968: pp. 1-21.

Uses a follow-up survey of clinic clients to compare their characteristics with that of the general population and with earlier survey results from 1961.

893

Eberhard, W. and Eberhard, A.

"Family Planning in a Taiwan Town." In *Settlement and Social Change in Asia.* Berkeley: University of California Press, 1967: pp. 204-221.

Indicates that characteristics of acceptors of a private family planning program in a Taiwanese town differ from those found in the larger government program.

894

Faundes-Latham, A. et al.

"Effects of a Family Planning Program on the Fertility of a Marginal Working-Class Community in Santiago." *Demography* 5(1), 1967: pp. 122-137.

Description of pilot program and estimation of fertility rates using retrospective pregnancy histories.

895

Faundes-Latham, A. et al.

"The San Gregorio Experimental Family Planning Program: Changes Observed in Fertility and Abortion Rates." *Demography* 5(2), 1968: pp. 836-845.

Survey data for 1964 and 1966 document a substantial decline in fertility and an even larger decline in induced abortion in an area of Santiago, Chile, following an intensive program integrated with a well-staffed maternal and child health program.

896

Fawcett, J.T. and Sam Boonsuk, A.

"Thailand: Using Family Planning Acceptors to Recruit New Cases." *Studies in Family Planning* 1(39), Mar. 1969: pp. 1-3.

An apparently successful experiment, with control areas, to recruit new IUD cases by asking clinic cases to distribute cards to friends, promising free and preferential service at a crowded clinic.

897
Freedman, R. and Takeshita, J.Y.
"Studies of Fertility and Family Limitation in Taiwan." In Sheps and Ridley, eds. (*see* 73): pp. 174-197.

Report on the background, conduct, and findings of field research and action program in Taichung, Taiwan, 1962-65.

898
Gandotra, M.M.
"Standardised Birth Rate of Greater Bombay." *Journal of Family Welfare* 13(4), June 1967: pp. 1-5.

Examination of Bombay birth rate trends to estimate relative influences of changes in age-sex-marital status, of registration efficiency, or of genuine changes in fertility associated with family planning program.

899
Green, L.W. and Krotki, K.J.
Demographic Implications of the First Six Years of Family Planning in Karachi, 1958-1964. Research Report 55. Karachi: Institute of Development Economics, 1966; 49p.

900
Green, L.W. and Krotki, K.J.
"Class and Parity Biases in Family-Planning Programs: The Case of Karachi." *Eugenics Quarterly* 15(4), Dec. 1968: pp. 235-251.

Discusses program implications of differences between the socioeconomic distribution and parity of family planning clients with the distributions for the whole population.

901
Hawley, A.H. and Prachuabmoh, V.
"Family Growth and Family Planning: Responses to a Family-Planning Action Program in a Rural District of Thailand." *Demography* 3(2), 1966: pp. 319-331.

Follow-up survey of family planning knowledge, attitudes, and practice after initiation of family planning action program. (For the initial benchmark preprogram survey see 828.)

902
Hermalin, A.I.
"Taiwan: An Area Analysis of the Effect of Acceptances on Fertility." *Studies in Family Planning* 1(33), Aug. 1968: pp. 7-11.

903
Koya, Y.
"Does the Effect of a Family Planning Program Continue?" *Eugenics Quarterly* 11(3), Sept. 1964: pp. 141-147.

An attempt to assess the continuing effect of a family planning program after seven years by internal comparison and by comparison with national data; inability to control for out-migration and age changes makes interpretation of fertility decline difficult.

904
Kwon, E. H. et al.
A Study on Urban-Population Control: Sungdong Gu Action-Research Project on Family Planning and Fertility. Seoul: College of Medicine and School of Public Health, Seoul National University, 1967; 149p.

Patient records and survey data used to study the effect of the consultation stations, the acceptability of various contraceptives, and a coupon system.

905
Lee, B.M. and Isbister, J.
"The Impact of Birth Control Programs on Fertility." In Berelson et al., eds. (*see* 53): pp. 737-758.
An attempt to assess the impact of program acceptances on birth rate in Korea.

906
Okada, L.M.
"Use of Matched Pairs in Evaluation of a Birth Control Program." *Public Health Reports* 84(5), May 1969: pp. 445-450.
Comparison of samples of U.S. Negro women who participated in a postpartum birth control program with matched nonparticipants.

907
Potter, R.G., Jr. et al.
"Taiwan's Family Planning Program." *Science* 160(3840), May 1968: pp. 848-853.
Considers arguments against the claimed success of the Taiwan and Korean programs and provides a selective documentation of points favoring the view that the programs do enable those who participate to prevent a substantial number of births.

908
Ross, J.A.
"Predicting the Adoption of Family Planning." *Studies in Family Planning* 1(9), Jan. 1966: pp. 8-12.

909
Sheikh, M.H.
"Review Article: Projections of the Population of Pakistan by Age and Sex: 1965-1986, a Measure of the Potential Impact of a Family Planning Programme." *Pakistan Development Review* (Karachi) 7(2), Summer 1967: pp. 260-270.
Critique of the Brackett-Akers projections (see 793) as a suitable basis for measuring potential success of family planning program.

910
Srinivasan, K. et al.
"Analysis of the Declining Fertility in Athoor Block." *Bulletin* of the Institute of Rural Health and Family Planning (Gandhigram) 4(3), June 1969: pp. 28-58.
An important analysis of the apparently declining birth rates in a rural block where the well-known intensive Gandhigram family planning program operated; may be one of the few places in India where a fertility decline associated with a program effect is carefully analyzed; methodological problems and solutions are instructive.

911
Takeshita, J.Y. et al.
"A Study of the Effectiveness of the Pre-Pregnancy Health Program in Taiwan." *Eugenics Quarterly* 11(4), Dec. 1964: pp. 222-233.
Compares changes in fertility of couples in a family planning program with matched couples not in the program.

912
Takeshita, J.Y. et al.
"West Malaysia: 1969 Family Planning Acceptor Follow-up Survey." *Studies in Family Planning* 1(51), Mar. 1970: pp. 18-23.
A follow-up of a sample of acceptors compared with the general population of married women of childbearing age interviewed earlier in KAP survey; covers termination rates, later pregnancy, later birth control practice in relation to demographic and social characteristics.

913
Wolfers, D.
"The Demographic Effects of a Contraceptive Programme." *Population Studies* 23(1), Mar. 1969: pp. 111-140.

Using Singapore data, examines the program effect by measures of mean live birth interval, controlled for postpartum sterility, and other sterility, and extraprogram contraception use.

VI.B.3.f Cost-benefit studies
See also: 208.

914
Agarwala, S.N.
"The Arithmetic of Sterilization in India." *Eugenics Quarterly* 13(3), Sept. 1966: pp. 209-213.
Examines cost-benefit aspects and the effect on the birth rate.

915
Basu, R.N.
"Cost-Benefit Analysis of Family Planning Programme." *Family Planning News* Dec. 1968: pp. 2-6.
Very rough estimates of the unit cost of a birth prevented by IUD or sterilization in the Indian program, 1965-68.

916
Campbell, A.A.
"The Role of Family Planning in the Reduction of Poverty." *Journal of Marriage and the Family* 30(2), 1968: pp. 236-245.
Estimates the number of poor families with unwanted children, the costs of reaching them with contraceptives, and the benefits to the family and society.

917
Enke, S.
"Fewer Births—Better Living." *Tempo.* TMP-34. Santa Barbara, Calif: Center for Advanced Studies, General Electric, 1968; 15p.

Reviews government costs involved in excess childbearing among the poor and raises questions about how to obtain useful cost-benefit ratios for different possible types of family planning services for the U.S. poor.

918
Enke, S.
"Raising Per Capita Income through Fewer Births." *Tempo.* TMP-9. Santa Barbara, Calif.: Center for Advanced Studies, General Electric, 1968; 19p.
Economic-demographic relationships used to develop model for analyzing the rate of return of a program of birth prevention; policy implications.

919
Leasure, J.W.
"Some Economic Benefits of Birth Prevention." *Milbank Memorial Fund Quarterly* 45(4), Oct. 1967: pp. 417-425.
Interesting public-cost-benefit analysis of preventing a birth; used to estimate level of payments for proposed family-limitation program based on incentives for periods without births.

920
Leibenstein, H.
"Pitfalls in Benefit-Cost Analysis of Birth Prevention." *Population Studies* 23(2), July 1969: pp. 161-170.
Interesting critique of the applicability of benefit-cost analysis in estimating the economic value of a prevented birth. [For a comment by S. Enke and a rejoinder see Population Studies 24(1), Mar. 1970: pp. 115-119.]

921
Repetto, R.
"India: A Case Study of the Madras Vasectomy Program." *Studies in Family Planning* 1(31), May 1968: pp. 8-16.

Benefit-cost analysis of the vasectomy program; includes descriptions of promoters' activities and social "intangible costs" involved; brief comparison with programs in other Indian states.

VI.B.3.g Combinations of these
See also: 357, 1508, 1511.

922
Abhayaratne, O.E.R. and Jayewardene, C.H.S.
Family Planning in Ceylon. Colombo: Colombo Apothecaries, 1968; 188p.
Survey of the development of population policy, a follow-up survey of acceptors in Greater Colombo, and an action program to test the relative efficacy of male- and female-oriented propaganda; relevant background in item 1493.

923
Berelson, B.
"KAP Studies on Fertility." In Berelson et al., eds. (*see* 53): pp. 655-668.
Summarizes results of surveys on knowledge, attitudes, and practice of family planning with special reference to program implications.

924
Berelson, B. and Freedman, R.
"A Study in Fertility Control." *Scientific American* 210, May 1964: pp. 29-37.
Nontechnical report on the background, purpose, methods, and results of the experimental pilot project in accelerated dissemination of family planning information conducted in Taichung, Taiwan, in 1963.

925
Chandrasekaran, C.
"Recent Trends in Family Planning Research in India." In Berelson et al., eds. (*see* 53): pp. 545-559.

Summarizes Indian studies measuring attitude and knowledge and assesses changes associated with action programs.

926
Chow, L.P.
"A Programme to Control Fertility in Taiwan: Setting, Accomplishment and Evaluation." *Population Studies* 19(2), Nov. 1965: pp. 155-166.
Statistical report of the first year of Taiwan's family planning program.

927
Chow, L.P.
"Evaluation Procedures for a Family Planning Program." In Berelson et al., eds. (*see* 53): pp. 675-689.
Description of variety of procedures used in the Taiwan program.

928
Chow, L.P.
"Evaluation of the Family Planning Program in Taiwan, Republic of China." *Journal of the Formosan Medical Association* (Taipei) 67(7), July 1968: pp. 280-308.

929
Freedman, R. et al.
"Hong Kong: The Continuing Fertility Decline, 1967." *Studies in Family Planning* 1(44), Aug. 1969: pp. 8-15.
Analyzes effects of age structure and nuptiality trends on the birth rate and speculatively relates changes to program activity.

930
Hawley, A.H. et al.
"Thailand: Family Growth in Pho-tharam District." *Studies in Family Planning* 1(8), Oct. 1965: pp. 1-7.

931
Kantner, J.F.
"Pakistan: The Medical Social Research Project at Lulliani." *Studies in Family Planning* 1(4), Aug. 1964: pp. 5-10.

Summary of various efforts to introduce the IUD and the pill in the area of Lulliani, with some detail about the comparative results of different approaches.

932
Koya, Y.
Pioneering in Family Planning: A Collection of Papers on the Family Planning Programs and Research Conducted in Japan. Tokyo: Japan Medical Publishers with the assistance of The Population Council, 1963; 173p.

933
***Koya, Y. et al.**
"Seven Years of a Family Planning Program in Three Typical Japanese Villages." *Milbank Memorial Quarterly* 34(4), Oct. 1958: pp. 363-372.

An apparently successful attempt to decrease fertility and substitute contraception for abortion in Japan.

934
***Koya, Y. et al.**
"Five-Year Experiment on Family Planning among Coal Miners in Japan." *Population Studies* 13(2), Nov. 1959: pp. 157-163.

Evaluates success of a program to reduce fertility and substitute contraception for abortion.

935
Mauldin, W.P.
"Measurement and Evaluation of National Family Planning Programs." *Demography* 4(1), 1967: pp. 71-80.

936
Requena, B. and Monreal, T.
"Evaluation of Induced Abortion Control and Family Planning Programs in Chile." *Milbank Memorial Fund Quarterly* 46(3, Part 2), July 1968: pp. 191-218.

937
Saunders, L.
"Research and Evaluation: Needs for the Future." In Berelson et al., eds. (*see* 53): pp. 779-788.

Review of wide range of evaluation methods and purposes.

VI.C Governmental policies or programs that go beyond birth-control services

See also: 648, 649, 656, 665, 1048, 1086, 1284.

938
Berelson, B.
"Beyond Family Planning." *Science* 163(3867), Feb. 1969: pp. 533-543. [Also in *Studies in Family Planning* 1(38), Feb. 1969: pp. 1-16.]

Important analysis of recent proposals for governmental actions that extend beyond the traditional family planning approach to lowering the birth rate; with extensive references.

VI.D Religious organizations

VI.D.1 Statements of doctrine and belief

See also: 657, 827, 977, 1470.

939
Barrett, D.N., ed.
The Problem of Population: Moral and Theological Considerations. Notre Dame, Ind.: University of Notre Dame Press, 1964; 161p.

940
Burch, T.K.
"A Demographic Prospective." In *The Challenge of Mater and Magistra.* Edited by J.N. Moody and J.G. Lawler. New York: Herder and Herder, 1963: pp. 222-237.

> *Description and comment on the papal encyclical and related aspects of fertility control and population growth.*

941
Birmington, W., ed.
What Modern Catholics Think about Birth Control: A New Symposium. Signet Books T2577. New York: New American Library, 1964; 256p.

942
Callahan, D.
The Catholic Case for Contraception. New York: Macmillan, 1969; 240p.

> *Collection of articles and documents by prominent Catholic theologians and laymen who have argued for a change in Catholic teaching.*

943
Fagley, R.M.
"Doctrine and Attitudes of Major Religions in Regard to Fertility." In *Proceedings of the World Population Conference, 1965 (see* 44): pp. 78-84.

944
Feldman, D.M.
Birth Control in Jewish Law: Marital Relations, Contraception, and Abortion as Set Forth in the Classic Texts of Jewish Law. New York: New York University Press, 1968; 322p.

945
Grisez, G.G.
Contraception and the Natural Law. Milwaukee: Bruce, 1964; 245p.

946
Kelly, G.A.
Birth Control and Catholics. Garden City, N.Y.: Doubleday, 1963; 264p.

947
Kirk, D.
"Factors Affecting Moslem Natality." In Berelson et al., eds. (*see* 53): pp. 561-579. [Summary in *Proceedings of the World Population Conference, 1965 (see* 44): pp. 149-154.]

> *Survey of Moslem doctrine and cultural values causing high fertility, together with a review of data where available on Moslem fertility and family planning.*

948
Ling, T.O.
"Buddhist Factors in Population Growth and Control: A Survey Based on Thailand and Ceylon." *Population Studies* 23(1), Mar. 1969: pp. 53-60.

> *Examines religious teachings and survey results to assess the impact of Buddhist doctrine on fertility.*

949
Noonan, J.T., Jr.
Contraception: A History of Its Treatment by the Catholic Theologians and

Canonists. Cambridge, Mass.: Belknap Press of Harvard University Press, 1965; 561p.

Traces the history of and compares various views of the Catholic position on contraceptive use.

950
Noonan, J.T., Jr.
The Church and Contraception: The Issues at Stake. New York: Paulist Press, Deus Books, 1967; 84p.

951
Pyle, L., ed.
The Pill and Birth Regulations: The Catholic Debate, Including Statements, Articles, and letters from the Pope, Bishops, Priests, and Married and Unmarried Laity. Baltimore: Helicon Press, 1964; 225p.

952
Reiterman, C.
"Birth Control and Catholics." *Journal for the Scientific Study of Religion* 4(2), Spring 1965: pp. 213-233.

An analysis of 2,863 issues of the Jesuit weekly, America, to investigate the extent to which the birth control controversy represented a historical internal conflict within the Catholic church.

953
Roberts, T.D., ed.
Contraception and Holiness: The Catholic Predicament. New York: Herder and Herder, 1964; 346p.

954
Rock, J.
The Time Has Come: A Catholic Doctor's Proposal to End the Battle over Birth Control. New York: Alfred A. Knopf, 1963; 204p.

An unorthodox statement by a distinguished Catholic doctor active in the development of the contraceptive pill.

955
Schieffelin, O., ed.
Muslim Attitudes toward Family Planning. New York: Population Council, 1967; 134p.

A collection of documents and statements by Muslim political and religious leaders, together with commentary on factors affecting Muslim fertility.

956
Valsecchi, A.M.
Controversy: The Birth Control Debate 1958-1968. London: Geoffrey Chapman, 1968; 235p.

Documents the conflicting views in Catholic church up to the release of the papal encyclical Humanae Vitae.

957
Wilson, G.B.
"Christian Conjugal Morality and Contraception." In *Population Ethics.* Edited by E.X. Quinn. Washington: Corpus Books, 1968: pp. 98-108.

Presents the Christian ethical basis of marriage and relates this to the question of contraception.

VI.D.2 Empirical studies of religious differentials

958
Ahmed, M.
"Rates and Levels of Mortality and Fertility in Pakistan." *Population Review* (Madras) 10(1), Jan. 1966: pp. 44-60.

Muslim and non-Muslim fertility and mortality differentials analyzed by stable population analysis for 1951.

959
Attal, R.
"The Statistics of North African Jewry." *Jewish Journal of Sociology* 5(1), June 1963: pp. 27-34.

960
Bachi, R.
"The Demographic Development of Italian Jewry from the Seventeenth Century." *Jewish Journal of Sociology* 4(2), Dec. 1962: pp. 172-190.

Demographic history of Italian Jewry, their social characteristics and location in Rome or elsewhere, 1600-1953.

961
Balasubramanian, N.S.
"Sociological Aspects of High Birth Rate in India." *AICC Economic Review* (New Delhi) 17(19), Apr. 1966: pp. 15-18.

Discusses large family norms of religious groups in India and suggests ways for change.

962
Blake, J.
"The Americanization of Catholic Reproductive Ideals." *Population Studies* 20(1), July 1966: pp. 27-43.

Analyzes how the Catholic and non-Catholic differentials in family size values are related to the values of the Catholic church.

963
Burch, T.R.
"The Fertility of North American Cath-

olics: A Comparative Overview." *Demography* 3(1), 1966: pp. 174-187.

Examines fertility and nuptiality patterns of Canadian and U.S. Catholics, including ethnic differentials.

964
Chou, R.C. and Brown, S.
"A Comparison of the Size of Families of Roman Catholics and Non-Catholics in Great Britain." *Population Studies* 22(1), Mar. 1968: pp. 51-60.

Compares desired and actual fertility of Catholics and non-Catholics taking into account husband's occupation, age at marriage, and wife's age.

965
Day, L.H.
"Fertility Differentials Among Catholics in Australia." *Milbank Memorial Fund Quarterly* 42(2, Part 1), Apr. 1964: pp. 57-83.

Describes fertility differentials for Catholics by age, marriage cohorts, rural-urban residence, and country of birth, from 1954 survey.

966
Day, L.H.
"Family Size and Fertility." In *Australian Society: A Sociological Introduction.* Edited by A.F. Davies and S. Encel. New York: Atherton, 1965: pp. 156-167.

Based on an analysis of a special 20 percent sample of the women over age 40, currently married and living with husband for at least 15 years; establishes by multivariate analyses that fertility is higher for Catholics than others, for rural rather than urban, and for certain ethnic groups; also indicates trends for fertility decline and changing family size distributions over time.

967
Day, L.H.
"Natality and Ethnocentrism: Some Re-

lationships Suggested by an Analysis of Catholic-Protestant Differentials." *Population Studies* 22(10), Mar. 1968: pp. 27-50.

Comparative study of fertility rates and associated socioeconomic indexes for selected countries of "controlled" natality, classified by proportion Catholic.

968
Goering, J.M.
"The Structure and Processes of Ethnicity: Catholic Family Size in Providence, Rhode Island." *Sociological Analysis* 26(3), Fall 1965: pp. 129-136.

Fertility differentials between Irish and Italian Catholics related to age at marriage and occupational status.

969
*Freedman, R. et al.
"Socio-Economic Factors in Religious Differentials in Fertility." *American Sociological Review* 26(4), Aug. 1961: pp. 608-614.

Matches Catholics, Jews, and Protestants from a national U.S. sample to demonstrate that socioeconomic factors controlled do not account for the distinctive Catholic fertility values.

970
Goldscheider, C.
"Ideological Factors in Jewish Fertility Differentials." *Jewish Journal of Sociology* 7(1), June 1965: pp. 92-105.

An analysis of the effect of ideological differentials on Jewish fertility, controlling for social class differences.

971
Goldscheider, C.
"Nativity, Generation and Jewish Fertility." *Sociological Analysis* 26(3), Fall 1965: pp. 137-147.

Study of fertility differentials of Jewish couples by immigrant generation.

972
Goldscheider, C.
"Socio-Economic Status and Jewish Fertility." *Jewish Journal of Sociology* 7(2), Dec. 1965: pp. 221-237.

Uses sample survey of Jewish population in Providence, Rhode Island, to explore intergenerational changes in fertility behavior, considering social status variability.

973
Goldschieder, C.
"Trends in Jewish Fertility." *Sociology and Social Research* 50(2), Jan. 1966: pp. 173-186.

Based on Providence, Rhode Island, social survey and deals with generational changes.

974
Goldscheider, C.
"Fertility of the Jews." *Demography* 4(1), 1967; pp. 196-209.

Reviews previous studies' findings and examines Providence, Rhode Island, survey results; presents hypothesis relating fertility patterns to minority status and process of acculturation.

975
Harter, C.L. and Roussel, J.
"The Fertility of White Females in New Orleans: A Comparison of Protestants and Parochial—and Secular—Educated Catholics." *Milbank Memorial Fund Quarterly* 47(1, Part 1), Jan. 1969: pp. 39-53.

976
Higgens, E.
"Differential Fertility, Outlook and Patterns among Major Religious Groups in Johannesburg." *Social Compass* (Rotterdam) 11(1), 1964: pp. 23-62.

Detailed analysis from 1957-58 survey of interrelation of social and demographic variables, attitudes, and birth control practices of Afrikaans Protestant, English Protestant, Jewish, and Catholic groups.

Fertility differences among members of Roman Catholic and Pentecostal Holiness churches in a Negro ghetto related to differences in church membership status of husbands.

977

Jones, G.W. and Nortman, D.
"Roman Catholic Fertility and Family Planning: A Comparative Review of Research Literature." *Studies in Family Planning* 1(34), Oct. 1968: pp. 1-27.

Extensive collection of results of empirical studies concerning the levels of Catholic fertility, attitudes, knowledge, and practice of birth control; long reference section.

978

Matras, J.
"Religious Observance and Family Formation in Israel; Some Intergenerational Changes." *American Journal of Sociology* 69(5), Mar. 1964: pp. 464-475.

Relates intergenerational change in religious observance to changes in family formation patterns on basis of survey of maternity cases.

979

Matras, J. and Auerbach, C.
"On Rationalization of Family Formation in Israel." *Milbank Memorial Fund Quarterly* 40(4), Oct. 1962: pp. 453-480.

Role of religious commitment, ethnic background, social status, and accessibility in affecting use of contraception and responsiveness to interviews about it in a sample of Israeli Jews.

980

Mayhew, B.H., Jr.
"Behavioral Observability and Compliance with Religious Proscriptions on Birth Control." *Social Forces* 47(1), Sept. 1968: pp. 60-70.

981

Nuesse, C.J.
"Recent Catholic Fertility in Rural Wisconsin." *Rural Sociology* 28(4), Dec. 1963: pp. 379-393.

Child-woman ratios indicate the maintenance and probable recent increase in religious differentials, with higher fertility for Catholics.

982

Potvin, R.H. and Burch, T.K.
"Fertility, Ideal Family-Size and Religious Orientation among U.S. Catholics." *Sociological Analysis* 29(1), Spring 1968: pp. 28-34.

Relates fertility values and behavior to indexes of religiosity, derived by factor analysis of sample survey.

983

Potvin, R.H. and Westoff, C.F.
"Higher Education and the Family Normative beliefs of Catholic Women." *Sociological Analysis* 28(1), Spring 1967: pp. 14-21.

Large sample used to analyze the effect of attendance at sectarian and nonsectarian colleges on familial attitudes.

984

Potvin, R.H. et al.
"Factors Affecting Catholic Wives' Conformity to Their Church Magisterium's Position on Birth Control." *Journal of Marriage and the Family* 30(2), May 1968: pp. 263-272.

Examines socioeconomic, religiosity, and nuptiality differentials in the contraceptive practice of Catholic women.

985
Schmelz, U.O. and Glikson, P., eds.
Jewish Population Studies 1961-1968. Institute of Contemporary Jewry, Hebrew University of Jerusalem, London: Institute of Jewish Affairs, 1970; 174p.

Survey research in Jewish populations; current research reports on studies in various developed nations; a selected bibliography, 1961-68.

987
Stycos, J.M.
"Contraception and Catholicism in Latin America." *Journal of Social Issues* 23(4), Oct. 1967: pp. 115-133.

Survey results from eight Latin American cities used to related religiosity of Catholic women to ideal family size and birth-control attitudes.

987
*Van Heek, F.
"Roman Catholicism and Fertility in the Netherlands: Demographic Aspects of Minority Status." *Population Studies* 10(2), Nov. 1956: pp. 125-138.

Important attempt to explain why Catholic fertility rates are uniquely high in the Netherlands.

988
Westoff, C.F. and Potvin, R.H.
"Higher Education, Religion and Women's Family-Size Orientations." *American Sociological Review* 31(4), Aug. 1966: pp. 489-496.

Summary of the first part of a larger study on the influence of college education, particularly in Catholic schools, on the family size goals of the students.

989
Zimmer, B.G. and Goldscheider, C.
"A Further Look at Catholic Fertility." *Demography* 3(2), 1966: pp. 462-469.

Finds that traditional Catholic-Protestant fertility differentials in the U.S. are much less in the surburban than in the metropolitan central cities.

VI.E Other institutions: the private market, the medical profession, international agencies, etc.
See also: 50, 223, 379, 660, 883, 884.

990
The following articles about the role of private and governmental agencies in international work on family planning in relation to population appeared in *Demography* 5(2), 1968:

Chandrasekaran, C. "The ECAFE Program to Assist Fertility Control": pp. 651-668.

Deverell, C. "The IPPF—Its Role in Developing Countries": pp. 574-577.

Harkavy, O. et al. "An Overview of the Ford Foundation's Strategy for Population Work": pp. 541-552.

Notestein, F.W. "The Population Council and the Demographic Crisis of the Less Developed World": pp. 553-560.

Ravenholt, R.T. "The A.I.D. Population and Family Planning Program—Goals, Scope, and Progress": pp. 561-573.

991
American Medical Association. Committee on Human Reproduction.
"The Control of Fertility." *Journal of the*

American Medical Association 194(4), Oct. 1965: pp. 230-470.

Manual for American physicians describing their role in family planning and technical information on medical practice.

992
Blacker, C.P.
"The International Planned Parenthood Federation: Aspects of Its History." *Eugenics Review* 56(3), Oct. 1964: pp. 135-142.

993
Cartwright, A.
"England and Wales: General Practioners and Family Planning." *Studies in Family Planning* 1(32), June 1968: pp. 10-15.

Results of a survey concerning knowledge and attitudes of doctors toward presenting birth control information to patients; religious differentials examined.

994
Cornish, M.J. et al.
Doctors and Family Planning. No. 19. New York: National Committee on Maternal Health, 1963; 100p.

Results of 1957 interview survey of the attitudes of American doctors toward family planning and counseling, distribution of contraceptives, and related subjects.

995
Eliot, J.W. and Meier, G.
"Fertility Control in Hospitals with Residencies in Obstetrics and Gynecology: An Exploratory Study." *Obstetrics and Gynecology* 28, Oct. 1966: pp. 582-591.

996
Eliot, J.W. and Meier, G.
"Estimation of Family Planning Assist-ance Available to Low Income Patients through Hospital Obstetric and Gynecology Services." *American Journal of Public Health and the Nation's Health* 56(1), Nov. 1966: pp. 1858-1865.

997
Farley, J.U. and Leavitt, H.J.
"Jamaica: Private Sector Distribution of Contraceptives." *Studies in Family Planning* 1(33), Aug. 1968: pp. 11-12.

Econometric analysis on an area basis of the factors that affect the sale of condoms, including the religious and income distribution, an earlier experimental program, and the distribution of other consumer goods.

998
Farley, J.U. and Leavitt, H.J.
"Private-Sector Logistics in Population Control: A Case in Jamaica." *Demography* 5(1), 1968: pp. 449-459.

Studies distribution, importation, and sale of commercial contraceptives and suggests policies for developing private-sector distribution.

999
Fawcett, J.T. et al.
"Thailand: Monitoring the Commercial Distribution of Oral Contraceptives." *Studies in Family Planning* 1(48), Dec. 1969: pp. 10-12.

Description of a program for obtaining data on commercial distribution of contraceptives through private channels.

1000
Gille, H.
"The Role of the United Nations Family in Action Programmes in the Field of Population." In Szabady et al., eds. (*see* 40): pp. 97-103.

Brief history of U.N. population organizations and their assistance to national programs.

1001

Guttmacher, A.F.

"The United States Medical Profession and Family Planning." In Berelson et al., eds. (*see* 53): pp. 455-463.

Discusses how to overcome barriers to involvement of doctors in family planning in the U.S.

1002

Khan, A.H. and Choldin, H.M.

"A Commercial System for Introducing Family Planning in Comilla, Pakistan." In Berelson et al., eds. (*see* 53): pp. 477-485.

Sums up experimental distribution of contraceptives through local agents, especially shopkeepers.

1003

Levin, H.L.

"Distribution of Contraceptive Supplies through Commercial Channels." In Berelson et al., eds. (*see* 53): pp. 487-495.

Estimates some present patterns and recommends changes for higher distribution rates.

1004

Levin, H.

"Commercial Distribution of Contraceptives in Developing Countries: Past, Present, and Future." *Demography* 5(2), 1968: pp. 941-946.

1005

Miller, R.A. et al.

"Survey of the Sales of Contraceptives by Pharmacies of Dacca, East Pakistan." *Public Health Reports* 83(1), Jan. 1968: pp. 49-52.

Examines availability, price, and selection of different contraceptive methods; characteristics of customers.

1006

Peel, J.

"Contraception and the Medical Profession." *Population Studies* 18(2), Nov. 1964: pp. 133-145.

History of changing attitudes in Great Britain in the nineteenth and twentieth centuries.

1007

Rettie, J.

"Problems and Progress in Family Planning in Europe and the Near East." In Szabady et al., eds. (*see* 40): pp. 253-258.

Traces the increasing role of the International Planned Parenthood Federation in national activities of Europe and the Near East.

1008

Siegel, E. and Dillehay, R.C.

"Some Approaches to Family Planning Counseling in Local Health Departments: A Survey of Public Health Nurses and Physicians." *American Journal of Public Health and the Nation's Health* 56(11), Nov. 1966: pp. 1840-1846.

1009

Simon, J.L.

"A Huge Marketing Research Task— Birth Control." *Journal of Marketing Research* 5, Feb. 1968: pp. 21-27.

1010

Taylor, C.E. and Hall, M.F.

"Health, Population and Economic Development: International Health Programs Have an Important Role in Promoting Economic Development and Population Control." *Science* Aug. 1967: pp. 651-657.

General discussion of the effect of health programs on mortality and fertility and of the interrelations between health and socioeconomic development.

1011

United Nations. Children's Fund. Executive Board.

Family Planning: Report of the Executive Director on the Possible Role of UNICEF. New York: 1966; 2 vols.

1012

United Nations. Trust Fund for Population Activities.

Report on the United Nations Trust Fund for Population Activities and the Role of the United Nations in Population Action Programmes. SOA/Ser. 5/10. New York: 1969; 35p.

1013

United States Office of the War on Hunger. Population Service.

Population Program Assistance: Aid to Developing Nations by the United States, Other Nations, and International and Private Agencies. Washington: Government Printing Office, 1968; 175p.

Descriptive summaries of external aid provided to developing nations and the programs in this area.

VII. STUDIES RELATING OTHER GENERAL CHARACTERISTICS OF THE SOCIETY OR THE SUBGROUP TO FERTILITY OR FERTILITY NORMS

VII.A Urbanization and density (e.g., urban-rural differences, form, and character of urbanization, suburbanization)

See also: 1, 56, 64, 129, 130, 132, 133, 136, 138, 302, 303, 310, 349, 356, 358, 378, 429, 432, 446, 516, 521, 537, 547, 548, 550, 551, 552, 554, 563, 564, 565, 567, 569, 570, 576, 582, 583, 587, 965, 966, 989, 1041, 1049, 1069, 1070, 1088, 1102, 1106, 1107, 1143, 1145, 1228, 1229, 1247, 1493, 1494, 1497, 1499, 1504, 1506, 1510, 1512, 1519, 1521, 1523, 1527, 1531, 1533, 1534, 1537, 1538, 1539, 1616.

1014
*Burnight, R.G. et al.
"Differential Rural-Urban Fertility in Mexico." *American Sociological Review* 21(1), Feb. 1956: pp. 3-8.

In 1950 fertility ratios in Mexican municipios negatively related to city size and to urbanization.

1015
Caldwell, J.C.
"Fertility Differentials as Evidence of Incipient Fertility Decline in a Developing Country: The Case of Ghana." *Population Studies* 21(1), July 1967: pp. 5-21.

Rural-urban fertility differentials presented and interpreted by estimates of influence of other factors (mortality, nuptiality, education, religion).

1016
Duncan, O.D.
"Farm Background and Differential Fertility." *Demography* 2, 1965: pp. 240-249.

An important multivariate analysis of interacting effect on fertility of farm background and education in the U.S., indicating that educational differentials are very small for couples without a farm background.

1017
Duza, M.B. and Husain, I.
"Differential Fertility in Pakistan." In *Studies in the Demography of Pakistan.* Edited by W.C. Robinson. Karachi:

Pakistan Institute of Development Economics, Dec. 1967: pp. 93-137.

Examines urban-rural, socioeconomic, nuptiality, and religious fertility differentials.

1018
Farley, R.
"Recent Changes in Negro Fertility." *Demography* 3(1), 1966: pp. 188-203.

Discusses the effect of urbanization and family planning on Negro fertility.

1019
Goldstein, S. and Mayer, K.B.
"Illegitimacy, Residence, and Status." *Social Problems* 12(4), Spring 1965: pp. 428-436.

Analyzes the relation of various factors to illegitimacy in Rhode Island and concludes that relationships differ radically in city and suburbs.

1020
Goldstein, S. and Mayer, K.B.
"Residence and Status Differences in Fertility." *Milbank Memorial Fund Quarterly* 43(3), July 1965: pp. 291-310.

A study of the relative influence on fertility of socioeconomic status of small areas and their classification as urban or suburban.

1021
Matras, J.
"Strategies of Family Formation: Urban Rural, Size-of-City, Provincial and Major City Variations among Canadian Female Cohorts." *Canadian Review of Sociology and Anthropology* 3(3), Aug. 1966: pp. 132-144.

See item 565.

1022
Nazaret, F.
"Fertility Survey of 1963 in the Philip-

pines." *Philippine Sociological Review* (Quezon City) 12(1-2), 1964: pp. 5-16.

1963 sample survey on labor force used to relate fertility and desired family size to husband's occupation, wife's education, urban-rural residence, and religion.

1023
***Okun, B.**
Trends in Birth Rates in the United States since 1870. Baltimore: Johns Hopkins Press, 1958; 236p.

Analysis of comparative historical fertility trends in the urban and rural sectors, indicating parallel movements.

1024
Olusanya, P.O.
"Rural-Urban Fertility Differentials in Western Nigeria." *Population Studies* 23(3), Nov. 1969: pp. 363-378.

Comparison of attitudes toward family size and actual fertility, based on sample surveys in two cities and five villages; city samples preferred somewhat smaller families, but preferred size is large in all subsamples; no actual consistent urban-rural fertility differentials emerged.

1025
Paulus, C.R.
The Impact of Urbanization on Fertility in India. Mysore: University of Mysore, 1966; 106p.

1931-51 examination through the intermediate variables of migration, occupation, levels of living, and literacy.

1026
Pool, D.I.
"Post-war Trends in Maori Population Growth." *Population Studies* 21(2), Sept. 1967: pp. 87-98.

Reviews trends of differentials in fertility and other vital rates, including urban-rural differentials.

1027
*Robinson, W.C.
"Urban-Rural Differences in Indian Fertility." *Population Studies* 14(3), Mar. 1961: pp. 218-234.
An evaluation of the evidence concerning urban-rural fertility differentials.

1028
Robinson, W.C.
"Urbanization and Fertility: The Non-Western Experience." *Milbank Memorial Fund Quarterly* 41(3), July 1963: pp. 291-308.
Comparative analysis concluding that higher rural than urban fertility is not universal, that it has grown less with decreasing differentials in infant mortality, and that where it is found an important cause is differential nuptiality.

1029
Rosset, E.
"New Tendencies in the Reproduction of the Population in Poland." In Szabady et al., eds. (*see* 39): pp. 105-111.
Reports on changes in reproduction rates since 1931, with special emphasis on the effects of mortality change on rural-urban differentials.

1030
Sabagh, G. and Van Arsdol, M.D., Jr.
"Suburban Transition and Fertility Changes: An Illustrative Analysis." In *International Population Conference. New York, 1961.* London: U.N.E.S.C.O., 1963: pp. 128-137.

1031
Somoza, J.L.
"Fertility Levels and Differentials in Argentina in the Nineteenth Century." *Milbank Memorial Fund Quarterly* 46(3, Part 2), July 1968: pp. 53-71.
Variety of data estimate historical trends, urban-rural, and educational differentials.

1032
Teper, S.
Patterns of Fertility in Greater London: A Comparative Study. London: Greater London Council, Research and Intelligence Unit, Occasional Paper No. 1, 1968; 31p.
Summarizes data on total and age-specific fertility in Greater London as compared with England and Wales and with other conurbations and at the borough level; effects of age, marital status, migration, and other variables.

1033
Thanawalla, Y. et al.
"Residential Differentials in Fertility." *Michigan State University Quarterly Bulletin* 48(4), May 1966: pp. 529-537.
Analysis of fertility ratios for 1960 by economic areas of Michigan, classified by metropolitan-nonmetropolitan status and by urban, rural, and farm residence.

1034
Theissen, D.
"Population Density and Behavior: A Review of Theoretical and Physiological Contributions." *Texas Reports on Biology and Medicine* 22, Summer 1964: pp. 266-314.
Physiological and behavioral consequences of increasing population density in animal populations other than human; bears on the question of whether increasing population density associated with high fertility may have harmful consequences.

1035
Ueda, K.
"Fertility Differentials and Trends in Japan." In 1967 I.U.S.S.P. (*see* 21): pp. 256-265.

Analysis of differential fertility in Japan taking into account a grouping of prefectures by percentage in primary industry, educational attainment of husband, and whether husband is in agriculture; considerable convergence in the postwar period to 1963, but origin is from a complex of balancing factors.

Correlation of fertility to city size, urban growth, sex ratio in reproductive ages, and nuptiality for 23 urban and rural areas.

1036
Vávra, Z.
"Changes in the Birth Rates of the Urban and Rural Population." In Szabady et al., eds. (*see* 39) pp. 206-213.
Data on recent changes in birth rates of Czech and Slovak urban and rural populations.

1037
Williamson, R.C.
"Some Factors in Urbanism in a Quasi-Rural Setting: San Salvador and San Jose." *Sociology and Social Research* 47(2), Jan. 1963: pp. 187-200.
Urban-rural differences in fertility and attitudes to birth control compared with an attempt to explain why differences are greater for Costa Rica than for El Salvador.

1038
Yamamoto, M.
"Trend in the Prefectural Dispersion of Age-Specific Fertility of Married Women in Japan, 1930-1960." In *Annual Reports of the Institute of Population Problems* No. 11. Tokyo: Institute of Population Problems, 1966: pp. 43-46, 87.

1039
Zarate, A.O.
"Some Factors Associated with Urban-Rural Fertility Differentials in Mexico." *Population Studies* 21(3), Nov. 1967: pp. 283-293.

VII.B Migration and physical mobility
See also: 64, 358, 426, 432, 521, 551, 552, 633, 641, 1025, 1032, 1070, 1102, 1145, 1407, 1506, 1516, 1534, 1537.

1040
Alstrom, C.H. and Lindeluis, R.
"A Study of the Population Movement in Nine Swedish Subpopulations in 1800-1849 from the Genetic-Statistical Viewpoint." Translated by E. Odelberg. *Supplementum ad Acta Genetica et Statistica Medica* 16, 1966; 44p.
Studies spatial distance between parents' birthplace and birthplace of children.

1041
De Jong, G.F.
Appalachian Fertility Decline: A Demographic and Sociological Analysis. Lexington: University of Kentucky Press, 1968; 138p.
Examines 1930-60 trends in fertility affected by net migration, changing attitudes, and urban-rural differences; general economic and social development discussed; appendix includes measurements of fertility indexes.

1042
Henin, R.A.
"Fertility Differentials in the Sudan (with Reference to the Nomadic and Settled Population)." *Population Studies* 22(1), Mar. 1968: pp. 147-164.

Examines differentials in average number of births reported among settled and nomadic tribes. (For a more complete analysis see 1043.)

1043
Henin, R.A.
"The Patterns and Causes of Fertility Differentials in the Sudan." *Population Studies* 23(2), July 1969: pp. 171-198.

Fertility differentials of settled and nomadic populations related to age at marriage, marital stability, polygamy, fetal death, and morbidity.

1044
Macisco, J.J., Jr.
"Fertility of White Migrant Women, U.S. 1960: A Stream Analysis." *Rural Sociology* 33(4), Dec. 1968: pp. 474-479.

Analysis of migration fertility differentials for movements to different kinds of metropolitan areas.

1045
Macisco, J.J., Jr. et al.
"Migration Status, Education and Fertility in Puerto Rico, 1960." *Milbank Memorial Fund Quarterly* 47(2), Apr. 1969: pp. 167-187.

Examines relation of migration to fertility, controlling for educational differentials.

1046
Myers, G.C. and Morris, E.W.
"Migration and Fertility in Puerto Rico." *Population Studies* 20(1), July 1966: pp. 85-96.

Analysis for relation for migration status and fertility for 25-percent sample of ever-married women from 1960 census.

VII.C Economic Variables

VII.C.1 Macroeconomic (e. g., the effect of economic growth, cyclical fluctuations, structural economic change)
See also: 64, 66, 100, 129, 133, 310, 362, 365, 433, 434, 440, 495, 497, 705, 707, 708, 709, 721, 728, 869, 1050, 1145, 1147, 1410, 1549, 1559, 1561, 1569, 1584.

1047
*Banks, J.A.
Prosperity and Parenthood. London: Routledge & Kegan Paul, 1954; 240p.

A historical analysis of the interaction of changing living standards and general economic conditions in fertility decline in the nineteenth century in England.

1048
Branson, W.H.
"Social Legislation and the Birth Rate in Nineteenth Century Britain." *Western Economic Journal* 6(2), Mar. 1968: pp. 133-144.

Constructs a simple model connecting the birth rate to economic variables and applies the model to nineteenth-century Britain; argues that a key factor is social legislation affecting both the cost of raising children and the income they contribute to the family.

1049
Caldwell, J.C.
"Fertility Attitudes in Three Economically Contrasting Rural Regions of Ghana." *Economic Development and Cultural Change* 15(2), Jan. 1967: pp. 217-238.

Results of a survey on desired family size, value of children, and attitude toward contraception in three areas of Ghana in different stages of development.

1050
Easterlin, R.A.
"The American Baby Boom in Historical Perspective." *The American Economic Review* 51(5), Dec. 1961: pp. 869-911.

The postwar fertility experience of the U.S. viewed in the context of Kuznets' cycles; relates cyclical variations to employment and income changes in the urban and rural sectors.

1051
Easterlin, R.A.
"On the Relation of Economic Factors to Recent and Projected Fertility Changes." *Demography* 3(1), 1966: pp. 131-153.

Important theory relating variations in number of young men in the labor force, their experience, the demand for their services, and their own expectations to fertility changes.

1052
Easterlin, R.A.
"Economic Demographic Interactions and Long Swings in Economic Growth." *American Economic Review* 56(5), Dec. 1966: pp. 1063-1104.

Discusses possible interrelation for long-run economic swings and demographic factors, presenting both a theory and empirical tests.

1053
Easterlin, R.A.
Population, Labor Force, and Long Swings in Economic Growth: The American Experience. National Bureau of Economic Research, General Series, 86. New York: Columbia University Press, 1968; 298p.

Historical analysis of interaction between long swings in economic activity, fertility, age structure, and labor-force participation rates; important contribution both in developing theories and assembling important sets of data.

1054
***Eversley, D.E.C.**
"Population and Economic Growth in England before the 'Take-Off.'" In *Contributions and Communications to the First International Conference of Economic History* (Stockholm). Paris and The Hague: Mouton, 1960: pp. 457-473.

1055
Ferenbac, I.
"The Impact of the Technical Development and the New Socialist Relations of Production on the Birth and Death Rates in the Romanian People's Republic." In Szabady et al., eds. (*see* 39): pp. 135-140.

1056
***Galbraith, V. and Thomas, D.S.**
"Birth Rates and Inter-War Business Cycles." *Journal of American Statistical Association* 36(216), Dec. 1941: pp. 465-476.

Shows the positive relation over time between economic conditions on the one hand and period marriages and birth rates on the other.

1057
Hanley, S.B.
"Population Trends and Economic Development in Tokugawa Japan: The Case of Bizen Province in Okayama." *Daedalus* 97(2), Spring 1968: pp. 622-635.

Historical trends in district population growth related to agricultural and commercial development.

1058
Heer, D.M.
"Economic Development and the Fertility Transition." *Daedalus* 97(2), Spring 1968: pp. 447-462.

Causal factors in the historical relationship of economic development and fertility in developed countries.

1059
* Hyrenius, H.
"The Relation between Birth Rates and Economic Activity in Sweden, 1920-1944." *Bulletin of Oxford University, Institute of Statistics* 8(1), Jan. 1946: pp. 14-21.

1060
*Kirk, D.
"The Influence of Business Cycles on Marriage and Birth Rates." In *Demographic and Economic Change in Developed Countries.* Princeton: Princeton University Press, 1960: pp. 241-260.

1061
Krishnamurty, K.
"Economic Development in Low Income Countries: An Empirical Study for India." *Economic Development and Cultural Change* 15(1), Oct. 1966: pp. 70-75.

Regression analysis of the effect of changes of per-capita income on birth rate and the effect of per-capita income changes and government welfare expenditures on death rate.

1062
Kvasna, A.IA.
"Some Problems of the Demography of the Developing Countries of Asia and Africa." *Soviet Sociology* 4(4), Spring 1966: pp. 3-11.

Critical review of the "Neo-Malthusian" position, contrasting favorably with the Marxist emphasis on increasing production as compared with other approaches.

1063
Livi Bacci, M.
"Modernization and Tradition in the Recent History of Italian Fertility." *Demography* 4(2), 1967: pp. 657-672.

Examines regional fertility differentials (1931-66) in relation to net per-capita income, national fertility trends as related to business cycle fluctuations, and cohort fertility differentials as related to educational level in Florence.

1064
Lowry, I.S.
Population Policy, Welfare, and Regional Development. Paper prepared for the Conference on Regional Development Planning, University of Puerto Rico, 29-31 Mar. 1967. Santa Monica, Calif.: RAND Corporation, 1968; 41p.

Optimum model for population and labor force and various alternative policies to manipulate demographic variables, including birth rate, to achieve optimal size.

1065
Rao, S.V. et al.
"Birth Rates and Economic Development: Some Observations from Japanese Data." *Sankhyā* (Calcutta) (Series B) June 1968: pp. 149-156.

Three models based on Japanese data for examining the relation of economic growth to birth rate changes: a cross-sectional model involving income, proportion rural, and infant mortality; a time-series model involving income and marriage rates; and a third model including an index based on induced abortion data.

1066
Saunders, J.V.D. and Reinhart, G.R.
"Demographic and Economic Correlates of Development as Measured by Energy Consumption." *Demography* 4(2), 1967: pp. 773-779.

Per-capita energy consumption for 112 countries related to four economic variables and four demographic variables.

1067
Silver, M.
"Births, Marriages, and Income Fluctuations in the United Kingdom and Japan." *Economic Development and Cultural Change* 14(3), Apr. 1966: pp. 302-315.

Evidence of relation of birth and marriage trends to ordinary and Kuznets' business cycles.

1068
Stockwell, E.G.
"Some Demographic Correlates of Economic Development." *Rural Sociology* 31(2), June 1966: pp. 216-224.

Correlations of indexes of economic development and several demographic variables on a national level.

1069
Weintraub, R.
"The Birth Rate and Economic Development." *Econometrica* 30(4), Oct. 1962: pp. 812-817.

Brief cross-sectional regression analysis of the relation of income, proportion of population in farming, and infant mortality to fertility.

1070
Yasuba, Y.
Birth Rates of the White Population in the United States, 1800-1860: An Economic Study. The Johns Hopkins University Studies in Historical and Political Science, Series 79, 2. Baltimore: Johns Hopkins Press, 1962; 198p.

Regional and state trends in birth and death rates, including consideration of related demographic and socioeconomic factors; methodology for estimating rates from incomplete historical data.

1071
Zaidan, G.C.
"Population Growth and Economic Development." *Studies in Family Planning* 1(42), May 1969: pp. 1-6.

Schematic model of the effect of population growth on per-capita income growth.

VII.C.2 Microeconomic (e.g., the effect on individuals of income, wealth, labor-force participation, economic policies without a specific pro- or antinatalist primary purpose)
See also: 83, 313, 377, 504, 607, 678, 787, 997, 1512, 1532, 1565.

1072
Blake, J.
"Are Babies Consumer Durables?" *Population Studies* 22(1), Mar. 1968: pp. 5-25.

Argues against the view attributed to Becker (see 494) that children are valued by the same processes as consumer goods.

1073
Carleton, R.O.
"Labor Force Participation: A Stimulus to Fertility in Puerto Rico?" *Demography* 2, 1965: pp. 233-239.

1074
Deutsch, A.
Income Redistribution through Canadian Federal Family Allowances and Old Age Benefits. Queen's University Papers in Taxation and Public Finance, 4. Toronto: Canadian Tax Foundation, 1968; 133p.

1075

Freedman, R. and Coombs, L.
"Economic Considerations in Family Growth Decisions." *Population Studies* 20(2), Nov. 1966: pp. 197-222.

Studies the effect of current income, family income streams, and family expenditure allocations on childspacing.

1076

Heer, D.M. and Bryden, J.G.
"Family Allowances and Population Policy in the U.S.S.R." *Journal of Marriage and the Family* 28(4), Nov. 1966: pp. 514-519.

Assembles data on the operation of the family allowance program and monetary awards to mothers of large families at various times 1944-64, with international comparisons.

1077

Higgins, E.
"The Bearing of Family Allowances on Family Size in an Urban White Population." *Tydskrif vir Maatskaplike Navorsing* (Pretoria) 12(2), May 1962: pp. 165-176.

Study of reproductive facts, norms, and attitudes among socioeconomic groups in Johannesburg.

1078

Kamerschen, D.R.
"Socio-economic Determinants of Fertility Patterns." *Population Review* (Madras) 11(1), Jan. 1967: pp. 24-29.

Proposed modifications of models by Becker (see 494) and Adelman (see 128).

1079

Madison, B.
"Canadian Family Allowances and Their Major Social Implications." *Journal of Marriage and the Family* 26(2), May 1964: pp. 134-141.

Description of allowance system; effect on family income, birth rate, infant mortality, and family size.

1080

Rimashevskalia, N.
"Studying the Income and Structure of Families with Children." *Soviet Sociology* 1(2), Fall 1962: pp. 53-56.

Information on the number of children by income and the average age of children in a Soviet survey sample.

1081

Schorr, A.L.
"Income Maintenance and the Birth Rate." *Social Security Bulletin* 28(12), Dec. 1965: pp. 22-30.

Considers possible effects of an income-maintenance program on the U.S. birth rate by reviewing experience in other countries and factors that might affect U.S. experience.

1082

Schorr, A.L.
Poor Kids: A Report on Children in Poverty. New York: Basic Books, 1966; 205p.

Possible effects on fertility of income maintenance programs and how need for programs is related to family size.

1083

Simon, J.L.
"The Effect of Income on Fertility." *Population Studies* 23(3), Nov. 1969: pp. 327-341.

Develops a model to account for the different relationship of income to fertility in cross-sectional and time-series studies.

1084

Stewart, C.M.
"Family Allowances Statistics in Great Britain." *Population Studies* 16(3), Mar. 1963: pp. 210-218.

Illustrates possible use of data from 1946 family allowance law to study fertility effects on birth cohorts.

1085
Vadakin, J.C.
Children, Poverty, and Family Allowances. New York: Basic Books, 1968; 222p.
Survey of family allowance plans throughout the world and review of proposed plans for the U.S.

1086
Whitney, V.H.
"Fertility Trends and Children's Allowance Programs." In *Children.'s Allowances and Economic Welfare of Children.* Edited by E.M. Burns. *The Report of a Conference.* Children's Allowances Conference Warrenton, Va., 22-24 Oct. 1967. New York: Citizen's Committee for Children of New York, 1968: pp. 123-139.
Why a system of low or moderate allowance payments is ineffectual in affecting fertility.

VII.D Ethnic, regional, and racial classifications
See also: 64, 132, 214, 263, 303, 446, 518, 526, 548, 549, 556, 557, 559, 566, 583, 965, 966, 968, 972, 980, 1018, 1036, 1041, 1049, 1145, 1199, 1200, 1202, 1220, 1228, 1236, 1356, 1453, 1493, 1499, 1516, 1537.

1087
Beaujeu-Garnier, J.
Geography of Population. Translated by S.H. Beaver. Geographies for Advanced Study Series. London: Longmans, Green, 1966; 386p.
General work on population geography with section on areal differences in birth rates.

1088
Breznik, D.
"Fertility of the Yugoslav Population." In Szabady et al., eds. (*see* 40): pp. 53-67.
On the differential timing of fertility declines among regions for the period 1921-66; reports on 1961-62 regional differentials and relation of fertility to illiteracy, income, education, urbanization, and ethnic composition.

1089
Campbell, A.A.
"Fertility and Family Planning among Non-White Married Couples in the United States." *Eugenics Quarterly* 12(3), Sept. 1965: pp. 124-131.
A summary of data in the 1960 Growth of American Families study on white-nonwhite differences in facts and norms about fertility, fecundity, and contraception. (See also more complete treatment in item 1537.)

1090
Campbell, A.A.
"White-nonwhite Differences in Family Planning in the United States." *Health, Education, and Welfare Indicators* Feb. 1966: pp. 13-21.
Family size, fecundity, and contraceptive use and success differentials.

1091
Chai, C.K.
Taiwan Aborigines. Cambridge, Mass.: Harvard University Press; London: Oxford University Press, 1967; 238p.
Anthropologic study of genetics of Taiwanese aborigines; discussion of demographic and family structure variables.

1092
Farley, R.
"The Demographic Rates and Social Institutions of the Nineteenth-Century Negro Population: A Stable Population Analysis." *Demography* 2, 1965: pp. 386-398.
Analysis of demographic rates for Negroes using quas´-stable population techniques on U.S. census data 1830-1910.

1093
Goldscheider, C. and Uhlenberg, P.R.
"Minority Group Status and Fertility." *American Journal of Sociology* 74(4), Jan. 1969: pp. 361-372.
Examines religious and ethnic group fertility differentials and presents hypothesis relating fertility behavior to group status and isolation.

1094
Heer, D.
"Fertility Differences between Indian and Spanish-Speaking Parts of Andean Countries." *Population Studies* 18(1), July 1964: pp. 71-84.
Alternative explanation to fertility differentials presented by Stycos (see 1107).

1095
Huyck, E.E.
"White Non-White Differentials: Overview and Implications." *Demography* 3(2), 1966: pp. 548-565.

1096
Hyrenius, H.
The Reindeer-Farming Population in Sweden. Reports, 7a. Goteborg, Sweden: Demographic Institute, University of Goteborg, 1969; 31p.
Nuptiality, migratory, and reproductive patterns of a small Lapp community in northern Scandinavia.

1097
Kiser, C.V. and Frank, M.E.
"Factors Associated with the Low Fertility of Nonwhite Women of College Attainment." *Milbank Memorial Fund Quarterly* 45(4), Oct. 1967: pp. 427-449.
Considers age at marriage, marital stability, and female employment status as basis for racial fertility differentials at different socioeconomic levels.

1098
Kitagawa, E.M. and Hauser, P.M.
"Trends in Differential Fertility and Mortality in a Metropolis." In *Contributions to Urban Sociology.* Edited by E.W. Burgess and D.J. Bogue. Chicago: University of Chicago Press, 1964: pp. 59-85.
Changing Negro-white fertility differentials between 1920 and 1960, taking into account the effect of socioeconomic status on a local-area basis in Chicago.

1099
Leasure, J.W. and Shrock, N.W.
"White and Non-White Fertility by Census Tract for 1960." *Eugenics Quarterly* 11(3), Sept. 1964: pp. 148-153.
Interaction of socioeconomic and racial fertility differentials based on census tract measures in selected metropolitan areas.

1100
Lunde, A.S.
"White-Nonwhite Fertility Differentials in the U.S." *Health, Education, and Welfare Indicators* Sept. 1965: pp. 23-38.
Socioeconomic and demographic factors affecting trends in differential fertility.

1101
Mazur, D.P.
"Fertility among Ethnic Groups in the USSR." *Demography* 4(1), 1967: pp. 172-195.

1102
Mitchell, J.C.
"Differential Fertility amongst Urban Africans in Northern Rhodesia." *Central African Journal of Medicine* (Salisbury) 10(6), June 1964: pp. 195-211.

Fertility differentials in relation to tribal categories, urbanization, mobility, religion, and other variables.

1103
Mitchell, J.C.
"Differential Fertility among Africans in Zambia." *Rhodes-Livingstone Journal* 37, June 1965; 25p.

Report on a 1951-54 survey among urban Africans indicating that fertility varied significantly with religion (Christian and other), and by tribal grouping (Bemba and other), but not by urbanization or status; use of the child-woman ratio as fertility measure may not adequately allow for mortality differential.

1104
Muhsam, H.V.
Beduin of the Negev: Eight Demographic Studies. Eliezer Kaplan School of Economics and Social Sciences, Hebrew University of Jerusalem. Jerusalem: Jerusalem Academic Press, 1966; 123p.

Studies, using 1946 data, of the tribal and family structure, marriage habits, and fertility patterns of the Beduin.

1105
Pavlik, Z.
"Demographic Differences in the Development of the Population of Czeck Regions and Slovakia." In Szabady et al., eds. (*see* 39): pp. 196-200.

Analyzes persistent Czeck-Slovak differences in fertility, even when socioeconomic factors are taken into account.

1106
Saw, S.H.
"Fertility Differentials in Early Postwar Malaya." *Demography* 4(2), 1967: pp. 641-656.

Presents interstate, racial, and urban-rural gross reproduction rate differentials based on census data from 1947 and 1957.

1107
Stycos, J.M.
"Culture and Differential Fertility in Peru." *Population Studies* 16(3), Mar. 1963: pp. 257-270.

Analyzes unexploited regional data from the 1940 census to study the impact of urbanization, literacy, and Indian or Spanish culture on fertility.

1108
Taagepera, R.
"National Differences within Soviet Demographic Trends." *Soviet Studies* 20(4), Apr. 1969: pp. 478-489.

Inference from available data about ethnic differentials in fertility in the Soviet Union; data on incidence of "Heroine Mother" awards.

1109
Taeuber, I.B.
"Demographic Modernization: Continuities and Transitions." *Demography* 3(1), 1966: pp. 90-108.

Study of U.S. ethnic groups to test structural relationships of demographic transition in modern urban setting.

1110
Zelnik, M.
"Fertility of the American Negro in 1830 and 1850." *Population Studies* 20(1), July 1966: pp. 77-83.

1111
Zelnik, M.
"The Level of Nonwhite Fertility in the United States, 1930 and 1920." *Eugenics Quarterly* 14(4), Dec. 1967: pp. 265-270.

> *Presents estimates for the nonwhite population paralleling in part those for the white population, 1855-1960, as cited in item 430.*

VII.E The nature and audience of the mass media

See also: 82, 133, 1533.

1112
Cornell University. International Population. Program.
Latin American Newspaper Coverage of Population and Family Planning. No. 1. Ithaca, N.Y.: Cornell University, 1967; 27p.

> *Initial report of experiment coding articles concerning population in Latin American newspapers.*

VII.F Health, mortality, genetics, nutrition, and other physiological factors

See also: 133, 138, 453, 595, 637, 1010, 1043, 1069, 1091, 1165, 1173, 1178, 1340, 1512, 1631.

1113
Arriaga, E.
"The Effect of a Decline in Mortality on

the Gross Reproduction Rate." *Milbank Memorial Fund Quarterly* 45(3), July 1967: pp. 333-352.

1114
Bacola, E.
"Reproductive Rates in Families of Children with Idiopathic Mental Retardation." *Pediatrics* 37(4), 1966: pp. 675-677.

1115
Baird, D.
"Variations in Fertility Associated with Changes in Health Status." In Sheps and Ridley, eds. (*see* 73): pp. 353-376.

> *Review of health and biosocial factors related to fertility, with special reference to studies in Aberdeen, Scotland.*

1116
Banik, N.D. et al.
"A Study of Birth Weight of Indian Infants and Its Relationship to Sex, Period of Gestation, Maternal Age, Parity, and Socio-Economic Classes." *Indian Journal of Medical Research* (Calcutta) 55, Dec. 1967: pp. 1378-1386.

1117
Bradshaw, B.S.
"Fertility Differences in Peru: A Reconsideration." *Population Studies* 23(1), Mar. 1969: pp. 5-19.

> *Suggests that fertility differentials estimated by Stycos, Heer, and James fail to account for the impact of child mortality; indicates Indian fertility comparable to that in the better developed Spanish-speaking areas.*

1118
Czeizel, A. and Bene, E.
"Studies on the Fertility of Radiolo-

gists." *Journal of Biosocial Science* 1(2), Apr. 1969: pp. 145-151.

Possible genetic effects of exposure to radiation on fertility.

1119
Davis, K.
"Sociological Aspects of Genetic Control." In *Genetics and the Future of Man.* Proceedings of the Nobel Conference, 1965. Amsterdam: North-Holland, 1966: pp. 174-204.

Sociological factors that impede eugenics and possible effects genetic control might have on society.

1120
Griffith, H.B.
"Gonorrhea and Fertility in Uganda." *Eugenics Review* 55(2), July 1963: pp. 103-108.

On basis of rates of male acute gonorrhea and urethral stricture compared with female fertility rate, concludes that gonorrhea was one of the major determinants of fertility in Uganda.

1121
Heer, D.M.
"Fertility Differences in Andean Countries: A Reply to W.H. James." *Population Studies* 21(1), July 1967: pp. 71-73.

A reply to item 1124.

1122
Heuser, R.L.
"Multiple Births, United States—1964." *Vital and Health Statistics* (Series 21) 14, Oct. 1967: 50p.

Statistics on multiple live births related to age of mother, race, and parity.

1123
Horwitz, A. and Burke, M.H.
"Health, Population and Development."

In *Population Dilemma in Latin America.* Edited by J.M. Stycos and J. Arias. Washington: American Assembly, 1966: pp. 145-195.

Reviews demographic trends and the development of health facilities in Latin America.

1124
James, W.H.
"The Effect of Altitude on Fertility in Andean Countries." *Population Studies* 20(1), July 1966: pp. 97-101.

A comment on articles by Heer (see 1094) and Stycos (see 1107).

1125
Johnston, F.E. et al.
"The Population Structure of the Peruvian Cashinahua: Demographic, Genetic and Cultural Interrelationships." *Human Biology* 41(1), 1969: pp. 29-41.

Examines the genetic implication of a high fertility isolated village with changing marriage patterns.

1126
Kirk, D.
"Demographic Factors Affecting the Opportunity for Natural Selection in the United States." *Eugenics Quarterly* 13(3), Sept. 1966: pp. 270-273.

Traces changes in fertility, mortality, and nuptiality patterns that have a potential effect on genetic selectivity.

1127
Lewontin, R.C., ed.
Population Biology and Evolution: Proceedings of the International Symposium Sponsored by Syracuse University and the New York State Science and Technology Foundation, 7-9 June 1967. Syracuse, N.Y.: Syracuse University Press, 1968; 205p.

1128
MacSorley, K.
"An Investigation into the Fertility Rates of Mentally Ill Patients." *Annals of Human Genetics* 27(3), Mar. 1964: pp. 247-254.

Compares the fertility of mentally ill patients with that of their siblings and of hospital control group.

1129
Neel, J.V. and Chagnon, N.A.
"The Demography of Two Tribes of Primitive, Relatively Unacculturated Indians." *Proceedings of the National Academy of Sciences* 59(3), Mar. 1968: pp. 680-689.

Fertility and mortality estimates for two primitive Soutk American Indian tribes used to develop an index of selection intensity for comparison with other primitive and modern societies; suggests the existence of a continuing potential for genetic change.

1130
Newman, P.
Malaria Eradication and Population Growth. Research Series, 10. Ann Arbor: Bureau of Public Health Economics, University of Michigan, 1965; 259p.

Analysis of the impact of malaria eradication on fertility and demographic change, with reference to Ceylon and British Guiana.

1131
Odegard, O.
"Marriage Rate and Fertility in Psychotic Patients before Hospital Admission and after Discharge." *International Journal of Social Psychiatry* 6(1-2), Summer 1960: pp. 25-33.

Study of patients in Norwegian hospitals over the period 1936-55.

1132
Pringle, G.
"Malaria and Vital Rates in Three East African Bantu Communities. I. Initial Demographical Survey." *British Journal of Preventive and Social Medicine* 18(1), Jan. 1964: pp. 43-51.

Preliminary report on a five-year study of how fertility and mortality are related to malaria control in three Bantu communities.

1133
Ridley, J.C. et al.
"The Effects of Changing Mortality on Natality: Some Estimates from a Simulation Model." *Milbank Memorial Fund Quarterly* 45(1), Jan. 1967: pp. 77-97.

Description of the model and presentation of results with varying survival rates and length of postpartum subfecundity.

1134
Schull, W.J. et al.
"Hirado: Temporal Trends in Inbreeding and Fertility." *Proceedings of the National Academy of Sciences of the United States of America* 59(3), Mar. 1968: pp. 671-679.

Examination of the fertility levels, reproductive behavior, and characteristics of children of consanguineous marriages.

1135
Waldrop, M.F. and Bell, R.Q.
"Effects of Family Size and Density on Newborn Characteristics." *American Journal of Orthopsychiatry* 36, Apr. 1966: pp. 544-550.

1136
Whitehead, L.
"Altitude, Fertility and Mortality in Andean Countries." *Population Studies* 22(3), Nov. 1968: pp. 335-346.

Argues that previous studies finding low fertility for Andean highland populations are incorrect because they fail to measure and control for high infant mortality, which distorts measures based on ratios of young children in the population.

Analysis of the cultural factors facilitating social changes under modernization, with emphasis on the role of rising expectations in urban areas.

VII.G General cultural values and other cultural traits not listed elsewhere

See also: 129, 595, 623, 1227, 1545.

1137
Azumi, K.
"The Mysterious Drop in the Japanese Birth Rate." *Transaction* 5(6), May 1968: pp. 46-49.

Unusual one-year drop in birth rates in 1906 and 1966 traced to actions based on persistent fear that girls born in those years will produce misfortunes; action in 1906 was to misrepresent birth years and in 1966 was to end pregnancies with induced abortion.

1138
Douglas, M.
"Population Control in Primitive Groups." *British Journal of Sociology* 17(3), Sept. 1966: pp. 263-273.

Presents thesis that populations act to control their growth in relation to general optima relating to certain values such as prestige, rather than subsistence alone.

1139
Dubois, C.A.
"Socio-Cultural Aspects of Population Growth." In *Human Fertility and Population Problems.* Edited by R.O. Greep. Cambridge, Mass.: Schenkman, 1963: pp. 251-265.

1140
Gould, K.H.
"Sex and Contraception in Sherupur." *Economic and Political Weekly* 6 Dec. 1969: pp. 1887-1892.

Typical cycle of sexual activity in family life stages of an Uttar Pradesh village, the roles of men and women, and cultural attitudes; makes a number of recommendations about family planning programs including greater emphasis on approaching men, use of simple methods such as coitus interruptus, and the value of stressing spacing.

1141
Kahl, J.A.
The Measurement of Modernism—A Study of Values in Brazil and Mexico. Austin: University of Texas Press, 1968; 210p.

A chapter relating fertility ideals to occupation, education, location and an index of modern values.

1142
* Miller, D.R. and Swanson, G.E.
The Changing American Parent. New York: John Wiley & Sons, 1958; 302p.

Chapter eight includes a speculative theory about the relation between bureaucratic employment and family size, with some empirical data.

1143
* Tambiah, S.J. and Ryan, B.
"Secularization of Family Values in Ceylon." *American Sociological Review* 22(3), June 1957: pp. 292-299.

Secularizing influences, which affect other areas of life, are not related to change in traditional familial values because of counteracting economic changes.

VII.H Combinations of a number of different societal characteristics

See also: 129, 130, 137, 349, 360, 384, 420, 459, 1511, 1535, 1563.

1144
Day, L.H. and Day, A.T.
"Family Size in Industrialized Countries: An Inquiry into the Socio-Cultural Determinants of Levels of Childbearing." *Journal of Marriage and the Family* 31(2), 1969: pp. 242-251.

Examination of sociocultural determinants in 20 low mortality, controlled natality countries; tests hypothesis of alternative roles to childbearing.

1145
Ford, T.R. and DeJong, G.F.
"The Decline of Fertility in Southern Appalachian Mountain Region." *Social Forces* 42(1), Oct. 1963: pp. 89-96.

Analysis of fertility decline in 190 countries, including measures of the effect of economic change, geographical diffusion, and migration.

1146
Freedman, R. et al.
"Fertility Trends in Taiwan: Tradition and Change." *Population Studies* 16(3), Mar. 1963: pp. 219-236.

Presents data from population register and from surveys bearing on the changing fertility trends in Taiwan affected both by tradition and modernization.

1147
Leasure, J.W.
"Factors Involved in the Decline of Fertility in Spain, 1900-1950." *Population Studies* 16(3), Mar. 1963: pp. 271-285.

Analysis of the interrelation of time series by region on marital fertility and socioeconomic status, casting doubt on the primacy of development factors on fertility decline.

1148
Peper, B.
"Population Growth in Java in the Nineteenth Century." *Population Studies* 24(1), Mar. 1970: pp. 71-84.

Examines the impact of changes in the standard of living and the colonial experience on the rapid population growth in Java; comments on the reliability of early population data and estimates.

1149
Samuel, T.J.
"Social Factors Affecting Fertility in India." *Eugenics Review* 57(1), Mar. 1965: pp. 5-15.

Discussion of the possible effect of various marriage practices, social attitudes, and societal characteristics on the Indian birth rate.

VIII. SOCIAL-PSYCHOLOGICAL VARIABLES

VIII.A The socialization process: how fertility behavior is learned and controlled (reference and membership groups, opinion leaders, and informal communication channels)

See also: 82, 98, 528, 657, 789, 821, 827, 846, 853, 854, 864, 1190, 1204, 1498, 1501, 1508, 1512, 1527.

1150
Berelson, B.
"On Family Planning Communication."
Demography 1(1), 1964: pp. 94-105.
> The role of various aspects of communication in relation to the effectiveness of available contraception, the traditional character of society, and the goal of making an impact first where motivation is strong.

1151
Chandrasekaran, C. and Bebarta, P.G.
"The Relative Role of Information Sources in the Dissemination of Knowledge of Family Planning Methods in Bombay City." *Journal of Family Welfare* (Bombay) 9(4), June 1963: pp. 5-14.
> Sources of information about family planning as reported by a sample of mothers chosen from birth registration files.

1152
Fawcett, J.T. et al.
Diffusion of Family Planning Information by Word of Mouth Communication: An Analysis of Time and Distance Factors at an IUD Clinic in Bangkok. Bangkok: National Research Council, 1966; 19p.

1153
Fryer, P.
The Birth Controllers. London: Martin Secker & Warburg, 1965; New York: Stein & Day, 1966; 384p.
> History of the development of family planning leadership.

1154
Gustavus, S.O. and Nam, C.B.
"The Formation and Stability of Ideal Family Size among Young People." *Demography* 7(1), Feb. 1970: pp. 43-51.
> Interview results for young school children suggest family size ideals are formed at a young age.

1155
Hoagland, H.
"Cybernetics of Population Control." In

Human Fertility and Population Problems. Edited by R.O. Greep. Cambridge, Mass.: Schenkman, 1963; pp. 5-20.

Social pathologies found in overcrowded animal populations related to potential human population problems.

1156
Palmore, J.A.
"Awareness Sources and Stages in the Adoption of Specific Contraceptives." *Demography* 5(2), 1968: pp. 960-972.

Analyzes interaction of sources of information, type of contraception, and stages in adoption before and during a family planning program.

1157
Poffenberger, T.
"Two Thousand Voluntary Vasectomies Performed in California: Background Factors and Comments." *Marriage and Family Living* 25(4), Nov. 1963: pp. 469-474.

Characteristics and information source of 2,000 men vasectomized by one doctor in California.

1158
Poffenberger, T.
"Social and Psychological Aspects of Diffusion and Adoption of Family Planning in India." *Social Work Forum* 4(4), Oct. 1966: pp. 8-15.

Develops theoretical framework for tracing the family planning change agent through social and psychological barriers in India.

1159
Shinozaki, N.
"Mutual Connection and Diffusion of Contraception, Abortion, and Sterilization." In *Archives of the Population Association of Japan* No. 4. Tokyo: Population Association of Japan, 1963: pp. 63-80. [English edition.]

1160
Stycos, J.M.
"Opinions of Latin-American Intellectuals on Population and Birth Control." *Annals of the American Academy of Political and Social Science* 360, July 1965: pp. 11-26.

Attitudes of opinion leaders of various ideologies on birth-control practices and programs.

1161
Stycos, J.M.
"Public and Private Opinion on Population and Family Planning." *Studies in Family Planning* 51, Mar. 1970: pp. 10-17.

Compares publicly expressed opinions and statements from the general population and elites (in confidential survey interviews) in countries at different development levels; uses material from the mass media, observations, and surveys to estimate attitudes toward population growth and family planning in the respondent's country and the world as a whole; crossnational correlations of attitudes and actual growth rates.

VIII.B Psychological and social-psychological variables related to fertility: feelings of insecurity, aspiration levels, neuroticism, impulse control, attitude toward sexuality, need to achieve, deferred gratification, apathy and fatalism, personal inadequacy, etc.

See also: 98, 587, 596, 1327, 1512.

1162
Back, K.W.
"New Frontiers in Demography and Social Psychology." *Demography* 4(1), 1967: pp. 90-97.

Suggests productive possibilities in interaction of demographic and psychological research.

1163
Bakker, C.B. and Dightman, C.R.
"Psychological Factors in Fertility Control." *Fertility and Sterility* 15(5), Sept.-Oct. 1964: pp. 559-567.

Personality characteristics of couples as measured by psychological tests related to efficiency of oral contraception.

1164
Barglow, P. et al.
"Hysterectomy and Tubal Ligation: A Psychiatric Comparison." *Obstetrics and Gynecology* 25, Apr. 1965: pp. 520-527.

1165
Bean, L.L.
"The Fertility of Former Mental Patients." *Eugenics Quarterly* 13(1), Mar. 1966: pp. 34-39.

Fertility experience of discharged female mental patients compared to matched never-treated females.

1166
***Centers, R. and Blumberg, G.**
"Social and Psychological Factors in Human Procreation: A Survey Approach." *Journal of Social Psychology* 40, Nov. 1954: pp. 245-257.

Compares small group of couples who do not want children with larger group who do and reports that psychological differences, rather than sociological, are significant.

1167
Christensen, H.T.
"Scandinavian and American Sex Norms: Some Comparisons, with Sociological Implications." *Journal of Social Issues* 22(2), Apr. 1966: pp. 60-75.

Comparison of norms relating to sexual permissiveness; attempt to develop sociological framework for a theory of normative morality.

1168
Ekbald, M.
"Social-Psychiatric Prognosis after Sterilization of Women without Children: A Follow-up Study of 60 Women." *Acta Psychiatrica Scandinavica* (Copenhagen) 39, 1963: pp. 481-514.

1169
Erlenmeyer-Kimling, L. et al.
"Current Reproductive Trends in Schizophrenia." In *Psychopathology of Schizophrenia.* Edited by P.H. Hoch and J. Zurbin. New York: Grune & Stratton, 1966: pp. 252-276.

1170
Ferber, A.S. et al.
"Men with Vasectomies: A Study of Medical, Sexual, and Psychosocial Changes." *Psychosomatic Medicine* 29(4), July-Aug. 1967: pp. 354-366.

Small sample survey of U.S. males used to analyze health effects, social, and psychological adjustment to vasectomies.

1171
Goshen-Gottstein, E.R.
Marriage and First Pregnancy: Cultural Influences on Attitudes of Israeli Women. Mind and Medicine Monographs, 11. London: Tavistock, 1966; 141p.

Unusual study of how the cultural-psychological set associated with traditional-modern background differences influence such matters as symptoms during first pregnancy, sex preference, breast feeding and its actual practice, birth-control attitudes, and communication with husband concerning family growth.

1172
Groat, H.T. and Neal, A.G.
"Social Psychological Correlates of Urban Fertility." *American Sociological Review* 32(6), Dec. 1967: pp. 945-959.

Study of the relation of various aspects of alienation scales to actual and desired fertility, with controls for education, religion, race, and age.

1173
Hopkinson, G.
"Celibacy and Marital Fertility in Manic-Depressive Patients." *Acta Psychiatrica Scandinavica* (Copenhagen) 39, 1963: pp. 473-476.

1174
Johnson, M.H.
"Social and Psychological Effects of Vasectomy." *American Journal of Psychiatry* 121, Nov. 1964: pp. 482-486.

1175
Kiser, C.V.
"Psychological Factors in Infertility—a Demographic Appraisal." *Journal of the Indian Medical Profession* 11(3), June 1964: pp. 4927-4929.

Trends and differentials in childlessness and the types of data needed to judge the importance of psychological factors.

1176
Landis, J.T. and Poffenberger, T.
"The Marital and Sexual Adjustment of 330 Couples Who Chose Vasectomy as a Form of Birth Control." *Journal of Marriage and the Family* 27(1), Feb. 1965: pp. 57-58.

Based on 50-percent questionnaire response among clients of one physician.

1177
Lehfeldt, H.
"Willful Exposure to Unwanted Pregnancy (WEUP): Psychological Explanation for Patient Failures in Contraception." *Sixth International Conference on Planned Parenthood*, 1959: pp. 110-114. [Also in *American Journal of Obstetrics and Gynecology* 78, Sept. 1959: pp. 661-665.]

1178
Lieberman, E.J.
"Preventive Psychiatry and Family Planning." *Journal of Marriage and the Family* 26(4), Nov. 1964: pp. 471-477.

1179
Marshall, J.F.
"A Neglected Area of Family Planning Research." *Population Review* (Madras) 11(1), Jan. 1967: pp. 30-37.

Suggests a conceptual framework for research on psychological and cultural factors affecting attitudes toward family planning.

1180
Metzner, R.J. and Golden, J.S.
"Psychological Factors Influencing Female Patients in the Selection of Contraceptive Devices." *Fertility and Sterility* 18(6), Nov.-Dec. 1967: pp. 845-856.

1181
Paniagua, M.E. et al.
"Medical and Psychological Sequelae of

Surgical Sterilization of Women." *American Journal of Obstetrics and Gynecology* 90(4), Oct. 1964: pp. 421-430.

Based on a sample of 519 Puerto Rican cases.

1182
Pohlman, E.
"Results of Unwanted Conceptions: Some Hypotheses Up for Adoption." *Eugenics Quarterly,* 12(1), Mar. 1965: pp. 11-18.

Develops hypotheses, many from psychoanalytic theory, to deal with the effects of unwanted conceptions on parents and children.

1183
Pohlman, E.
"Birth Control: Independent and Dependent Variables for Psychological Research." *American Psychologist* 21, Oct. 1966: pp. 967-970.

Suggested research on relation of psychological variables to fertility and family planning.

1184
Pohlman, E.
"A Psychologist's Introduction to the Birth Planning Literature." *Journal of Social Issues* 23(4), Oct. 1967: pp. 13-27.

1185
***Rainwater, L.**
And the Poor Get Children. Chicago: Quadrangle Books, 1960; 202p.

The social-psychological and situational factors preventing efficient family planning, based on intensive study of a small purposive sample of low-status couples.

1186
Rainwater, L.
"Attitudes of Patients Affecting Contraceptive Practice." In *Manual of Contraceptive Practice.* Edited by M.S. Calderone. Baltimore: Williams & Wilkins, 1964: pp. 87-95.

Discusses possible emotional barriers to contraceptive practices among different social and religious groups.

1187
Rainwater, L.
Family Design: Marital Sexuality, Family Size, and Contraception. Social Research Studies in Contemporary Life. Chicago: Aldine, 1965; 349p.

Examination of the sociopsychological and socioeconomic factors that determine family size goals and the use of family limitation methods.

1188
Rock, J. et al.
"Effect of Adoption on Infertility." *Fertility and Sterility* 16(3), May-June 1965: pp. 305-312.

Controlled experiment to study effect of adoption on fertility of previously barren couples.

1189
Shearer, M.L. et al.
"Unexpected Effects of an "Open Door" Policy on Birth Rates of Women in State Hospitals." *American Journal of Orthopsychiatry* 38(3), Apr. 1968: pp. 413-417.

1190
Smith, M.B.
"Motivation, Communications Research, and Family Planning." In Sheps and Ridley, eds. (*see* 73): pp. 70-89.

Surveys possibilities for the application of communications and motivation research to the promotion of effective birth control practices.

1191

Stevens, B.C.

Marriage and Fertility of Women Suffering from Schizophrenia or Affective Disorders. London: Oxford University Press, 1969; 188p.

1192

Stevens, B.C.

"Probability of Marriage and Fertility of Women Suffering from Schizophrenia or Affective Disorders." *Population Studies* 23(3), Nov. 1969: pp. 435-454.

> British sample of schizophrenic cases has lower marriage probabilities and lower fertility before marriage than normal population; no such difference is related to affective disorders; in posthospitalization period similar marriage differentials but not fertility differentials.

1193

Thomas, J.L.

"Issues, Facts, and Population Policy Re-examined." In *Population Ethics.* Edited by E.X. Quinn. Washington: Corpus Books, 1968: pp. 58-77.

> A Catholic priest calls for a new view of population policy in light of societal changes in human sexuality.

1194

Waldrop, M.F. and Bell, R.Q.

"Relation of Preschool Dependency Behavior and Family Size and Density." *Child Development* 35, 1964: pp. 1187-1195.

> Psychological analysis of the effect of family size and age of sibs to nursery school behavior.

1195

Wallach, E.E. and Garcia, C.R.

"Psychodynamic Aspects of Oral Contraception: A Review." *Journal of the American Medical Association* 203(11), Mar. 1968: pp. 927-931.

> Emotional factors that may affect acceptance of oral contraception.

1196

*Westoff, C.F. et al.

"Fertility through Twenty Years of Marriage: A Study in Predictive Possibilities." *American Sociological Review* 23(5), Oct. 1958: pp. 549-556.

> Unique 20-year follow-up study of a sample of couples originally interviewed and tested when they were engaged to be married; compares original statements of desired family size with performance after 20 years and relations of values and performance to a battery of social and psychological variables.

1197

Wyatt, F.

"Clinical Notes on the Motives of Reproduction." *Journal of Social Issues* 23(4), Oct. 1967: pp. 29-56.

IX. SOCIAL AND DEMOGRAPHIC FACTORS AFFECTING LEVELS OR NORMS FOR IMPORTANT INTERMEDIATE VARIABLES

IX.A Contraception and family planning

See also: 49, 81, 89, 204, 317, 377, 463, 464, 466, 503, 525, 534, 536, 543, 562, 566, 569, 571, 576, 580, 582, 586, 587, 597, 623, 632, 672, 683, 701, 719, 774, 789, 806, 828, 830, 835, 848, 852, 856, 859, 860, 867, 883, 897, 922, 933, 976, 984, 997, 1037, 1090, 1094, 1171, 1180, 1181, 1185, 1186, 1187, 1195, 1313, 1314, 1497, 1498, 1501, 1502, 1503, 1504, 1506, 1512, 1519, 1520, 1522, 1523, 1525, 1527, 1528, 1529, 1531, 1532, 1534, 1535, 1538, 1644.

1198
Ahmed, M. and Ahmed, F.
"Male Attitudes toward Family Limitation in East Pakistan." *Eugenics Quarterly* 12(4), Dec. 1965: pp. 209-226.

> Based on a 1963 study of a small nonrandom sample of married males to determine their attitudes toward birth control.

1199
Bachi, R. and Matras, J.
"Contraception and Induced Abortions among Jewish Maternity Cases in Israel." *Milbank Memorial Fund Quarterly* 40(2), Apr. 1962: pp. 207-229.

> A preliminary report on ethnic, demographic, and socioeconomic factors affecting birth control practices in a good sample of Israeli maternity cases in 1959-60.

1200
Bachi, R. and Matras, J.
"Family Size Preferences of Jewish Maternity Cases in Israel." *Milbank Memorial Fund Quarterly* 42(2, Part 1), Apr. 1964: pp. 38-56.

> Family-size preferences and contraceptive use related to ethnic and socioeconomic group status.

1201
Badenhorst, L.T.
"Family Limitation and Methods of Contraception in an Urban Population." *Population Studies* 16(3), Mar. 1963: pp. 286-301.

> Differentials of contraceptive use by age, income, religion, education, and language spoken for a stratified sample of urban and suburban white women in Johannesburg.

1202
Beasley, J.D. et al.
"Attitudes and Knowledge Relevant to

Family Planning among New Orleans Negro Women." *American Journal of Public Health and the Nation's Health* 56(11), Nov. 1966: pp. 1847-1857.

Women exhibit lack of knowledge of aspects of reproductive physiology relevant to family planning and a desire to have contraceptive methods and to limit family size; educational, religious, age, and parity differentials.

1203
Caldwell, J.C. and Igun, A.
"The Spread of Anti-Natal Knowledge and Practice in Nigeria." *Population Studies* 24(1), Mar. 1970: pp. 21-34.

Report on a survey of source and timing of knowledge and use of contraception and abortion; urban-rural, income, religious, and age-sex differentials.

1204
Carlsson, G.
"The Decline of Fertility: Innovation or Adjustment Process." *Population Studies* 20(2), Nov. 1966: pp. 149-174.

Raises and partially tests important theoretical questions as to whether birth control in marriage existed on a fairly wide scale before modern secular fertility decline and whether the spread of birth control follows the hypothesis of a lag.

1205
Coughlin, R.J. and Coughlin, M.M.
"Fertility and Birth Control among Low Income Chinese Families in Hong Kong." *Marriage and Family Living* 25(2), May 1963: pp. 171-177.

Interviews with 300 women voluntarily participating in a family planning program showed little knowledge about, but little resistance to, birth control.

1206
Dandekar, K.
"Vasectomy Camps in Maharashtra."

Population Studies 17(2), Nov. 1963: pp. 147-154.

Characteristics of males who underwent vasectomy in 42 government-sponsored camps in Maharashtra 1959-62.

1207
Demeny, P.
"Early Fertility Decline in Austria-Hungary: A Lesson in Demographic Transition." *Daedalus* 97(2), Spring 1968: pp. 502-522.

Relates provincial fertility differentials to development; suggests evidence reveals marital fertility control before general fertility decline and areal fertility declines do not follow the pattern of demographic transition theory.

1208
Dow, T.E., Jr.
"Attitudes toward Family Planning in Nairobi." *Demography* 4(2), 1967: pp. 780-797.

KAP survey of contraceptive methods; acceptance differentials by education, hospital use, parental and spouse approval.

1209
Draper, E.
Birth Control in the Modern World. London: George Allen & Unwin, 1965; 275p.

Survey of the history and prospects for birth control discussing in a general way many of the facts and their actual or presumed correlates.

1210
Hall, M.F.
"Family Planning in Lima, Peru." *Milbank Memorial Fund Quarterly* 43(4, Part 2), Oct. 1965: pp. 100-116.

Survey results used to estimate incidence of abortion, level and methods of contraceptive use, and attitudes toward family limitation; socioeconomic status differentials.

1211
Hong, S.B. and Yoon, J.H.
"Male Attitudes toward Family Planning on the Island of Kangwha-Gun, Korea." *Milbank Memorial Fund Quarterly* 40(4), Oct. 1962: pp. 443-452.

Male attitudes to family size and contraception in a small Korean sample.

1212
India. Cabinet Secretariat.
The National Sample Survey, Sixteenth Round: July 1960-June 1961. No. 116. Tables with notes on family planning. Calcutta: Eka Press; Delhi: Manager of Publications, Civil Lines, 1967; 164p.

Report on an all-India urban survey; contains mainly tabulations and relatively little

1213
India. Kerala. Demographic Research Center (Travandrum).
"A Study of Persons Who Have Undergone Sterilization Operations in Kerala." *Population Review* (Madras) 6(2), July 1962: pp. 137-142.

Demographic and socioeconomic characteristics of a large sample of hospital patients in India.

1214
Institute of Economic Growth. Demographic Section.
Family Planning in Selected Villages (Awareness, Belief, Knowledge and Practice). Institute of Economic Growth, Occasional Papers, 6. Bombay: Asia Publishing House, 1962; 88p.

1215
Jain, S.P.
"Fertility Trends in Greater Bombay." In 1967 I.U.S.S.P. (*see* 21): pp. 325-336.

Some preliminary results of the Greater Bombay fertility survey of 1966, indicating that knowledge and practice of contraception were still at a rather low level at that time, but with marked class differentials; especially documented with reference to education.

1216
Kurup, R.S. and Mathen, T.K.
"Sterilization as a Method of Family Limitation in Kerala State." *Population Review* (Madras) 10(2), July 1966: pp. 61-68.

Statistical report on demographic characteristics of sterilization cases.

1217
Langford, C.M.
"Birth Control Practice in Britain." *Family Planning* 17(4), Jan. 1969: pp. 89-92.

Marriage-cohort trends in extent and type of contraceptive practice and source of information.

1218
*Lewis-Faning, E.
Report on an Inquiry into Family Limitation and Its Influence on Human Fertility During the Past Fifty Years. Papers of the Royal Commission on Population, 1. London: H.M.S.O., 1949; 202p.

Unique work in presenting national statistical estimates of the use of contraception on a historical basis for major social classes that can be related to actual changes in fertility by social class.

1219
Madras. Superintendent of Census.
Family Planning Attitude in Madras City. Census of India, 9(10-F). 1966; 52p.

A KAP study.

1220
Molnos, A.
Attitudes towards Family Planning in

East Africa: An Investigation in Schools around Lake Victoria and in Nairobi. IFO-Institute for Economic Research Afrika-Studien, 26. Munich: Weltforum Verlag, 1968; 414p.

Reports on surveys of students' attitudes and sets forth suggestions for a psychological approach to family planning promotion.

1221
*Morrison, W.A.
"Attitude of Males toward Family Planning in a Western Indian Village." *Milbank Memorial Fund Quarterly* 25(1), Jan. 1957: pp. 67-81.

Desire for more children and expressed unwillingness to use contraception negatively related to number of living sons and to educational and caste status.

1222
Novak, F.
"Why Does Contraception Meet So Many Difficulties in Superseding Abortion?" *Seventh International Conference on Planned Parenthood*, 1963; pp. 634-637.

1223
Pacheco, A. and Osteria, T.
"Some Findings on the Attitudes toward Family Size Preferences and Family Limitation." *Statistical Reporter* (Manila) 10(3), July-Sept. 1966: pp. 1-8.

Philippine town study of family size preferences, knowledge and use of contraception by family size, education, husband's occupation, and duration of marriage.

1224
Pareek, U. and Kothandapani, V.
"Modernization and Attitude toward Family Size and Family Planning: Analysis of Some Data from India." *Social Biology* 16 (1) , Mar. 1969: pp. 44-48.

Reports correlations between family size preference and family planning attitudes and 33 socioeconomic and attitudinal variables for a sample of 1,300 respondents in a tribal belt in Bihar.

1225
Pathfinder Fund. International IUD Programme.
The following are part of a continuing series of reports from public and private clinic sources on the demographic and socioeconomic correlates of IUD acceptance and termination:

Geographic Series No. 1: The Yugoslavia Multi-Clinic Trial (Oct. 1969).

Geographic Series No. 1A: The Dubrovnik Luncheon (n.d.).

Geographic Series No. 2: The Israel Multi-Clinic Trial (Nov. 1969).

Geographic Series No. 3: The Clarence J. Gamble International IUD Baseline: Asia and Far East (Dec. 1969).

Geographic Series No. 4: The Clarence J. Gamble International IUD Baseline: Europe and Near East (Apr. 1970).

Geographic Series No. 5: The Hong Kong Multi-Clinic Trial (n.d.)

"Factors Governing IUD Performance." *American Journal of Public Health* 60(10), Oct. 1970.

"The M-211 Device: Possible Turning Point in Approach." *Advances in Planned Parenthood* 5, 1969: pp. 100-109.

1226
Poffenberger, T.
"Age of Wives and Number of Living Children of a Sample of Men Who Had the Vasectomy in Meerut District, U.P." *Journal of Family Welfare* (Bombay) 13(4), June 1967: pp. 48-51.

1227
Poffenberger, T. and Patel, H.G.
"The Effect of Local Beliefs on Attitudes toward Vasectomy in Two Indian Villages in Gujarat State." *Population Review* (Madras) 8(2), July 1964: pp. 37-44.

Survey on how specific cultural values affect attitudes toward vasectomy.

1228
Pool, D.I.
"Ghana: A Survey on Fertility and Attitudes toward Family Limitation." *Studies in Family Planning* 1(25), Dec. 1967: pp. 10-15.

Analysis of response patterns shows widespread lack of concern on family limitation and generally favorable attitude toward large families; educational, urban-rural, and tribal differentials.

1229
*Poti, S.J.
"An Enquiry into the Prevalence of Contraceptive Practices in Calcutta City." In *Sixth International Conference on Planned Parenthood.* London: International Planned Parenthood Federation, 1959: pp. 52-60.

Early study of the simultaneous interrelation of social status, family planning, and fertility in a developing country; shows significant use of contraception in Calcutta.

1230
Potter, R.G., Jr. et al.
"Knowledge of the Ovulatory Cycle and Coital Frequency as Factors Affecting Conception and Contraception." *Milbank Memorial Fund Quarterly* 40(1) Jan. 1962: pp. 46-58.

U.S. metropolitan sample survey of relation between contraceptive knowledge and coital frequency on contraceptive effectiveness, with controls for socioeconomic and religious factors.

1231
Raman, M.V.
"Knowledge and Practice of Contraception in India: A Survey of Some Recent Studies." *Artha Vijñāna* (Poona) 5(2), June 1963: pp. 81-96.

Regional variations compared on basis of review of local studies.

1232
*Riley, J.W. and White, M.
"The Use of Various Methods of Contraception." *American Sociological Review* 5(6), Dec. 1940: pp. 890-903.

First major empirical national study of the use of contraception in relation to social class, religion, and urbanization.

1233
Roberts, G.W. et al.
"Knowledge and Use of Birth Control in Barbados." *Demography* 4(2), 1967: pp. 576-600.

A 1964 sample survey on levels and correlates of knowledge, practice, and information on sources in family planning.

1234
Rowntree, G. and Pierce, R.M.
"Birth Control in Britain, Part 1." *Population Studies* 15(1), July 1961: pp. 3-31.

First national representative study in England on correlates of attitudes toward and use of contraception.

1235
Ryder, N.B. and Westoff, C.F.
"Use of Oral Contraception in the United States, 1965." *Science* 153(3741), Sept. 1966: pp. 1199-1205.

An early report from the 1965 national fertility study of the level and correlates of use of oral contraception in the U.S. from 1960-65; considers parity, age, education, and religion.

1236

Ryder, N.B. and Westoff, C.F.

"Fertility Planning Status: United States, 1965." *Demography* 6(4), Nov. 1969: pp. 435-444.

Rather high failure rates in the U.S. in planning number and, especially, timing of pregnancies are estimated from 1965 national fertility study; shows more success for educated, Protestants, and whites, but failure rates high in all strata; significant discussion of methodological problems of measuring success and failure.

1237

*Sagi, P.C. et al.

"Contraceptive Effectiveness as a Function of Desired Family Size." *Population Studies* 15(3), Mar. 1962: pp. 291-296.

Use of contraception increases and rate of unplanned pregnancies decreases as the desired family size is approached in metropolitan U.S.

1238

San, M. and Sen, D.K.

"Family Planning Practice of Couples of Reproductive Age Group in a Selected Locality in Calcutta—June 1965." *Journal of Family Welfare* (Bombay) 14(1), Sept. 1967: pp. 13-24.

Survey data on contraceptive practice as related to education, family size, income, and age for a sample of the couples in service area of a health and family planning clinic.

1239

Sarupria, S.L.

"Attitudes towards Family Planning in a Small Urban Community." *Indian Journal of Social Work* (Bombay) 25(1), Apr. 1964: pp. 79-87.

Small sample survey indicating that higher status respondents are more favorable in principle but not in action.

1240

Stoeckel, J. and Choudhury, M.A.

"Factors Related to Knowledge and Practice of Family Planning in East Pakistan Villages." *Social Biology* 16 (1), Mar. 1969: pp. 29-38.

KAP study of 2,008 respondents relates socioeconomic correlates to family planning.

1241

*Valien, P. and Fitzgerald, A.P.

"Attitudes of the Negro Mother towards Birth Control." *American Journal of Sociology* 55(3), Nov. 1949: pp. 279-283.

1242

Westoff, C.F. and Ryder, N.B.

"United States: Methods of Fertility Control, 1955, 1960, and 1965." *Studies in Family Planning* 1(17), Feb. 1967: pp. 1-5.

On the basis of the 1965 national fertility study, steady increase is shown in the proportions using contraception (especially among those with low rates of use earlier) and a shift toward the pill from the condom, diaphragm, and nonuse; an increasing proportion of Catholics are shown to be using methods not approved by the church.

1243

Westoff, C.F. and Ryder, N.B.

"Duration of Use of Oral Contraception in the United States, 1960-65." *Public Health Reports* 83(4), Apr. 1968: pp. 277-287.

On basis of the 1965 national fertility study, estimates discontinuation rates in use of oral contraceptives by age, parity, race, education, and reasons stated for terminatiom.

1244

Westoff, C.F. and Ryder, N.B.

"Experience with Oral Contraception in the United States, 1960-65." *Clinical Obstetrics and Gynecology* 11(3), Sept. 1968: pp. 734-752.

Draws on earlier reports (see 1235, 1242, 1645) to describe the remarkably rapid diffusion of the use of contraception in the U.S., its relation to age, marriage duration, parity, education, and religion and its possible connection to the birth rate decline during this period.

1245
Westoff, C.F. and Ryder, N.B.
"Recent Trends in Attitudes toward Fertility Control and in the Practice of Contraception in the United States." In Behrman et al., eds: (*see* 51): pp. 388-412.
Report based on the 1965 national fertility study.

IX.B Fecundity (including postpartum amenorrhea)
See also: 81, 1506, 1512, 1634, 1652, 1655.

1246
Ber, A. and Brociner, C.
"Age of Puberty in Israeli Girls." *Fertility and Sterility* 15(6), Nov.-Dec. 1964: pp. 640-647.
Age at menarche related to ethnic origin and social status of father.

1247
Berquo, E.S. et al.
"Levels and Variations in Fertility in Sao Paulo." *Milbank Memorial Fund Quarterly* 46(3, Part 2), July 1968: pp. 167-185.
Special emphasis on estimates of fecundability and on comparisons of desired and actual fertility in Sao Paulo districts central and rural zones.

1248
Bonte, M. and van Balen, H.
"Prolonged Lactation and Family Spacing in Rwanda." *Journal of Biosocial Science* 1(2), Apr. 1969: pp. 97-100.

1249
Buck, C. and Stavraky, K.
"The Relationship between Age at Menarche and Age at Marriage among Childbearing Women." *Human Biology* 39(2), May 1967: pp. 93-102.
Contingency analysis of data on mother's age at marriage, at menarche, and at maternity obtained from birth records in hospitals.

1250
Chang, K.S.F. et al.
"Climate and Conception Rates in Hong Kong." *Human Biology* 35 (3), Sept. 1963: pp. 366-376.
Finds seasonal variations in conception rates related to temperature but is unable to distinguish the effects of climate on fertility as distinguished from general social links to seasons.

1251
Glaser, J.H. and Lachenbruch, P.A.
"Observations on the Relationship between Frequency and Timing of Intercourse and the Probability of Conception." *Population Studies* 22(3), Nov. 1968: pp. 399-407.
Illustrates a simplified model in which frequency of intercourse is assumed to be subject to chance fluctuations.

1252
Jain, A.K.
"Socio-Economic Correlates of Fecundability in a Sample of Taiwanese Women." *Demography* 6(1), Feb. 1969: pp. 75-90.

1253

Jain, A.K.

"Fecundability and Its Relation to Age in a Sample of Taiwanese Women." *Population Studies* 23(1), Mar. 1969: pp. 69-85.

Presents estimates of mean fecundability at marriage, including analyses of memory and truncation bias.

1254

Jain, A.K.

"Relative Fecundability of Users and Non-Users of Contraception." *Social Biology* 16(1), Mar. 1969: pp. 39-43.

Data from Taichung study (see 1508).

1255

Jain, S.P.

"Post-partum Amenorrhea in Indian Women." In 1967 I.U.S.S.P. (*see* 21): pp. 378-388.

A longitudinal study relating age, parity, and extent of breast feeding to length of amenorrhea, with comparisons to other studies.

1256

Lachenbruch, P.A.

"Frequency and Timing of Intercourse: Its Relation to the Probability of Conception." *Population Studies* 21(1), July 1967: pp. 23-31.

1257

MacMahon, B. and Worchester, J.

"Age at Menopause, United States, 1960-1962." *Vital and Health Statistics* 19, Oct. 1966; 20p.

Age at menopause in relation to family life cycle, economic, and physiological characteristics.

1258

Potter, R.G., Jr. et al.

"Applications of Field Studies to Research on the Physiology of Human Reproduction: Lactation and Its Effects upon Birth Intervals in Eleven Punjab Villages, India." In Sheps and Ridley, eds. (*see* 73): pp. 377-399.

Relation of pregnancy outcomes, lactation, postpartum amenorrhea, and age of mother to length of birth interval in an Indian village sample.

1259

Ridley, J.C. et al.

"On the Apparent Subfecundity of Non-Family Planners." *Social Biology* 16(1), Mar. 1969: pp. 24-28.

Report on experiments using simulation model described in item 320.

1260

Salber, E.J. et al.

"The Duration of Postpartum Amenorrhea." *American Journal of Epidemiology* 82(3), 1966: pp. 347-358.

Length of postpartum amenorrhea related to length of lactation and other variables for a sample of U.S. women.

1261

Salber, E.J. et al.

"Duration of Postpartum Amenorrhea in Successive Pregnancies." *American Journal of Obstetrics and Gynecology* 100, 1 Jan. 1968: pp. 24-29.

Finds a consistent pattern in length of postpartum amenorrhea for successive pregnancies after adjusting for the effect of lactation in a sample of 80 women.

1262

Sehgal, B.S. and Singh, R.

"Breast Feeding, Amenorrhea and Rates of Conception in Women." *Journal of Family Welfare* (Bombay) 14(1), Sept. 1967: pp. 44-49.

Relation of lactation and amenorrhea to conception rates in 12 Indian villages.

1263
Sheps, M.C.
"An Analysis of Reproductive Patterns in an American Isolate." *Population Studies* 19(1), July 1965: pp. 65-80.

Reproductive patterns of a high-fertility religious sect; examines the intermediate effects of lactation and postpartum amenorrhea on birth intervals.

1264
Singer, K.
"Duration of Post-Partum Amenorrhea in Indian Women." *Journal of Family Welfare* (Bombay) 13(4), June 1967: pp. 27-35.

Longitudinal survey data on lactation, nutrition, amenorrhea, infant mortality.

1265
Stukovský, R. et al.
"Family Size and Menarcheal Age in Constanza, Roumania." *Human Biology* 39 (3), Sept. 1967: pp. 277-283.

Proportions menstruating by age and number of siblings in family.

1266
Tietze, C.
"The Effect of Breastfeeding on the Rate of Conception." In *International Population Conference.* New York, 1961. London: U.N.E.S.C.O., 1963: pp. 129-136.

1267
Treloar, A.E. et al.
"Variation of the Human Menstrual Cycle through Reproductive Life." *International Journal of Fertility* 12(Part 2, No. 1) Jan.-Mar. 1967: pp. 77-126.

IX.C Nuptiality

See also: 56, 81, 130, 234, 303, 358, 395, 507, 508, 509, 557, 625, 1017, 1107, 1149, 1169, 1173, 1192, 1249, 1486, 1502, 1504, 1506, 1510, 1511, 1519, 1520, 1531, 1612, 1616, 1617, 1624.

1268
Agarwala, S.N.
Age at Marriage in India. Allahabad: Kitab Mahal, 1962; 296p.

A wide-ranging analysis of the historical trends in age at marriage in India and its relation to caste, religion, migration, mortality, and region; discusses in detail methodological problems of indirect estimates of age at marriage from census and other sources.

1269
Agarwala, S.N.
"Widow Remarriages in Some Rural Areas of Northern India." *Demography* 4(1), 1967: pp. 126-134.

Survey results on social and demographic characteristics of widows and their pattern of remarriage.

1270
Akers, D.S.
"On Measuring the Marriage Squeeze." *Demography* 4(2), 1967: pp. 907-924.

How the age distribution of men and women affects the potentials for marriage and the age at marriage.

1271
*Berent, J. et al.
"Social Mobility and Marriage: A Study of Trends in England and Wales." In *Social Mobility in Britain.* Edited by D.V. Glass. London: Routledge & Kegan Paul, 1954: pp. 321-348.

1272

Bernard, J.

"Marital Stability and Patterns of Status Variables." *Journal of Marriage and the Family* 28(4), Nov. 1966: pp. 421-439.

Relationship of income, occupation, and education to marital stability for white and nonwhite population.

1273

Blake, J.

"Parental Control, Delayed Marriage, and Population Policy." In *Proceedings of the World Population Conference, 1965* (*see* 44): pp. 132-136.

Discusses the effect of arranged marriages on age at marriage; examines data from Asian countries and historical Western experience.

1274

Burchinal, L.G.

"Trends and Prospects for Young Marriages in the United States." *Journal of Marriage and the Family* 27(2), May 1965: pp. 243-254.

Based on historical review of rates, considers factors affecting decisions to marry at young ages, and the relation of such characteristics to marriage success.

1275

Christensen, H.T.

"Timing of First Pregnancy as a Factor in Divorce: A Cross-Cultural Analysis." *Eugenics Quarterly* 10(3), Sept. 1963: pp. 119-129.

Analysis of data from three populations to support the hypothesis that premarital pregnancy increases the probability of divorce and that this relationship is strongest where sex mores are most restrictive.

1276

Clignet, R.

"Urbanization and Family Structure in the Ivory Coast." *Comparative Studies in Society and History* 8(4), July 1966: pp. 385-401.

A field survey serves as a basis for relating urbanization to changes in marriage and family.

1277

Glick, P.C.

"Marriage Instability: Variations by Size of Place and Region." *Milbank Memorial Fund Quarterly* 41(1), Jan. 1963: pp. 43-55.

Analysis of variance of factors affecting rates of separation and divorce based on 1960 census.

1278

Glick, P.C.

"Permanence of Marriage." *Population Index* 33(4), Oct.-Dec. 1967: pp. 517-526.

1279

Grønseth, E., ed.

"Approaches to the Study of the Decision to Marry." *Acta Sociologica* (Copenhagen) 8(1-2), 1964: pp. 1-176.

Collection of papers from many countries on the factors affecting who marries, when, and with what motives.

1280

Hair, P.E.H.

"Bridal Pregnancy in Rural England in Earlier Centuries." *Population Studies* 20(2), Nov. 1966: pp. 233-243.

1281

Hair, P.E.H.

"Bridal Pregnancy in Earlier Rural England Further Examined." *Population Studies* 24(1), Mar. 1970: pp. 59-70.

Continuation of an earlier study (see 1280) concerning bridal pregnancy in the sixteenth and nineteenth centuries; courting and nuptial factors in early pregnancy and seasonal periods for forbidding marriage are considered.

1282
Kharchev, A.G.
"On Some Results of a Study of the Motives for Marriage." *Soviet Sociology* 2(4), Spring 1964: pp. 41-51.

Results of a 1962 opinion survey in Leningrad includes age at marriage distributions and ratio of ages of brides and grooms; comparison of results with a 1959 survey.

1283
Kharchev, A.G.
"Marriage in the USSR." *Soviet Sociology* 5(4), Spring 1967: pp. 3-24.

Discusses empirical data from sample surveys, official registers, and secondary sources on attitudes toward marriage, age at marriage, mixed marriages, abortion by age groups, and divorce.

1284
Knodel, J.
"Law, Marriage and Illegitimacy in Nineteenth-Century Germany." *Population Studies* 20(3), Mar. 1967: pp. 279-294.

Examines the effect of legal restrictions on marriage or marriage patterns, illegitimacy, and fertility, with some discussion of implications for population policy.

1285
Korson, J.H.
"Age and Social Status at Marriage: Karachi, 1961-64." *Pakistan Development Review* (Karachi) 5(4), Winter 1965: pp. 586-600.

Muslim marriage register data used to relate couples' age at marriage to social status.

1286
Leplae, C.
"Celibacy in Belgium: A Preliminary Study." *Acta Sociologica* (Copenhagen) 8(1-2) 1964: pp. 15-26.

Elaborates on sociological definition of celibacy and analyzes factors affecting it.

1287
Lungwitz, K.
"Divorces by Age of Divorced Persons (with Respect to the Impact of Decreasing Age at Marriage on Its Development in the German Democratic Republic)." In Szabady et al., eds. (*see* 39): pp. 295-297.

On the interdependence of declining age at marriage and higher divorce rates in East Germany and their relation to social change.

1288
Mitchell, J.C.
"Marriage Stability and Social Structure in Bantu Africa." In *International Population Conference.* New York, 1961. London: U.N.E.S.C.O., 1963: pp. 255-263.

How family type interacts with urbanization to affect marital stability, based on limited data and plausible interpretations.

1289
Moss, J.J.
"Teenage Marriage: Cross National Trends and Sociological Factors in the Decision of When to Marry." *Acta Sociological* (Copenhagen) 8(1-2), Aug. 1964: pp. 98-117.

Summarizes findings of papers at 1963 international family research seminar on differential levels of teenage marriage rates for Sweden, U.S., Norway, Finland, and Yugoslavia.

1290
Obaidullah, M. and Rahman, K.F.
"Mean Duration of Married Fertile

Union in East Pakistan." *Journal of the Pakiston Academy for Rural Development* (Comilla) 5(1), July 1964: pp. 33-39.

Estimates derived from the 1961 Pakistan census and from sample survey in 1960-61.

1291
Ortmeyer, C.E.
"Educational Attainment as a Selective Factor in Marital Status Transitions in the United States." *Demography* 4(1), 1967: pp. 108-125.

Census data (1940-60) used to analyze trends in nuptial status by age and education of husbands and wives.

1292
Rele, J.R.
"Trends and Differentials in the American Age at Marriage." *Milbank Memorial Fund Quarterly* 43(2), Apr. 1965: pp. 219-234.

Reviews trends 1890-1960 and analyzes in detail social differentials in the decline in age at marriage 1940-60.

1293
Rosenwaike, I.
"Differentials in Divorce in Maryland." *Demography* 6(2), May 1969: pp. 151-159.

Record linkage study relates divorce risks by race, age at marriage, and previous marital status.

1294
Sadiq, N.M.
"Estimation of Nuptiality and Its Analysis from Census Data of Pakistan." *Pakistan Development Review* (Karachi) 5(2), Summer 1965: pp. 229-248.

Estimates time trends in mean age at marriage and differentials by region, rural-urban, and religion.

1295
Saveland, W. and Glick, P.C.
"First-Marriage Decrement Tables by Color and Sex for the United States in 1958-60." *Demography* 6(3), Aug. 1969: pp. 243-260.

Important set of data based primarily on the 1960 census, providing by age, sex, and race, life-table probabilities for first marriage taking mortality and marriage probabilities into account, probabilities of remaining single, proportions marrying at various time periods after age 14.

1296
Stone, L.
The Crisis of the Aristocracy, 1558-1641. Oxford: Clarendon Press, 1965; 841p.

Study of social change based on personal histories of the 382 English noblemen of this period; data on family life cycle, especially as affected by marriage patterns.

1297
*Tella, A.
"The Economic Cycle in Marriages." *National Industrial Conference Board Business Record* 17(11), Nov. 1960: pp. 20-22.

Demonstrates a large correlation between short-term fluctuations in employment rate and hours worked with marriage rate in U.S. for 1952-60.

1298
Udry, J.R.
"Marital Instability by Race, Sex, Education, and Occupation: Using 1960 Census Data." *American Journal of Sociology* 72(2), Sept. 1966: pp. 203-209.

1960 census data used to compute marriage disruption rates.

1299
Vukovich, G.
"Some Characteristics of Hungarian

Nuptiality." In *International Population Conference.* New York, 1961. London: U.N.E.S.CO., 1963: pp. 319-326.

Historical nuptiality rates and remarriage rates, by demographic variables and by broad occupational strata.

1300
Vukovich, G.
"Some Questions of Marriage Mobility in Budapest." In Szabady et al., eds. (*see* 39): pp. 302-306.

Degrees of homogamy for various occupational strata reported, showing little change over time.

IX.D Fetal mortality, including induced abortion

See also: 56, 81, 96, 236, 468, 489, 557, 582, 670, 671, 672, 681, 697, 722, 933, 1199, 1200, 1210, 1283, 1506, 1527, 1532.

1301
Agarwala, S.N.
"Abortion Rate among a Section of Delhi's Population." *Medical Digest* 30(1), Jan. 1962: pp. 1-7.

Relates abortion rates to age, income, education, and contraceptive use.

1302
Armijo, R. and Monreal, T.
"The Problem of Induced Abortion in Chile." *Milbank Memorial Fund Quarterly* 43(4, Part 2), Oct. 1965: pp. 263-280.

On the high incidence and the social and economic correlates of illegal induced abortion in Santiago.

1303
Bates, J.E. and Zawadaski, E.S.
Criminal Abortion: A Study in Medical Sociology. Springfield, Ill.: Charles C Thomas, 1964; 250p.

An attempt to describe the subculture of criminal abortion in the U.S. on the basis of scattered evidence from doctors, abortionists, clients, case histories, statistical and legal records.

1304
Borell, U.
"Abortion for Controlled Medico-Social Indications in Sweden." *Medical Gynaecology and Sociology* 3(4), Apr. 1968: pp. 90-95.

Incidence of legal abortion in Sweden, 1938-64, including foreign applications for the period 1962-65, socioeconomic, and health aspects.

1305
Coombs, L. et al.
"Inferences about Abortion from Foetal Mortality Data." *Population Studies* 23(2), July 1969: pp. 247-265.

1306
*Devereux, G.
A Study of Abortion in Primitive Societies: A Typological, Distributional and Dynamic Analysis of the Prevention of Birth in 400 Preindustrial Societies. New York: Julian Press, 1955; 394p.

1307
Douglas, C.A.
"Infant and Perinatal Mortality in Scotland." *Vital and Health Statistics* 5, Nov. 1966: 44p.

Analysis of Scottish infant and perinatal mortality in various socioeconomic, physiological, ecological, and marital status groups with discussion of effects of maternal and child welfare policies.

1308
Erhardt, C.L.
"Pregnancy Losses in New York City, 1960." *American Journal of Public Health and the Nation's Health* 53(9), Sept. 1963: pp. 1337-1352.
Estimation of pregnancy loss rates from data of hospitals, clinics, private physicians, and nurses.

1309
Family Planning Association.
Abortion in Britain. Proceedings of a conference held by the Family Planning Association at the University of London Union on 22 Apr. 1966. London: Pitman Medical Publishing, 1966; 125p.
Texts of papers, summary of discussion, and resolutions concerning abortion and its role in health services.

1310
Feldstein, M.S.
"A Binary Variable Multiple Regression Method of Analysing Factors Affecting Peri-natal Mortality and Other Outcomes of Pregnancy." *Journal of the Royal Statistical Society* (Series A, General) 129(1), 1966: pp. 61-73.
Multivariate analysis of factors affecting pregnancy outcomes in Great Britain.

1311
Freedman, R. et al.
"Social Correlates of Fetal Mortality." *Milbank Memorial Fund Quarterly* 44(3, Part 1), July 1966: pp. 327-344.
Relating fetal mortality to age, parity, socioeconomic status, and child spacing in Detroit.

1312
Gold, E.M. et al.
"Therapeutic Abortions in New York City: A 20-Year ReviPw." *American Journal of Public Health and the Nation's Health* 55(7), July 1965: pp. 964-972.
Statistics on the frequency of therapeutic abortion for 1951-62 compared with earlier report for 1943-47; indicates persistent ethnic and racial differences but lower rates.

1313
Hall, M.F.
"Birth Control in Lima, Peru: Attitudes and Practices." *Milbank Memorial Fund Quarterly* 43(4, Part 2), Oct. 1965: pp. 409-438.
Relation of social status to use of contraception or induced abortion in Lima, Peru.

1314
Hall, R.E.
"Therapeutic Abortion, Sterilization, and Contraception." *American Journal of Obstetrics and Gynecology* 91, 15 Feb. 1965: pp. 518-532.
Availability of abortion, sterilization, and contraception in a sample of American hospitals, indicating the greater availability for private patients.

1315
Harter, C.L. and Beasley, J.D.
"A Survey Concerning Induced Abortion in New Orleans." *American Journal of Public Health* 57(11), Nov. 1967: pp. 1937-1947.
Sample survey report on attitudes toward abortion and its reported incidence in relation to age, parity, race, religion, and social class.

1316
Hendricks, C.H.
"Delivery Patterns and Reproductive Efficiency among Groups of Differing Socio-Economic Status and Ethnic Origins." *American Journal of Obstetrics and Gynecology* 97, 1 Mar. 1967: pp. 608-624.
Comparison of pregnancy experience, including abortion and other complications among white and nonwhite patients receiving private or clinic care.

1317

Hong, S.B.

Induced Abortion in Seoul, Korea. Seoul: Dong-A Publishing, 1966; 9lp.

One of the best studies available of the incidence and correlates of illegal induced abortion in a probability sample of married women in a large city; material on the social and demographic correlates, the association with contraceptive practices, and some of the health aspects.

1318

Huldt, L.

"Outcome of Pregnancy When Legal Abortion Is Readily Available." *The Lancet* Mar. 1968: pp. 467-468.

Data on pregnancy outcome in Stockholm, 1950-65; incidence of deliveries was inversely related to incidence of legal abortion, with a slight decline in criminal abortions in last four years.

1319

India. Demographic Training and Research Centre (Chembur).

Demographic, Social and Medical Aspects of Abortion. Bombay: 1968; 116p.

1320

International Conference on Abortion.

The Terrible Choice: The Abortion Dilemma. New York: Bantam Books, 1968; 110p.

Based on the proceedings of the International Conference on Abortion, presents statistical data on abortions; discusses legal, ethical, and social aspects.

1321

Jain, A.K.

"Fetal Wastage in a Sample of Taiwanese Women." *Milbank Memorial Fund Quarterly* 47(3, Part 1), July 1969: pp. 297-306.

Fetal mortality by age of mother, prior contraceptive use, and pregnancy order; considers memory bias and compares results with other studies.

1322

James, W.H.

"Notes towards an Epidemiology of Spontaneous Abortion." *American Journal of Human Genetics* 15(3), Sept. 1963: pp. 223-240.

Analysis of some demographic correlates of abortion based on a nonprobability U.S. sample, following lines of Kinsey studies.

1323

James, W.H.

"Stillbirth and Birth Order." *Annals of Human Genetics* 32(2), Oct. 1968: pp. 151-162.

Model for the relations between birth order and the occurrence of fetal losses of more than 5 months gestation, taking into account alternatives of birth limitation or birth compensation by couples after a fetal loss and of differential fertility.

1324

James, W.H.

"The Causes of Induced Abortion." *Population Studies* 23(1), Mar. 1969: pp. 105-109.

Critique of article by Treffers (see 1345).

1325

Klinger, A.

"Abortion Programs." In Berelson et al., eds. (*see* 53): pp. 465-476.

Relation of legal abortions in Eastern Europe to parity, age, use of contraception, and health.

1326

Kučera, M.

"The Abortion Rate in Czechoslovakia." In *Czechoslovak Population Prob-*

195

lems. Prague: Czechoslovak State Population Committee, 1968: pp. 40-54.

Data on level of and differentials in spontaneous and induced abortion, 1958-67, by age, parity, reasons for abortion, urban-rural.

1327
Lee, N.H.
The Search for an Abortionist. Chicago: University of Chicago Press, 1969; 207p.

Social, psychological, medical, and legal factors of 114 women involved in obtaining an abortion.

1328
Lowe, D. and Lowe, H.V.H.
Abortion and the Law. New York: Pocket Books, 1966; 116p.

1329
Miltényi, K.
"Impact of Heterogeneous Marriages on Birth Control." In Szabady et al., eds. (*see* 39): pp. 153-158.

Effect of the relative occupational and class positions of a large sample of husbands and wives on the use of abortion to interrupt pregnancies.

1330
Niswander, K.R. et al.
"Changing Attitudes towards Therapeutic Abortion." *Journal of the American Medical Association* 196(13), June 1966: pp. 1140-1143.

Incidence of therapeutic abortions in two New York hospitals in relation to family life cycle, religion, and other characteristics.

1331
Pettersson, F.
Epidemiology of Early Pregnancy Wastage: Biological and Social Correlates of Abortion, and Investigation Based on Materials Collected within Uppsala, Sweden. Scandinavian University Books. Stockholm: Svenska Bokförlaget, 1968; 125p.

1332
Potter, R.G., Jr. et al.
"Fetal Wastage in Eleven Punjab Villages." *Human Biology* 3 (3), Sept. 1965: pp. 262-273.

Intensive program of regular home visits in rural India to obtain detailed menstrual and pregnancy histories; important analysis of problems of getting accurate information.

1333
Requena, B.M.
"Social and Economic Correlates of Induced Abortion in Santiago, Chile". *Demography* 2, 1965: pp. 33-49.

Data for working-class area based on sample survey.

1334
Requena, B.M.
"The Problem of Induced Abortion in Latin America." *Demography* 5(2), 1968: pp. 785-799.

Reviews the extent and correlates of induced abortion in Latin America; advances the thesis that an increase in contraception and abortion are likely to go together, since both are solutions to a similar problem in a transitional stage.

1335
Rice-Wray, E.
"The Provoked Abortion: A Major Public Health Problem." *American Journal of Public Health and the Nation's Health* 54(2), Feb. 1964: pp. 313-321.

Summary of findings of Mexican survey concerning socioeconomic and demographic correlates of induced abortion.

1336
Roberts, D.F.
"Probability of Spontaneous Abortion

in Multiparae." *Journal of Reproduction and Fertility* 7(1), Feb. 1964: pp. 89-97.

Data on relation of spontaneous abortion probabilities to pregnancy order.

1337
Robinson, D.
"Precedents of Foetal Death." *American Journal of Obstetrics and Gynecology* 97(7), 1967: pp. 936-942.

U.S. fetal mortality differentials by race, economic status, and prenatal care, based on a sample of fetal deaths and a control sample of live births.

1338
Russell, C. et al.
"Smoking in Pregnancy, Maternal Blood Pressure, Pregnancy Outcome, Baby Weight and Growth, and Other Related Factors. A Prospective Study." *British Journal of Preventive and Social Medicine* 22(3), July 1968: pp. 119-126.

1339
Shapiro, S. et al.
"A Life Table of Pregnancy Terminations and Correlates of Fetal Loss." *Milbank Memorial Fund Quarterly* 40(1), Jan. 1962: pp. 7-45.

Demographic factors affecting fetal mortality based on a large New York sample.

1340
Shapiro, S. et al.
Infant, Perinatal, Maternal, and Childhood Mortality in the United States. American Public Health Association, Vital and Health Statistics Monographs. Cambridge, Mass.: Harvard University Press, 1968; 388p.

1960 monograph examines trends and social and demographic correlates.

1341
Slatis, H.M. and De Cloux, R.
"Seasonal Variation in Stillbirth Frequencies." *Human Biology* 39(3), Sept. 1967: pp. 284-294.

Concurrent analysis of the frequency of stillbirths by month, state, and race; hypothesis to explain seasonal patterns.

1342
Smith, D.T., ed.
Abortion and the Law. Cleveland: Press of Western Reserve University, 1967; 237p.

Essays dealing with legal, medical, and religious aspects of abortion.

1343
Tietze, C.
"Therapeutic Abortions in the United States." *American Journal of Obstetrics and Gynecology* 101(6), July 1968: pp. 784-787.

Estimates of the number of therapautic abortions performed in the U.S., 1963-65, by geographic region, ethnic group, and type of hospital teaching program.

1344
Tietze, C.
"Abortion Laws and Abortion Practices in Europe." Medica International Congress Series, 207. In *Advances in Planned Parenthood—V* 1969; pp. 194-212.

Abortion rates for European countries over several decades, social and demographic correlates of abortion, legal and de-facto grounds for abortion, and incidence of medical complications from abortions.

1345
Treffers, P.E.
"Abortion in Amsterdam." *Population Studies* 20(3), Mar. 1967: pp. 295-309.

Abortion estimates in relation to social status, practice of contraception, and communication between patients for hospital sample.

1346
Valaoras, V.G. et al.
"Greece: Postwar Abortion Experience." *Studies in Family Planning* 46, Oct. 1969: pp. 10-16.

1347
Warburton, D. and Fraser, F.C.
"Spontaneous Abortion Risks in Man: Data from Reproductive Histories Collected in a Medical Genetics Unit." *American Journal of Human Genetics* 16(1), Mar. 1964: pp. 1-25.
Effect of demographic and physiological factors on the incidence of spontaneous abortions in samples used in genetic family history studies.

1348
Westoff, C. et al.
"The Structure of Attitudes toward Abortion." *Milbank Memorial Fund Quarterly* 47(1), Jan. 1969: pp. 11-37.
Clusters of abortion attitudes, derived by factor analysis, related to social and demographic categories.

1349
World Health Organization.
"Causes of Foetal Mortality." *Epidemiological and Vital Statistics Report* (Geneva) 19(6), 1966: pp. 262-334.
Statistical data on causes of fetal mortality, 1945-63.

IX.E Others:
prenuptial pregnancy,
frequency of
intercourse, etc
See also: 81, 1637, 1650.

1350
Chandrasekaran, C. and Talwar, P.P.
"Forms of Age-Specific Birth Rates by Orders of Birth in an Indian Community." *Eugenics Quarterly* 15(4), Dec. 1968: pp. 264-272.
Reproductive histories used to study the influence of age-specific fertility at one birth order on other birth orders and the effect of secondary sterility on the relationships.

1351
Christensen, H.T. and Carpenter, G.R.
"Value-Behavior Discrepancies Regarding Premarital Coitus in Three Western Cultures." *American Sociological Review* 27(1), Feb. 1962: pp. 66-74.
Comparative study of attitudes and reported behavior in the area of premarital coitus in small samples of university students (in Denmark, Utah, Indiana.).

1352
Coombs, L.G. et al.
"Premarital Pregnancy and Status before and after Marriage." *American Journal of Sociology* 75(5), Mar. 1970: pp. 800-820.
A Detroit longitudinal study based on repeated interviews and linked vital records shows that poor educational, occupational, and economic status after marriage of the premaritally pregnant is not a function of their low status origins; poor educational preparation explains much but not all of the postmarital disadvantage.

1353
Dooghe, G.
"Premarital Conceptions with Married Couples According to Socioprofessional Status." *Journal of Marriage and the Family* 30(2), May 1968: pp. 324-328.
Uses official population registers to study occupational differentials in age at marriage, fertility, and especially premarital conceptions.

1354
Goldstein, S.
"Premarital Pregnancies and Out-of-Wedlock Births in Denmark, 1960-65."
Demography 4(2), 1967: pp. 925-936.
  Estimates trends (1938-65) in premarital conceptions by age and rural-urban residence.

1355
Hartley, S.M.
"The Amazing Rise of Illegitimacy in Great Britain." *Social Forces* 44(4), June 1966: pp. 533-545.
  Presents and comments on statistics for England and Wales, 1938-62, on illegitimate and premaritally conceived legitimate materni-ties, with notes on comparable statistics for the United States.

1356
Henderson, M. and Kay, J.
"Differences in Duration of Pregnancy. Negro and White Women of Low Socio-economic Class." *Archives of Environmental Health* 14, June 1967: pp. 904-911.

1357
Lowrie, S.H.
"Early Marriage: Premarital Pregnancy and Associated Factors." *Journal of Marriage and the Family* 27(1), Feb. 1965: pp. 48-56.
  Ohio county study relates premarital preg-nancy to age of bride, length of employment, education and religion.

1358
Nieminen, A.
"Premarital Pregnancy in Finland." *Acta Sociologica* (Copenhagen) 7(4), 1964: pp. 225-228.
  Level, and some correlates of, premarital pregnancy in Finland, 1939-61.

1359
Wilson, K.
"Fertility in Newcastle-upon-Tyne." *Medical Gynaecology and Sociology* 3(8), Aug. 1968: pp. 246-251.
  Analysis of marriage-conception intervals 1960-64, by age at marriage, social class, and religion.

IX.F Combinations of any other intermediate variables without primary stress on any one (including interactions among them)

See also: 64, 98, 319, 560, 581, 587, 1089, 1493, 1494, 1505, 1508, 1509, 1516, 1518, 1531, 1537, 1538.

1360
Barrett, J.C. and Marshall, J.
"The Risk of Conception on Different Days of the Menstrual Cycle." *Population Studies* 23(3), Nov. 1969: pp. 455-461.
  Analyzes the experience of 241 British cou-ples as a basis for estimating the probability of conception in relation to days of menstrual cycle and as affected by coital frequency.

1361
Christensen, H.T.
"Child Spacing Analysis via Record Linkage: New Data Plus a Summing up from Earlier Reports." *Marriage and Family Living* 25(3), Aug. 1963: pp. 272-280.

Summary of four U.S. and one Danish record linkage studies relating child spacing (particularly pre- and early postmarital) to social status and divorce rates.

1362
Hutton, M.M.
"A Study of Social Factors Affecting Teen-Age Married Multiparae." *Canadian Journal of Public Health* 59(1), Jan. 1968: pp. 10-14.

Analyzes data collected in 1965 from 130 teenage married multiparae and from a control group aged 20-29; compares prematurity and perinatal mortality rates, socioeconomic and educational status of mothers, and pregnancy at the time of marriage.

1363
James, W.H.
"Stillbirth, Neonatal Death and Birth Interval." *Annals of Human Genetics* 32(2), Oct. 1968: pp. 163-172.

British data used to study the relationship between birth interval and perinatal death, controlling for results of prior pregnancies and parity.

1364
Mendoza-Hoyos, H.
"Research Studies on Abortion and Family Planning in Colombia." *Milbank Memorial Fund Quarterly* 46(3, Part 2) July 1968: pp. 223-234.

1365
Potter, R.G., Jr. et al.
"Variable Fecundability and the Timing of Births." *Eugenics Quarterly* 15(3), Sept. 1968: pp. 155-163.

Computer simulation model used to derive estimates of the distribution of fecundability of couples interrupting contraception and consequences for fertility.

1366
Rele, J.R.
"Some Correlates of the Age at Marriage in the United States." *Eugenics Quarterly* 12(1), Mar. 1965: pp. 1-6.

Implications of decline in the age at marriage for the rate of premarital conception, labor-force participation of women, education of women, and stability of marriage.

1367
Westoff, C.F. et al.
"Oral Contraception, Coital Frequency, and the Time Required to Conceive." *Social Biology* 16(1), Mar. 1969: pp. 1-10.

Interesting, elegantly reasoned analysis concluding that in the U.S. oral contraception is conducive to higher rates of coitus, but no difference in the time required to conceive when contraception is interrupted.

X. THE EFFECTS ON OTHER ASPECTS OF THE SOCIETY OF NORMS AND ACTUAL LEVELS AND PATTERNS OF FERTILITY, BIRTH SPACING, AND THE INTERMEDIATE VARIABLES

X.A Individual educational attainment and intelligence, aggregate effects on the educational system

See also: 572, 573, 1397, 1408, 1489.

1368
*Anastasi, A.
"Intelligence and Family Size." *Psychological Bulletin* 53(3), May 1956: pp. 187-209.
A review of the literature.

1369
Australia. Commonwealth Department of Education and Science.
"Problems Arising Out of the Post-War Rise in the Annual Birthrate as They Have Affected Australia's Primary, Secondary and Tertiary Education Systems." In 1967 I.U.S.S.P. (*see* 21): pp. 215-222.

1370
Brayer, F.T.
"Birth Order and College Attendance."
Journal of Marriage and the Family 28(4), Nov. 1966: pp. 480-484.
Finds that early parity children are more likely to attend college in a national sample of U.S. high school students; controls for socioeconomic status and family size. (For comment see 1374.)

1371
Chopra, S.L.
"Family Size and Sibling Position as Related to Measured Intelligence and Academic Achievement." *Journal of Social Psychology* 70, Oct. 1966: pp. 133-137.

1372
Folger, J.K. and Nam, C.B.
Education of the American Population. Washington: Government Printing Office, 1967; 290p.
General study of educational trends in the U.S.; analysis of the effect of changing composition of the population.

1373
Glass, D.V.
Differential Fertility, Ability and Educational Objectives: Problems for Study.
Godfrey Thomson Lecture. Edinburgh: Moray House, 1961; 27p.

1374
Hermalin, A.I.
"Birth Order and College Attendance: A Comment." *Journal of Marriage and the Family* 29(3), Aug. 1967: pp. 417-421.

A comment on item 1370.

1375
Higgins, J.V. et al.
"Intelligence and Family Size: A Paradox Resolved." *Eugenics Quarterly* 9(2), June 1962: pp. 84-90.

Empirical study in the U.S. which concludes that high reproduction rate of low I.Q. parents does not result in declining I.Q. rate because a large proportion of siblings of such parents do not marry or are childless.

1376
Lee, Y.J.
"Population Growth and the Problem of Education in Taiwan." Bank of China, *Economic Review* (Taipei) 101, Sept.-Oct. 1964: pp. 11-23.

1377
Malt, S.
"The Effect of Demographic Change on Public Education Expenditures." *Review of Social Economy* 26(2), Sept. 1968: pp. 118-129.

Examines the effect of population growth and changes in the age structure on public education expenditures.

1378
Mehta, P.
"Family Size and Intelligence of Gujarati Secondary School Pupils under Urban Conditions." *Indian Journal of Social Work* (Bombay) 21(1), June 1960: pp. 75-79.

Contradicts conclusions of Western studies of an inverse relation between family size, birth order, and intelligence.

1379
Nisbet, J.D. and Entwistle, N.J.
"Intelligence and Family Size, 1949-1965." *British Journal of Educational Psychology* 37: June 1967: pp. 188-193.

1380
***Quensel, C.T.E.**
"The Interrelations of Marital Status, Fertility, Family Size, and Intelligence Test Scores." *Population Studies* 11(3), Mar. 1958: pp. 234-250.

1381
Scott, J.A.
"Intelligence, Physique, and Family Size." *British Journal of Preventive and Social Medicine* 16(4), Oct. 1962: pp. 165-173.

Relates family size to reasoning test scores and physical development; considers social class factors.

X.B The economy

X.B.1 Macroeconomic (e.g., economic development, cyclical fluctuations, public costs)

See also: 362, 440, 618, 675, 684, 686, 917, 1051, 1053, 1539, 1559, 1567, 1569, 1584.

1382
Balakrishma, R.
Review of Economic Growth in India.
Bangalore City: Bangalore Press, 1961; 247p.
Includes discussions of effects on economic development of population trends, family structure, and the family planning programs.

1383
Cabello, O.
"Housing, Population Growth, and Economic Development." In *Population Dilemma in Latin America.* Edited by J.M. Stycos and J. Arias. Washington: American Assembly, 1966: pp. 101-122.

1384
Chilman, C.S.
"Population Dynamics and Poverty in the United States." *Welfare in Review* 4(6), June-July 1966: pp. 1-13.
General discussion of the possible relation of fertility trends to the incidence of poverty; illustrative statistics.

1385
Coale, A.J.
"The Economic Effects of Fertility Control in Undeveloped Areas." In *Human Fertility and Population Control.* Edited by R.O. Greep. Cambridge, Mass.: Schenkman, 1963; pp. 143-162.
A succinct statement of the argument that in less-developed countries a reduction of fertility has potentially favorable economic effects.

1386
*Coale, A.J. and Hoover, E.M.
Population Growth and Economic Development in Low-Income Countries. Princeton: Princeton University Press, 1958; 389p.
Historically important analysis of the consequences of high fertility and low fertility for development, with special reference to India and Mexico.

1387
David, A.S.
"Nepal: National Development, Population, and Family Planning." *Studies in Family Planning* 1(42), May 1969: pp. 6-16.
Examines impact of projected growth rates on gross domestic product, plans for elementary education, and cereal grain availability; briefly reviews history of family planning program and suggests greater development of organizational and administrative aspects.

1388
Demeny, P.
"Investment Allocation and Population Growth." *Demography* 2, 1965: pp. 203-232.
Important analysis of the short-run economic effects of investments in family limitation programs, using a model population with alternative population projections.

1389
Denison, E.F.
Why Growth Rates Differ. Washington: Brookings Institution, 1967; 494p.
Analysis of postwar economic growth in Western Europe and the U.S., including demographic factors.

1390
Easterlin, R.A.
"Long Swings in United States Demographic and Economic Growth: Some Findings on the Historical Pattern." *Demography* 2, 1965: pp. 490-507.

Examines factors in the relationship of Kuznets' cycles evident in demographic and labor-force growth.

1391
Easterlin, R.A.
"Effects of Population Growth on the Economic Development of Developing Countries." *Annals of the American Academy of Science* 369, Jan. 1967: pp. 98-108.

1392
Enke, S.
Economics for Development. Englewood Cliffs, N.J.: Prentice-Hall, 1963; 616p.
General text on developmental economics includes chapter on the demographic problems; suggests incentive payment scheme for vasectomy.

1393
Enke, S.
"Population and Development: A General Model." *Quarterly Journal of Economics* 77(1), Feb. 1963: pp. 55-70.
Population-investment growth model.

1394
Enke, S.
"The Economic Aspects of Slowing Population Growth." *The Economic Journal* 76(301), Mar. 1966: pp. 44-56.
Model for estimating high return in development of investments in birth prevention.

1395
Enke, S.
"Birth Control for Economic Development." *Science* 164(3881), May 1969: pp. 798-802.
Computer-model estimates of the effect of declining fertility on indexes of economic welfare.

1396
Enke, S. and Zind, R.G.
"Effect of Fewer Births on Average Income." *Journal of Biosocial Science* 1(1), Jan. 1969: pp. 41-55.
Model of the effect of fertility reduction on economic development, including consideration of changes in savings, investment, and labor force.

1397
Foster, P. and Yost, L.
"Uganda: Population Growth and Rural Development." *Studies in Family Planning* 1(43), June 1969: pp. 1-6.
Population projections for an African agricultural village used to assess the impact of population growth on per-capita income via its effect on educational attainment.

1398
Gendell, M.
"The Influence of Fertility Trends on the Potential for Domestic Capital Formation in Latin America." *Estadistica* (Washington) 23(89), Dec. 1965: pp. 675-686.
Discusses mechanisms by which declining fertility influences age structure, rate of saving, and allocation of investment.

1399
Habakkuk, J.
"Population Problems and European Economic Development in the Late Eighteenth and Nineteenth Centuries." *American Economic Review* 53(2), May 1963: pp. 607-618.

1400
Hamilton, F.E.I.
Yugoslavia: Patterns of Economic Activity. New York: Frederick A. Praeger, 1968; 384p.
Discusses demographic factors.

1401

Hansen, B. and Marzouk, G.A.
Development and Economic Policy in the U.A.R. (Egypt). Amsterdam: North-Holland, 1965; 333p.

Includes demographic and socioeconomic profile of U.A.R. and a discussion of population policies in the context of economic development.

1402

Hoover, E.M.
"Economic Consequences of Population Growth." *Indian Journal of Economics* (Allahabad) 47(184), July 1966: pp. 1-11. [Also in *Indian Journal of Public Health* 12, Jan. 1968: pp. 17-22.]

Examines briefly interrelationships of population growth and composition with per-capita economic growth.

1403

Hoover, E.M. and Perlman, M.
"Measuring the Effects of Population Control on Economic Development: A Case Study of Pakistan." *Pakistan Development Review* 6(4), Winter 1966: pp. 545-566.

Estimates the effect of mortality and fertility reductions on aggregate and per-capita income, savings, output, and the need for imported capital.

1404

Husain, I.Z.
"Population and Economic Development." *Indian Journal of Economics* (Allahabad) 44(172), July 1963: pp. 23-40.

Examines hypotheses about relation of fertility and other vital rates to socioeconomic factors from data on 19 countries at different per-capita income levels.

1405

Jones, E.L. and Mingay, G.E., eds.
Land, Labour and Population in the In-dustrial Revolution Essays Presented to J.D. Chambers, London: Edward Arnold; New York: Barnes & Noble, 1967; 286p.

Several essays on population growth and economic development in eighteenth- and nineteenth-century Britain.

1406

Jones, G.W. and Gingrich, P.
"The Effects of Differing Trends in Fertility and of Educational Advance on the Growth, Quality, and Turnover of the Labor Force." *Demography* 5(1), 1968: pp. 226-248.

Implications for developing countries of alternate assumptions about future fertility and educational inputs.

1407

Kelley, A.C.
"Demographic Change and Economic Growth: Australia, 1861-1911." *Explorations in Entrepreneurial History* 5, Spring-Summer 1968: pp. 207-277.

Economic analysis of the impact of demographic change on economic growth in Australia, trends in migration and their influence on age structure and fertility, labor-force growth and the dependency burden, residential development and life-cycle patterns of saving; analysis of correlation of cyclical fluctuations.

1408

Kuznets, S.
Modern Economic Growth: Rate, Structure, and Spread. Studies in Comparative Economics, 7. New Haven: Yale University Press, 1966; 529p.

A general work that discusses fertility and population growth in the context of economic growth.

1409

Kuznets, S.
"Population and Economic Growth."

Proceedings of the American Philosophical Society 111(3), June 1967: pp. 170-192.

Analysis, with illustrations, of how fertility change and other aspects of population growth may interact with other economic and cultural conditions in economic growth.

1410
Kuznets, S.
"Economic Aspects of Fertility Trends in the Less Developed Countries." In Behrman et al., eds. (*see* 51): pp. 157-179.

Key issues in the relation of economic development, fertility, and other demographic variables; gives more attention than most scholars to factors that may accentuate the relationship.

1411
Lakshman, T.K.
"Main Bottlenecks in the Growth of Indian Economy." *AICC Economic Review* (Delhi) 16(8), Sept. 1964: pp. 19-24.

Relation of population growth to future economic planning.

1412
Lampman, R.J.
"Some Interactions between Economic Growth and Population Change in the Philippines." *The Philippine Economic Journal* 6(1), no. 11, First Semester 1967: pp. 1-20.

Examines economic growth effects of alternative population growth rates.

1413
Lewis, W.A.
Development Planning: The Essentials of Economic Policy. London: George Allen & Unwin; New York: Harper & Row, 1966; 270p.

Examination of the process of development planning, including population growth factors.

1415
Linden, F.
"Consumer Markets: Marriages and Families." *Conference Board Business Management Record* Sept. 1963: pp. 56-58.

Significance of trends in family formation in the U.S. (1940-75) for marketing.

1416
Lipton, M.
"Population, Land, and Decreasing Returns to Agricultural Labor." Oxford University, Institute of Economics and Statistics *Bulletin* 26(2), May 1964: pp. 123-157.

Ricardian theory of diminishing returns to agricultural labor applied to South Asia; suggests need for birth control in reducing excess rural population.

1417
Meade, J.E.
"Population Explosion, the Standard of Living and Social Conflict." *Economic Journal* 77(306), June 1967: pp. 233-255.

Discussion of the economic problems of rapid population growth under conditions of high density, with illustrations from Mauritius.

1417
Okazaki, Y.
"Population, Labour Force and Economic Development in Japan." In 1967 I.U.S.S.P. (*see* 21): pp. 63-69.

Projections of labor force and productivity indicate that low fertility of recent years—even when combined with high recent productivity—will leave significant labor shortages in particular parts of Japanese economy requiring changes in present system of lifetime attachment to firms and industries.

1418
Ominde, S.H.
"The Population Factor in Kenya's

Economic Development." *Bulletin of the International Institute for Labour Studies* (Geneva) 3, Nov. 1967: pp. 14-28.

1419
Rau, B.R.K.
"Some Economic Aspects of the Population Problem in India." *AICC Economic Review* (Delhi) 17(3), July 1965: pp. 35-40.
Considers the effect of birth rate levels and trends on economic planning in India, with international comparison.

1420
Rivlin, A.M.
"Population Growth and the American Economy." In *Population Ethics*. Edited by E.X. Quinn. Washington: Corpus Books, 1968: pp. 43-57.
Impact of recent fertility trends on U.S. economy, considering both public and private cost of children.

1421
Rizk, H.
"Population Growth and Its Effect on Economic and Social Goals in the United Arab Republic." *Population Review* (Madras) 7(1), Jan. 1963: pp. 51-56.
History of accelerating Egyptian population growth 1800-1960 related to stagnant postwar per-capita national income.

1422
Robinson, J.
"Population and Development." *Pakistan Economic Journal* (Dacca) 10(1), Mar. 1960: pp. 1-7.
Outline of arguments on the effects of population size and rates of economic change.

1423
Ruprecht, T.K.
"Fertility Control and Per Capita Income in the Philippines: Some First Approximations." *Philippine Economic Journal* 6(1), no. 11, First Semester 1967: pp. 21-48.
Aggregate production function model used to analyze the effect of population growth on economic development.

1424
Ruprecht, T.K.
"Fertility Control, Investment and Per Capita Output: A Demographic-Econometric Model of the Philippines." In 1967 I.U.S.S.P. (*see* 21): pp. 98-107.
Regression model, based on historical economic relations, shows that without reduced fertility economic deterioration is likely to occur soon; with improved economic input conditions, fertility reduction will increase the resulting benefits considerably.

1425
Sheppard, H.L.
Effects of Family Planning on Poverty in the United States. Kalamazoo, Mich.: W.E. Upjohn Institute for Employment Research, 1967; 27p.
Discusses the potential impact of family planning on the reduction of poverty.

1426
Spengler, J.J.
"Population Movements and Economic Development in Nigeria." In *The Nigerian Political Scene*. Edited by R.O. Tilman and T. Cole. Durham: Duke University Press, 1962: pp. 147-197.
Considers economic effects, growth, and changes in composition of population.

1427
Spengler, J.J.
"Demographic Factors and Early Modern Economic Development." *Daedalus* 97(2), Spring 1968: pp. 433-446.

Examines the contribution of slow population in preindustrial Western Europe to economic growth.

1428
Strauss, C.B.
"Population Growth and Economic Developments." *South African Journal of Economics* 31(2), June 1963: pp. 138-148.
Outline of theory and application to South Africa.

1429
Tachi, M. and Okazaki, Y.
"Economic Development and Population Growth—with Special Reference to Southeast Asia." *The Developing Economies* (Tokyo) 3(4), Dec. 1965: pp. 497-515.
Comparative study of demographic situation of Japan and Southeast Asia.

1430
United Nations. Economic Commission for Africa.
"Demographic Factors Related to Social and Economic Development in Africa." *Economic Bulletin for Africa* (Addis Ababa) 2(2), June 1962: pp. 59-81.

1431
Walker, K.
"Ideology and Economic Discussion in China: Ma Yin-Ch'u on Development Strategy and His Critics." *Economic Development and Cultural Change* 11(2, Part 1), Jan. 1963: pp. 113-133.
Includes examination of the content articles between 1955 and 1960 on the interrelations of population and economic development.

1432
Yamaguchi, J.T.
"Recent Development in Employment and the Labour Force in Japan—Aspects of Trend in Labour Shortage." In 1967 I.U.S.S.P. (*see* 21): pp. 113-124.
Demonstrates how the age-structure effects of fertility trends have affected labor supply, sources of labor recruitment, and many aspects of labor market in Japan, with larger changes in prospect for rest of century.

X.B.2 Microeconomic (e.g., family expenditures, the economic position of the family)
See also: 83, 377, 501, 502, 655, 1352, 1532.

1433
David, M.H.
Family Composition and Consumption. Amsterdam: North-Holland, 1962; 109p.
U.S. survey data on family expenditures in relation to age, marital status, and family size.

1434
***Forsyth, F.G.**
"The Relationship between Family Size and Family Expenditure." *Journal of the Royal Statistical Society* (Series A) 123(4), 1960: pp. 367-397.

1435
Freedman, R. and Coombs, L.
"Childspacing and Family Economic Position." *American Sociological Review* 31(5), Oct. 1966: pp. 631-648.
Presents evidence that child spacing affects family income, assets, and income position, independently of actual and expected family size in Detroit, Michigan.

1436
*Henderson, A.M.
"The Cost of a Family." *Review of Economic Studies* 17(43), 1949-50: pp. 127-148.

1437
Lorimer, F.
"The Economics of Family Formation under Different Conditions." In *Proceedings of the World Population Conference, 1965. (see* 44): pp. 92-96.
Attempts to show how balance of production and consumption for families and societies is affected by variations in birth and death rates, which affect age and sex structures.

1438
Orshansky, M.
"More about the Poor in 1964." *Social Security Bulletin* 29(5), May 1966: pp. 3-38.
Relation of family size and poverty in detailed profile of the U.S. poor.

1439
Schorr, A.L.
"The Family Cycle and Income Development." *Social Security Bulletin* 29(2), Feb. 1966: pp. 14-25.
Compares the timing of stages of family growth, income, aspirations, and occupational choice as basis for considering conflict of aspiration and need, with relevance to proposed income maintenance programs.

X.C Social mobility
See also: 536.

1440
Tien, H.Y.
"Mobility, Non-Familial Activity, and Fertility." *Demography* 4(1), 1967: pp. 218-227.
Survey of the results of U.S. studies of the relationship of family size to social mobility and female nonfamilial activity.

X.D Employment status of women
See also: 598, 1302, 1440, 1650.

1441
Cain, G.G.
Married Women in the Labor Force. Chicago: University of Chicago Press, 1966; 159p.
Economic analysis of the labor-force participation of married women in the U.S.; basic model includes family-size variables.

1442
Dodge, N.T.
Women in the Soviet Economy: Their Role in Economic, Scientific, and Technical Development. Baltimore: Johns Hopkins Press, 1966; 331p.
Chapter on demographic factors affecting employment.

1443
Kučera, M.
"Employment of Women and Reproduction." *Czechoslovak Population Problems.* Prague: Digest Bulletin of the Czechoslovak State Population Committee, 1967: pp. 26-31.

1444

Michel, A.

"Needs and Aspirations of Married Women Workers in France." *International Labour Review* (Geneva) 94(1), July 1966: pp. 39-53.

> On the basis of a questionnaire survey, analyzes aspirations of women workers in relation to number of children, income, and other social factors.

X.E Individual health and physical development, effects on health services

See also: 490, 1381, 1470.

1445

Barker, J.S.F.

"The Effect of Partial Exclusion of Certain Matings and Restriction of Their Average Family Size on the Genetic Composition of a Population." *Annals of Human Genetics* 30(1), 1966: pp. 7-11.

> On the prevention and cure of genetic disease; examines consequences in the first and later generations of partial as opposed to total exclusion.

1446

Barker, D.J.P. and Record, R.G.

"The Relationship of the Presence of Disease to Birth Order and Maternal Age." *American Journal of Human Genetics* 19(3, Part 2) May 1967: pp. 433-

1447

Calderone, M.S.

"Public Health Aspects of Famly Plan-

ning." *Applied Therapeutics* (Toronto) 6, Apr. 1964: pp. 338-351.

1448

David, H.P., ed.

Population and Mental Health. Bern: Hans Huber; New York: Springer, 1964; 181p.

> Proceedings of the sixteenth annual meeting of the Federation for Mental Health, August 1963.

1449

Douglas, J.W.B. and Simpson, H.R.

"Height in Relation to Puberty, Family Size and Social Class: a Longitudinal Study." *Milbank Memorial Fund Quarterly* 42(3, Part 1), July 1964: pp. 20-35.

> Height and age at sexual maturation related to social class and number of siblings for 3,000 children born in Great Britain in 1946.

1450

German, J.

"Mongolism, Delayed Fertilization and Human Sexual Behavior." *Nature* 217, Feb. 1968: pp. 516-518.

> Examines the relation of coital frequency, duration of marriage, and maternal age to the incidence of mongoloid children.

1451

Goodman, L.A.

"Some Possible Effects of Birth Control on the Incidence of Disorders and on the Influence of Birth Order." *Annals of Human Genetics* 27(1), Aug. 1963: pp. 41-52.

> On the effect of the birth of a child with a particular disorder on further reproduction the relation to birth order.

1452

Grant, M.W.

"Rate of Growth in Relation to Birth

Rank and Family Size." *British Journal of Preventive and Social Medicine* 18(1), Jan. 1964: pp. 35-42.

Nine-year growth records of children in relation to birth order and number of siblings.

1453
Hill, A.C. and Jaffe, F.S.
"Negro Fertility and Family Size Preferences: Implication for Programming of Health and Social Services." In *The Negro American.* Edited by T. Parsons and K.B. Clark. Boston: Houghton Mifflin, 1966; pp. 205-224.

1454
Hunt, E.P.
Recent Demographic Trends and Their Effects on Maternal and Child Health Needs and Services. U.S. Children's Bureau. Washington: Government Printing Office, 1966; 20p.

1455
Illsley, R.
"Family Growth and Its Effect on the Relationship between Obstetric Factors and Child Functioning." In *Social and Genetic Influences on Life and Death.* Edited by R. Platt and A.S. Parkes. Eugenics Society Symposia, vol. 3. Edinburgh: Oliver & Boyd, 1967.

1456
Jayant, K.
"Effect of Parity on Optimal and Critical Birth Weights." *Annals of Human Genetics* 29(4), May 1966: pp. 363-365.

1457
Jennett, W.B. and Cross, J.N.
"Influence of Pregnancy and Oral Con-

traception on the Incidence of Strokes in Women of Childbearing Age." *Lancet* 7498, 1967: pp. 1010-1023.

Analysis by age, sex, pregnancy rate, mortality rate, use of orals, in comparison with controls of United Kingdom and Scottish populations.

1458
Lindsay, J.S. et al.
"Family Size and Admission to Psychiatric Hospitals." *Medical Journal of Australia* (Sydney) 2, Aug. 1964: pp. 262-264.

1459
Matsunaga, E.
"Possible Genetic Consequences of Family Planning" *Journal of the American Medical Association* 189(5), Oct. 1966: pp. 533-540.

The effects of fertility control in Japan on the incidence of congenital defects.

1460
Roberts, D.F. et al.
"Effects of Parity on Birth Weight and Other Variables in a Tanganyika Bantu Sample." *British Journal of Preventive and Social Medicine* 17, Oct. 1963: pp. 209-215.

1461
Robertson, I. et al.
"Child Health and Family Size. A Survey Relating to the Cape Coloured Population of Cape Town in the Years 1961-62." *South African Medical Journal* (Cape Town) 37, Aug. 1963: pp. 888-893.

1462
Rosa, F.W.
"Impact of New Family Planning Ap-

211

proaches on Rural Maternal and Child Health Coverage in Developing Countries: India's Example." *American Journal of Public Health and the Nation's Health* 57, Aug. 1967: pp. 1327-1332.

X.F Demographic variables: age, size, mortality, migration, sex ratos, population composition

See also: 1, 286, 305, 312, 358, 446, 583, 793, 1643.

1463
Berent, J.
"Causes of Fertility Decline in Eastern Europe and the Soviet Union." *Population Studies* 24(1), Mar. 1970: pp. 35-58.
First part of a larger study that examines the influence of purely demographic changes on the declines in fertility levels over 15 years; suggests that changes in age and sex structure and in nuptiality only partly explain lower fertility levels.

1464
Cann. H.M. and Cavalli-Sforza, L.L.
"Effects of Grandparental and Parental Age, Birth Order, and Geographic Variation on the Sex Ratio of Live-Born and Stillborn Infants." *American Journal of Human Genetics* 20(4), July 1968: pp. 381-391.
Data from a 1960 Italian study.

1465
Chow, L.P. et al.
"The Future Population of Taiwan Pro-

jected by Three Fertility Assumptions." *Journal of the Formosan Medical Association* (Taipei) 64, Sept. 1965: pp. 561-586.

1466
Coale, A.J.
"Birth Rates, Death Rates, and Rate of Growth in Human Population." In Sheps and Ridley, eds. (*see* 73): pp. 242-265.
On the interrelation of vital rates, age structure, and growth rates with special reference to stable population models.

1467
***Coale, A.J. and Tye, C.Y.**
"The Significance of Age-Patterns of Fertility in High Fertility Populations." *Milbank Memorial Fund Quarterly* 39(4), Oct. 1961: pp. 631-646.
Early, important demonstration that the age of parents when children are born, as well as the number of children, may affect population growth rates.

1468
Elliott-Jones, M.F.
"Population Growth and Fertility Behavior." *Conference Board Record* 5(9), Sept. 1968: pp. 34-43.
Examines determinants and implications of U.S. census projections and the relation to fertility behavior theory.

1469
Frejka, T.
"Reflections on the Demographic Conditions Needed to Establish a U.S. Stationary Population Growth." *Population Studies* 22(3), Nov. 1968: pp. 379-397.
Demonstrates the various demographic consequences of attaining a zero rate of population growth in the U.S. under various assumptions about fertility.

1470
Gastil, R.D. and Berry, P.C.
Alternative Birth Rate Projections to 1975 for Maternal and Child Health Planning. Harmon-on-Hudson, N.Y.: Hudson Institute, 1966; 127p.

Sets of projections based on trends in segments of the population; takes account of potential increase in contraception use, changes in age structure and marriage patterns, level of education, religious and racial composition.

1471
Glass, D.V.
"Fertility and Population Growth." In *Malthus Bicentenary Discussion on Fertility, Mortality and World Food Supplies.* Journal of the Royal Statistical Society (Series A) 129(2), 1966; pp. 210-248.

1472
Harewood, J.
"Population Growth in Grenada in the Twentieth Century." *Social and Economic Studies* (Jamaica) 15(2), June 1966: pp. 61-84.

Effect of demographic trends on age structure.

1473
Husain, I.Z.
Divisional Demographic Features and Projections of Uttar Pradesh, 1961-81. Lucknow: Demographic Research Centre, Lucknow University, 1967; 124p.

Fertility and mortality indexes used to project population growth and composition, and to relate differentials to socioeconomic correlates on the basis of division level rates.

1474
Ladinsky, J.
"Sources of Geographic Mobility among Professional Workers: A Multivariate Analysis." *Demography* 4(1), 1967: pp. 293-309.

Multiple regression analysis of the factors affecting migration of professional workers; marital status and family size variables.

1475
Lunde, A. et al.
"Marriages, Births, and Population Growth." *Health, Education, and Welfare Indicators* March 1963: pp. 17-30.

Effect of trends in nuptiality and natality on the growth and age composition of the population, 1920-62, and prospectively to 1975.

1476
Renkowen, K.O.
"The Sex of Live Births Born to Aged Women." *Annales Mediciane Experimentalis et Biologiae Fenniae* (Helsinki) 40(4), 1962: pp. 474-480.

Comparison of sex ratios of live births by age of mother and birth order for U.S. white population and Japan.

1477
Renkowen, K.O.
"Decreasing Sex-Ratio by Birth Order." *Lancet* 1, Jan. 1963: pp. 60.

Sex ratio of liveborns and late fetal deaths by birth order in white U.S. population related to maternal incompatibility, for male offspring with increasing birth order.

1478
Rubin, E.
"The Sex Ratio at Birth." *American Statistician* 21(4), Oct. 1967: pp. 45-48.

Considers variation in the sex ratio at birth by order of birth, by multiplicity of birth, and by age of the parents in U.S. data for 1964.

1479
Tietze, C.
"Mortality with Contraception and In-

duced Abortion." *Studies in Family Planning* 1(45), Sept. 1969: pp. 6-8.

Presents model and estimates of maternal mortality for induced abortion (in and out of hospital) and contraception.

1480
United Nations. Department of Economic and Social Affairs.
"World Population Prospects as Assessed in 1963." *Population Studies*, no. 41. New York: 1966; 149p.

Projections of fertility and mortality for the world and its regions, together with consequences for population size and age-sex distributions.

1481
Visaria, P.M.
"Fallacies in the Demographic Theory of Economic Stagnation." *Economic Weekly* 16(11), Mar. 1964: pp. 523-527.

Indian and model population data used to show the relative effects of mortality and fertility rate changes on labor-force size.

1482
Vukovich, G.
"Some Problems of Analysis of Reproduction." In Szabady et al., eds. (*see* 40): pp. 435-447.

Uses stable population model to estimate differences in actual and stable population age structures in Hungary.

X.G Others: general welfare, family life cycle, etc

See also: 606, 1439, 1529.

1483
Christensen, H.T.
"Children in the Family: Relationship of Number and Spacing to Marital Success." *Journal of Marriage and Family Living* 30(2), May 1968: pp. 283-289.

1484
***Douglas, J.W.B. and Blomfield, J.M.**
Children under Five. London: George Allen & Unwin, 1958; 177p.

Unique longitudinal study of a national sample of children that relates many aspects of their development and welfare to family size.

1485
Moller, H.
"Youth as a Force in the Modern World." *Comparative Studies in Society and History* (The Hague) 10(3), April 1968: pp. 237-260.

Examines the relation of the age distribution of populations to youth-motivated sociopolitical movements from 1750.

1486
Musgrove, F.
"Population Changes and the Status of the Young in England since the Eighteenth Century." *Sociological Review* 11(1), Mar. 1963: pp. 69-93.

Survey of possible effect of fertility and other demographic factors on freedom of population 10-20 years old, with respect to marriage and income.

1487
Osborn, F.H.
The Future of Human Heredity: An Introduction to Eugenics in Modern Society. New York: Weybright and Talley, 1968; 133p.

Overview of current eugenic thinking; analysis of historical demographic trends affecting the qualitative development of populations.

X.H Combinations of the other aspects of the society specified above
See also: 20, 413, 1564.

1488
Anderson, U.M. et al.
"The Medical, Social, and Educational Implications of the Increase in Out-of-Wedlock Births." *American Journal of Public Health and the Nation's Health* 56(11), Nov. 1966: pp. 1866-1873.

1489
Davis, K.
"The Population Impact on Children in the World's Agrarian Countries." *Population Review* (Madras) 9(1 and 2), Jan.-July 1965: pp. 17-31.

Considers impact of high fertility and growth rates on the welfare of children, with special reference to problems of education and potential for change through investments in education.

1490
Hillery, G.A.
"Navajos and Eastern Kentuckians: A Comparative Study in the Cultural Consequences of the Demographic Transition." *American Anthropologist* 68(1), Feb. 1966: pp. 52-70.

Empirical test for two culturally different populations of a series of hypotheses about changes that occur during the demographic transition (see 1543).

1491
Pohlman, E.
"Unwanted Conceptions: Research on Undesirable Consequences." *Eugenics Quarterly* 14(2), June 1967: pp. 143-154.

Presents hypothesis about causal links from unwanted pregnancies to undesirable consequences, indicating lack of evidence now to test them.

1492
Pohlman, E.
"The Timing of First Births: A Review of Effects." *Eugenics Quarterly* 15(4), Dec. 1968: pp. 252-263.

Reviews findings of various studies, 1939-68, and discusses the medical and demographic effects of strategies to raise age at first birth.

XI. MAJOR INTENSIVE SAMPLE SURVEYS DEALING SIMULTANEOUSLY WITH SOCIAL VARIABLES, SOCIAL NORMS, INTERMEDIATE VARIABLES, AND FERTILITY (ORIGINAL STUDIES AND CRITIQUES)

See also: 95, 525, 528, 923, 1224, 1233.

1493
Abhayaratne, O.E.R. and Jayewardene, C.H.S.
Fertility Trends in Ceylon. Colombo: Colombo Apothecaries, 1967; 421p.
> Uses both official demographic data and a special KAP survey to review trends, levels, and correlates of nuptiality, fertility, family size desires, attitudes, and practice of contraception; includes relationships to income, education, employment, ethnic-religious background, area regions, employment of wife, aspirations for children.

1494
Agualimpia, C. et al.
"Demographic Facts of Colombia. The National Investigation of Morbidity." *Milbank Memorial Fund Quarterly* 47(3, Part 1), July 1969: pp. 225-296.
> Results of a national survey including aspects of fertility, fetal mortality, and abortion; socioeconomic, urban-rural, and age differentials.

1495
Berelson, B.
"Turkey: National Survey on Population." *Studies in Family Planning* 1(5), Dec. 1964: pp. 1-5.
> A summary report of a 1963 survey on knowledge and practice of contraception, attitudes to contraception, desired family size, family planning programs, and population growth; differentials by education, sex, and place of residence.

1496
Byrue, J.
"A Fertility Survey in Barbados." *Social and Economic Studies* 15(4), Dec. 1966: pp. 368-378.
> A description of a Barbados KAP survey.

1497
Caldwell, J.C.
"The Control of Family Size in Tropical Africa." *Demography* 5(2), 1968: pp. 598-619.

General summary of the results of 18 KAP surveys bearing on levels and differentials of fertility, fertility norms, attitudes, and practice of family limitation and familial attitudes in relation to urban-rural differences, and various measures of modernization.

1498
Caldwell, J.C.
Population Growth and Family Change in Africa. The New Urban Elite in Ghana. Canberra: Australian National University Press, 1968; 222p.

Rather unique sample survey of wives and husbands in Ghana's urban elite, indicating that in various practices and attitudes they are changing toward Western models of family life, family planning, and views on population; evidence of considerable ambivalence and mixture of the traditional and modern is important.

1499
Chen, S. et al.
"Pattern of Fertility in Taiwan: Report of a Survey Made in 1957." *Journal of Social Science* (Taipei) 13, 1963; pp. 209-294.

Cohort analysis from four household surveys in villages and urban areas of Taiwanese, mainlanders, and mixed household; studies family size and fertility measures and their socioeconomic and cultural determinents.

1500
Cliquet, R.L.
"The Sociobiological Aspects of the National Survey on Fecundity and Fertility in Belgium." *Journal of Biosocial Science* 1, 1969: pp. 369-388.

General methods and selected results of the 1966 national survey on fecundity and fertility; important methodological problems in measuring both fecundity and contraception, with indications that gross underreporting of contraception can be corrected; indicates that "inefficient" contraceptive methods are widely used, although Belgium's fertility rates are low.

1501
Concepcion, M.B. and Flieger, W.
"Studies of Fertility and Fertility Planning in the Philippines." *Demography* 5(2), 1968: pp. 714-731.

Selected results of a variety of sample surveys bearing on such questions as validity of responses on desired number of children, knowledge, approval, practice of contraception and extent and reasons for discrepancies between these, age and education correlates shown for some data; stresses evidence for poor validity of attitude responses.

1502
*Dandekar, K.
Demographic Survey of Six Rural Communities. Bombay: Asia Publishing House, 1959; 142p.

Investigates the interrelation of social status variables with age at marriage, fertility, attitudes to family planning, and desired family size; finds essentially no relation between social factors and fertility.

1503
*Dandekar, V.M. and Dandekar, K.
Survey of Fertility and Mortality in Poona District. No. 27. Poona: Gokhale Institute of Politics and Economics, 1953; 191p.

1504
Driver, E.D.
Differential Fertility in Central India. Princeton: Princeton University Press, 1963; 191p.

KAP study for a sample in Nagpur district in 1958, which relates fertility, age at marriage, and child mortality to each other and to caste, income, education, rural-urban residence, occupation, and family type; finds generally small or no relationships to socioeconomic variables.

1505
Erlich, V. St.
Family in Transition: A Study of 300 Yugoslav Villages. Princeton: Princeton University Press, 1966; 489p.

A village-level study based on national sample of schoolteachers who answered questionnaires about the family structure, family and reproductive cycle, and social conditions in villages with which they are familiar.

1506
*Freedman, R. et al.
Family Planning, Sterility, and Population Growth. New York: McGraw-Hill, 1959; 515p.

The first of the Growth of American Families studies (1955), which involved a probability sample of white married women of childbearing age and related social and demographic variables to reports on actual fertility, expectations, desires, practice of contraception, and attitudes to it; includes among the social variables religion, education, income, occupation, city size, farm background.

1507
Freedman, R. et al.
"Fertility and Family Planning in Taiwan: A Case Study of the Demographic Transition." *American Journal of Sociology* 70(1), July 1964: pp. 16-27.

Early report on analysis in item 1508.

1508
Freedman, R. et al.
Family Planning in Taiwan: An Experiment in Social Change. Princeton: Princeton University Press, 1969; 501p.

Extensive analysis of a large-scale family planning action program in Taichung based on surveys before, during, and after the program, clinic records, and registration statistics; examines social and demographic correlates of fertility and birth control before and after; also a chapter on the larger, island-wide Taiwan program.

1509
Goyal, R.P. and Bisht, N.
Fertility and Family Planning in a Railway Workers Colony of Delhi. Delhi: Institute of Economic Growth, 1969; 96p.

Data from 1962 survey of fertility and family planning attitudes and use; socioeconomic, religious, caste, and family-size differentials.

1510
*Hatt, P.K.
Backgrounds of Human Fertility in Puerto Rico: A Sociological Survey. Princeton: Princeton University Press, 1952; 512p.

One of the first examples of use of a national sample survey to study the interrelation of social and economic variables, fertility norms, and fertility behavior.

1511
*Hill, R. et al.
The Family and Population Control: A Puerto Rican Experiment in Social Change. Chapel Hill: University of North Carolina Press, 1959; 481p.

Major survey and experiment studying the interrelation of social and economic variables, family structure, fertility norms, and fertility; places special emphasis on intrafamilial relations; tested various educational approaches for reducing the birth rate.

1512
* Kiser, C.V. and Whelpton, P.K. eds.
Social and Psychological Factors Affecting Fertility. 5 vols. New York: Milbank Memorial Fund, 1958.

Reports on the pioneering Indianapolis fertility study, one of the first intensive surveys to interrelate social norms about fertility and family planning to actual fertility and to a large number of demographic, social, and psychological variables; description of the basic study design and report analyses of specific hypotheses by many different authors.

(Only a few of the more important articles are individually listed.)

1513
Korea. Ministry of Health and Social Affairs.
The Findings of the National Survey on Family Planning, 1965. Seoul: 1965; 138p. [Text in Korean and English.]
Methodology and some of the results of major national benchmark KAP survey used to evaluate the Korean program for family planning.

1514
Korea. Ministry of Health and Social Affairs.
The Findings of the National Survey on Family Planning, 1966. Seoul: Planned Parenthood Federation of Korea, 1966; 221p. [Text in Korean and English.]
Presents findings of a nationwide field survey of a random sample of some 5,000 women; brief comparison with results of earlier surveys.

1515
Lopez, A.
"Some Notes on Fertility Problems in a Colombian Semi-urban Community." *Demography* 4(2), 1967: pp. 453-463.
Fragmentary data for sample of 100 women used to examine marriage and fertility patterns, birth spacing, coital frequency, contraceptive attitudes and use, and fecundability.

1516
Malaysia. National Family Planning Board.
Report on the West Malaysian Family Survey, 1966-1967. Kuala Lumpur: 1968; 534p.
Report on a national probability sample survey includes results on fertility, nuptiality, and family planning, socioeconomic, racial, and educational differentials; sections on methodology.

1517
Malta. Central Office of Statistics.
An Inquiry into Family Size in Malta and Gozo. Valletta: 1963; 305p.
Fairly extensive sample survey of married women in urban Malta and rural Gozo; detailed description of sampling procedures and characteristics of the sample, fertility rates, nuptiality patterns, age at marriage, child-spacing patterns, population projections.

1518
Miró, C.A.
"Some Misconceptions Disproved: A Program of Comparative Fertility Surveys in Latin America." In Berelson et al., eds. (*see* 53): pp. 615-634.
Report on seven-city comparative study of fertility that stresses the importance of demonstration of feasibility of such studies and presents preliminary results on social correlates of fertility and family planning.

1519
Miró, C.A. and Mertens, W.
"Influences Affecting Fertility in Urban and Rural Latin America." *Milbank Memorial Fund Quarterly* 46(3, Part 2), July 1968: pp. 89-117.
Reviews the major findings from the urban and rural fertility surveys coordinated by C.E.L.A.D.E. for many Latin American countries; demographic and social correlates of contraception, nuptiality, and fertility; urban-rural, educational, occupational, and demographic differentials.

1520
Miró, C.A. and Rath, F.
"Preliminary Findings of Comparative Fertility Surveys in Three Latin American Cities." *Milbank Memorial Fund Quarterly* 43(4, Part 2), Oct. 1965: pp. 36-68.

Results of a 1963 survey concerning pregnancy histories, attitudes toward ideal family size, ideal age at marriage, and family planning; differentials by age, marital status, place of birth, occupation, education, religion, and traditional values held.

1521
*Mukherjee, S.B.
Studies on Fertility Rates in Calcutta. Calcutta: Bookland Private, 1961; 143p.
Sample survey on fertility and family planning completed as part of a larger socioeconomic survey of Calcutta.

1522
Murphy, E.M., ed.
Four Fertility Surveys. Quezon City, Philippines: JMC Press, 1968; 134p.
Based on two masters' theses, measures of actual and desired fertility, knowledge, and practice of contraception, by age, marriage duration, education, occupation, and income for four Philippine municipalities.

1523
Otero, L.L.
"The Mexican Urbanization Process and Its Implications." *Demography* 5(2), 1968: pp. 866-873.
Preliminary results of a 1966-68 KAP survey with a national sample of 2,500 couples and 300 leaders in the social, political, and religious fields; knowledge, approval, and use of contraception related to type of rural-urban strata; joint decision making rather than male decision imposition more common in larger cities.

1524
Ozbay, F. and Shorter, F.C.
"Turkey: Changes in Birth Control Practices, 1963 to 1968." *Studies in Family Planning* 1(51), Mar. 1970: pp. 1-7.

Estimates the increase in practice of contraception, changes in attitudes and methods used by comparison of 1963 and 1968 KAP surveys; relates levels and changes to birth cohorts, age, urban, and regional status.

1525
*Pierce, R.M. and Rowntree, G.
"Birth Control in Britain. Part I: 'Attitudes and Practices'." *Population Studies* 15(1), July 1961: pp. 3-31. "Part II: 'Contraceptive Methods Used by Couples Married in the Last Thirty Years.'" *Population Studies* 15(2), Nov. 1961: pp. 121-160.
Reports on a national British KAP study.

1526
Poffenberger, T.
Husband-Wife Communication and Motivational Aspects of Population Control in an Indian Village. Monograph Series, 10. New Delhi: Central Family Planning Institute, 1969; 117p.
Based on five years of observation and interviewing; combines statistics on a small sample with individual case reports; concludes that patterns of communication, mother-in-law role, preference for sons, and family size and family planning values are rational in relation to need for protection of a son, especially for women in old age.

1527
Population Problems Research Council.
Summary of Ninth National Survey of Family Planning. Population Problems Series No. 20. Tokyo: Mainichi Newspapers, 1967; 69p.
Ninth in an extraordinary biennial series of surveys going back to 1950: Based on a multistage area sample survey with interviews covering postwar fertility, familisitic values, desired and actual family size, abortion, contraception, and demographic and social correlates; social correlates include education, occupation, wife's labor-force status, type of

community. (The eighth survey published in 1965 has an especially detailed and useful analysis.)

1528
*Singh, B.
Five Years of Family Planning in the Countryside. Lucknow: J.K. Institute of Sociology and Human Relations, Lucknow University, 1958; 118p.

1529
Srb, V.
"Research Regarding Marriage and Parenthood in Czechoslovakia." In *International Population Conference.* New York, 1961. London: U.N.E.S.C.O., 1963: pp. 138-148.

Survey based on the changing plans for numbers of children, on the use of contraception, on fear of becoming pregnant and sexual satisfaction, with relationships shown to demographic variables, wife's labor-force status, and family's occupational position.

1530
Stycos, J.M. and Back, K.W.
The Control of Fertility in Jamaica. Ithaca, N.Y.: Cornell University Press, 1964; 377p.

A study of the attitudes and reproductive behavior of a sample of "mated" lower class women, together with an experiment to change behavior by bringing information and service to ready but ambivalent elements in the population.

1531
*United Nations.
The Mysore Population Study. ST/SOA/ Ser.A/34. New York: 1961; 352p.

Still one of the most comprehensive studies of its kind available, coverage of a large number of social and economic variables in relation to marriage, fertility, mortality, and family planning; important methodological discussions.

1532
Visuri, E.
Poverty and Children. A Study in Family Planning. Transactions, 16. Helsinki: Westermarck Society, 1969; 154p.

Results from a 1965-66 survey of Helsinki welfare recipients concerning family size ideals and their demographic and socioeconomic correlates; attitudes, knowledge, and use of contraception and abortion; incidence of unwanted children; family size and contraceptive use related to incidence and regularity of public assistance needs.

1533
Waisenen, F.B. and Durlak, J.T.
A Survey of Attitudes Related to Costa Rican Population Dynamics. San José, Costa Rica: American International Association for Social and Economic Development, 1966, 189p.

Sample survey of attitudes of persons over age 20 toward family planning, abortion, ideal family size, and other attitudinal (not behavioral) aspects of fertility and family planning; relation tested by partial correlation to age, urbanism, education, use of mass media, and religiosity.

1534
*Westoff, C.F. et al.
Family Growth in Metropolitan America: Princeton: Princeton University Press, 1961; 433p.

The first report of the Princeton longitudinal fertility study, based on interviews with a sample of women who had recently had a second birth in the 10 largest metropolitan centers in the U.S.; covers a wide range of hypotheses and variables; distinctive in attention to social-psychological measures.

1535
Westoff, C.F. et al.
The Third Child: A Study in the Prediction of Fertility. Princeton: Princeton University Press, 1963; 293p.

Analytical report on findings of second stage of longitudinal study; data from interviews with 905 couples three years after the first interviews in 1957, with the objective being to explain why some couples stopped at two children while others had a third or fourth during this time interval.

1536
Westoff, C.F. et al.
"Some Selected Findings of the Princeton Fertility Study: 1963." *Demography* 1(1), 1964: pp. 130-135.
Survey of major findings with comparison of results with earlier studies.

1537
Whelpton, P.K. et al.
Fertility and Family Planning in the Unit-ed States. Princeton: Princeton University Press, 1966; 443p.
Major survey for a national sample of the U.S. in 1960 of fertility, family planning, fetal mortality, reproductive attitudes in relation to a wide range of social, economic, and demographic variables.

1538
*Yaukey, D.
Fertility Differences in a Modernizing Country. Princeton: Princeton University Press, 1961; 204p.
Pioneering fertility sample survey in Lebanon, with data on socioeconomic and religious correlates of fertility and of such intermediate variables as contraception, fetal mortality, intercourse, and marriage.

XII. DEMOGRAPHIC TRANSITION, OPTIMAL POPULATION, THE DEMOGRAPHIC BALANCE (AS AFFECTED BY THE RELATION OF FERTILITY TO MIGRATION, MORTALITY, AND RESOURCES)

See also: 13, 273, 281, 290, 330, 349, 358, 509, 657, 1028, 1064, 1109, 1134, 1147, 1207, 1416, 1466, 1475, 1490.

1539

Abu-Lughod, J.

"Urban-Rural Differences as a Function of the Demographic Transition: Egyptian Data and an Analytical Model." *American Journal of Sociology* 69(5), Mar. 1964: pp. 476-490.

> Model of demographic transition to predict changes in urban-rural differences for currently modernizing countries, after showing inadequacies of generalizations from Western experiences.

1540

Boserup, E.

Conditions of Agricultural Growth: The Economics of Agricultural Change Under Population Pressure. Chicago: Aldine, 1965; 124p.

> Departs from conventional analyses in emphasizing the role of population pressure in agricultural change, as well as reverse relation.

1541

Clark, C.

Population Growth and Land Use. London: Macmillan; New York: St. Martin's, 1967; 406p.

> Unorthodox view that population growth is associated with rapid increase of wealth and urbanization.

1542

Concepcion, M.B. and Murphy, E.M.

"Wanted: A Theory of the Demographic Transition." In 1967 I.U.S.S.P. (*see* 21): pp. 5-13.

> Review of some recent discussions of transition theory and some data for Asia; concludes that theories to explain the course of demographic transition are urgently needed but not available.

1543

Cowgill, D.O.

"Transition Theory as General Population Theory." *Social Forces* 41(3), Mar. 1963: pp. 270-274.

1544

Davis, K.

"The Theory of Change and Response

in Modern Demographic History." *Population Index* 29(4), Oct. 1963: pp. 345-366.

Important statement of the multiple alternate responses that a population can make to changes in basic social institutions and demographic pressures; based on a review of both contemporary and current evidence.

1545

Douglas, M.

"Population Control in Primitive Groups." *British Journal of Sociology* 17(3), Sept. 1966: pp. 263-273.

Four primitive groups illustrate thesis that indigenous population-control customs develop to try to attain optimum population related to standards of value and prestige that need not correspond to subsistence.

1546

Ehrlich, P.R.

The Population Bomb. New York: Ballantine, 1968; 223p.

A biologist's statement for a mass audience that overpopulation threatens imminent catastrophe for the world in terms of resource and ecological imbalance; stresses necessity of radical action both in population and resource fields.

1547

Feldt, A. and Weller, R.

"The Balance of Social, Economic, and Demographic Change in Puerto Rico 1950-1960." *Demography* 2, 1965: pp. 474-489.

1548

Frederiksen, H.

"Dynamic Equilibrium of Economic and Demographic Transition." *Economic Development and Cultural Change* 14(3), Apr. 1966: pp. 316-322.

Relationship of economic development and demographic transition in 21 countries.

1549

Frederiksen, H.

"Determinants and Consequences of Mortality and Fertility Trends." *Public Health Reports* 81(8), Aug. 1966: pp. 715-727.

Some empirical evidence for the thesis that fertility is more related to mortality decline than purely economic improvements.

1550

Frederiksen, H.

"Feedbacks in Economic and Demographic Transition." *Science* 166, Nov. 1969: pp. 837-847.

Two models of the demographic-economic relationship applied to empirical data.

1551

Friedlander, D.

"Demographic Responses and Population Change." *Demography* 6(4), Nov. 1969: pp. 359-381.

Tests in a preliminary way a theory that the nature of rural-urban fertility differentials in the demographic transition depend partly on internal and international migration opportunities.

1552

Gonzales, A.

"Some Effects of Population Growth on Latin America's Economy." *Journal of Inter-American Studies* 9(1), Jan. 1967: pp. 22-42.

Problems of population growth and resource allocation, with policy implications.

1553

Guzevaty, Y.

"Population Problems in Developing Countries." *International Affairs* (Moscow) 9, Sept. 1966: pp. 52-58.

A Soviet view of the population-development-resources problem.

1554

* Hatt, P.K. et al.

"Types of Population Balance." *American Sociological Review* 20(1), Feb. 1955: pp. 14-20.

Critique of the theory of demographic transition based on factor analysis of vital rates and indexes of modernization.

1555

Hauser, P.M.

"Population, Poverty, and World Politics." Edmund J. James lecture on government, *University of Illinois Bulletin* no. 97, 1965; 16p.

Traces interrelations of trends in population size, differential economic development, and bipolar political alignment.

1556

Heer, D.M.

"The Demographic Transition in the Russian Empire and the Soviet Union." *Journal of Social History* 1(3), Spring 1968: pp. 193-240.

Application of transition theory to Czarist Russia and the Soviet Union; considers the effects of urbanization, agrarian reforms, birth control, child welfare policies, the role of women, changes in the standard of living and in education; summary of estimates of demographic trends, 1861-1965.

1557

Kamerschen, D.R.

"On an Operational Index of 'Overpopulation'." *Economic Development and Cultural Change* 13(2), Jan. 1965: pp. 169-187.

Requirements for a satisfactory index and comments on current measures; suggests the total dependency ratio over 100 as the most useful index.

1558

Kirk, D.

"Natality in the Developing Countries: Recent Trends and Prospects." In *Fertility and Family Planning, A World View.* Edited by S.J. Behrman et al. Ann Arbor: University of Michigan Press, 1969: pp. 75-88.

Summary of recent trends, advancing the important thesis that the time required for the transition from high to low fertility is growing shorter.

1559

*Kuznets, S.

"Long Swings in the Growth of Population and in Related Economic Variables." *Proceedings of the American Philosophical Society* 102(1), Feb. 1958: pp. 25-52.

Important attempt to construct historical time series for the demographic components of population change and to analyze their interaction with long-term economic swings.

1560

Laffin, C.J.

The Hunger to Come. London: Abelard-Schuman, 1966; 207p.

Popular discussion of possibilities of large-scale food shortages and attempts to avert them by demographic means.

1561

Livi Bacci, M.

"Fertility and Nuptiality Changes in Spain from the Late 18th to the Early 20th Century." *Population Studies* 22(1, Part 1), Mar. 1968: pp. 83-102; and 22(2, Part 2), July 1968: pp. 211-234.

Historical analysis of national and regional trends in fertility and nuptiality; develops the thesis that fertility was already under control in eighteenth-century Spain and that its decline is not necessarily related to mortality decline or social development.

1562

Livi Bacci, M.

"Fertility and Population Growth in

Spain in the Eighteenth and Nineteenth Centuries." *Daedalus* 97(2), Spring 1968: pp. 523-535.

1563
McKeown, T.
"Medicine and World Population." In Sheps and Ridley, eds. (*see* 73): pp. 25-40.

On the relative contribution of medicine, other sources of mortality change, and changes in the birth rate to population growth trends through English history, with implications for other areas.

1564
*Meier, R.L.
Modern Science and the Human Fertility Problem. New York: John Wiley & Sons, 1959; 263p.

Natural scientist and planner discusses broad interrelations between past and probable future technological developments and fertility in relation to broad social and economic movements.

1565
*Ohlin, P.G.
"Mortality, Marriage, and Growth in Pre-Industrial Populations." *Population Studies* 14(3), Mar. 1961: pp. 190-197.

Develops theoretical model to demonstrate that if marriage was linked to inheritance and succession then fertility and mortality would tend to be negatively correlated in a balance-maintaining relation.

1566
Osvald, H.
The Earth Can Feed Us. Translated from the Swedish by B. Nesfield-Cookson. London: George Allen & Unwin, 1966; 141p.

Potentials for increased food production for projected population growth as an alternative of population control.

1567
Paddock, W. and Paddock, P.
Famine—1975! America's Decision: Who Will Survive? Boston: Little, Brown, 1967; 276p.

A much-cited, popular, and pessimistic discussion of demographic pressure on world food supplies, with suggested policy implications.

1568
* Petersen, W.
"The Demographic Transition in the Netherlands." *American Sociological Review* 25(3), June 1960: pp. 334-347.

1569
Podyashchikh, P.
"Impact of Demographic Policy on the Growth of the Population." In Szabady et al., eds. (*see* 40): pp. 231-258.

A Soviet demographer's critique of Western theories of the relation among population growth, fertility, and economic development; stresses the distinctive character of the demographic transition under a socialist economy.

1570
Population Reference Bureau.
"Low Birth Rates of European Catholic Countries." *Population Bulletin* 18(2), Mar. 1962: pp. 21-39.

Historical fertility transition in three predominately Catholic countries of Europe in an attempt to relate their experience to the current transition in Latin America.

1571
Roberts, G.W.
"Prospects for Population Growth in the West Indies." *Social and Economic Studies* (Jamaica) 11(4), Dec. 1962: pp. 333-350.

A review, before the dissolution of the Federation of West Indies, of current theories about demographic transition in relation to population development in the West Indies.

1572
* Ryder, N.B.
"The Conceptualization of the Transition in Fertility." Vol. 22. In *Cold Spring Harbor Symposia on Quantitative Biology.* Cold Spring Harbor, N.Y.: Long Island Biological Association, 1957: pp. 91-96.
A significant discussion of transition theory with emphasis on the role of changing patterns of nuptiality and mean age at childbearing.

1573
Satin, M.S.
"An Empirical Test of the Descriptive Validity of the Theory of Demographic Transition on a Fifty-three Nation Sample." *Sociological Quarterly* 10(2), Spring 1969: pp. 190-203.
Test of Cowgill's theory (see 1543).

1574
Shorter, F.C.
"The Application of Development Hypotheses in Middle Eastern Studies." *Economic Development and Cultural Change* 14(3), Apr. 1966: pp. 340-354.
Test of demographic transition and production structure transformation hypotheses using Middle East example.

1575
Solo, R.A.
Economic Organizations and Social Systems. New York: Bobbs-Merrill, 1967; 519p.
Chapter Eleven analyzes Malthusian theories.

1576
Spengler, J.J.
"Population Optima." In *The 99th Hour.* Edited by D.O. Price. Chapel Hill: University of North Carolina Press, 1967: pp. 29-50.
Alternative sets of criteria for evaluating optimum populations.

1577
*Taeuber, I.B.
"Japan's Demographic Transition Re-examined." *Population Studies* 14(1), July 1960: pp. 28-39.

1578
Van Bath, B.H.S.
"Historical Demography and the Social and Economic Development." *Daedalus* 97(2), Spring 1968: pp. 604-621.
Areal differences in population related to social and economic development.

1579
* Van Nort, L. and Karon, B.P.
"Demographic Transition Re-examined." *American Sociological Review* 20(5), Oct. 1955: pp. 523-527.
Critique of study by Hatt et al. (see 1554).

1580
Van de Walle, E. and Knodel, J.
"Demographic Transition and Fertility Decline: The European Case." In 1967 I.U.S.S.P. (*see* 21): pp. 47-55.
An empirical analysis that contradicts the traditional transition theory by showing that the beginning of a significant fertility decline began in various countries of Western Europe under quite different social, economic, and mortality conditions.

1581
Walsh, B.M.
"Another Look at the Concept of 'Over-Population.'" *Economic Development and Cultural Change* 17(1), Oct. 1968: pp. 95-98.
Comment on suggestions made in item 1557.

1582

*Weinstein, E.

"Comment on 'Demographic Transition Re-examined'." *American Sociological Review* 21(3), June 1956: pp. 369-371.

A rejoinder to Van Nort and Karon (see 1579).

1583

Wharton, C.R., Jr.

"The Green Revolution: Cornucopia or Pandora's Box?" *Foreign Affairs* 47(3), Apr. 1969: pp. 464-476.

Institutional adjustments required if the agricultural revolution is to make a significant contribution to the problem of population-food-economy balance.

1584

Wilkinson, M.

"Evidences of Long Swings in the Growth of Swedish Population and Related Economic Variables, 1860-1965." *Journal of Economic History* 27(1), Mar. 1967: pp. 17-38.

Tests the evidence of long Kuznets cycle swings in birth rates and other components of population growth as related especially to variations in economic indexes in Sweden, employment opportunities in the U.S., and internal and international migration streams.

XIII. BIOMEDICAL ASPECTS OF FERTILITY CONTROL

(Since this area is a large and complex literature in its own right, this category contains only an illustrative listing to indicate to the social science reader the kinds of literature available and specifically to make available some of the more important references on birth-control methods in use or under study and their biological consequences, effects, etc. Studies dealing with the field acceptance of various contraceptives by various social groups represent quite a different set of studies with social components, classified elsewhere.).
See also: 683, 684, 1127, 1309, 1479.

1585
Calderone, M.S., ed.
Manual of Contraceptive Practice. Baltimore: Williams & Wilkins, 1970; 491p.

1586
Corfman, P.A. and Segal, S.J.
"Biologic Effects of Intrauterine Devices." *American Journal of Obstetrics and Gynecology* 100, 1 Feb. 1968: pp. 448-459.

1587
Family Planning Federation of Japan. Sub-Committee on the Study of Induced Abortion.
Harmful Effects of Induced Abortion. Tokyo: Family Planning Federation of Japan, 1966; 97p.

1588
Food and Drug Administration. Advisory Committee on Obstetrics and Gynecology.
Second Report on the Oral Contraceptives. Washington: Government Printing Office, 1969; 88p.

1589
García, C.R., ed.
"Symposium on Oral Contraception." *Clinical Obstetrics and Gynecology* 11, Sept. 1968: pp. 623-752.

1590
Hartman, C.G.
Science and the Safe Period. Baltimore: Williams & Wilkins, 1962; 294p.

1591
Inman, W.H.W. and Vessey, M.P.
"Investigation of Deaths from Pulmonary, Coronary, and Cerebral Thrombosis and Embolism in Women of Child-Bearing Age." *British Medical Journal* 2, 27, Apr. 1968: pp. 193-199.

1592
Johnson, V.E. and Masters, W.H.
"Intravaginal Contraceptive Study: Anatomy." *Western Journal of Surgery, Obstetrics and Gynecology* 70, July-Aug. 1962: pp. 202-207.

1593
Johnson, V.E. and Masters, W.H.
"Intravaginal Contraceptive Study: Physiology." *Western Journal of Surgery, Obstetrics and Gynecology* 71, May-June 1963: pp. 144-153.

1594
Laurence, K.A.
"Current Laboratory Studies of Fertility Regulation: Evaluation of Their Possibilities." In Berelson et al., eds. (*see* 53): pp. 387-395.

1595
Pingus, G.
The Control of Fertility. New York: Academic Press, 1965; 360p.
A review, by the pioneer in the development of the pill, of the physiology of reproduction in higher animals, chemical methods of contraception, and their medical implications.

1596
Population Council.
Intrauterine Contraceptive Device. Preliminary Report on the Conference held in New York City, 30 Apr. and 1 May 1962. Prepared by W.O. Nelson et al. New York: 1962; 40p.
An early conference on new intrauterine devices, reviewing preliminary studies, and outlining recommendations for new studies.

1597
Sartwell, P.E. et al.
"Thromboembolism and Oral Contraceptives: An Epidemiologic Case-Control Study." *American Journal of Epidemiology* 90, Nov. 1969: pp. 365-380.

1598
Scott, R.B.
"Critical Illnesses and Deaths Associated with Intrauterine Devices." *Obstetrics and Gynecology* 31, Mar. 1968: pp. 322-327.

1599
Segal, S.J. et al., eds.
Intra-uterine Contraception: Proceedings of the Second International Conference. New York, 2-3 Oct., 1964. International Congress Series, 86. Amsterdam: Excerpta Medica, 1965; 250p.

1600
Segal, S.J. and Tietze, C.
"Contraceptive Technology: Current and Prospective Methods." *Reports on Population/Family Planning* Oct. 1969: pp. 1-20.

1601
Swyer, G.I.M., ed.
"Control of Human Fertility." *British Medical Journal* 26(1), Jan. 1970: pp. 1-97.
Fifteen papers on aspects of reproductive physiology, contraceptive pharmacology, and other medical aspects of contraception.

1602
Tietze, C.
The Condom as a Contraceptive. No. 5. New York: National Committee on Maternal Health, 1960; 44p.
Describes manufacture and testing procedures, sales, effectiveness, and correlates of use of condoms.

1603
Tietze, C. and Lewit, S.
"Evaluation of Intrauterine Devices: Ninth Progress Report of the Cooperative Statistical Program." *Studies in Family Planning* 1(55), July 1970: pp. 1-40.

1604

United States Food and Drug Administration. Advisory Committee on Obstetrics and Gynecology.

Report on Intrauterine Contraceptive Devices. Washington: Government Printing Office, 1968; 101p.

> Detailed report on the history, effectiveness, biologic action, side effects, and legislative proposals of the IUD; bibliography of clinical studies.

1605

Vessey, M.P. and Doll, R.

"Investigation of Relation between Use of Oral Contraceptives and Thromboembolic Disease: A Further Report." *British Medical Journal* 2(14), June 1969: pp. 651-657.

1606

World Health Organization.

Basic and Clinical Aspects of Intra-uterine Devices. Technical Report Series No. 332. Geneva: 1966; 25p.

1607

World Health Organization.

Biology of Fertility Control by Periodic Abstinence: Report of a WHO Scientific Group. Technical Report Series No. 360. Geneva: 1967; 20p.

1608

World Health Organization.

Hormonal Steriods in Contraception. Technical Report Series No. 386. Geneva: 1968; 28p.

1609

World Health Organization.

Intra-Uterine Devices: Physiological and Clinical Aspects Report of a WHO Scientific Group. Technical Report Series No. 397. Geneva: 1968; 32p.

XIV. THE EFFECTS OF VARIOUS INTERMEDIATE VARIABLES ON FERTILITY

XIV.A Nuptiality status and age at marriage

See also: 1, 136, 158, 303, 331, 362, 374, 377, 388, 395, 402, 435, 440, 504, 513, 518, 544, 559, 579, 625, 629, 858, 1039, 1043, 1065, 1281, 1284, 1463, 1516.

1610
Agarwala, S.N.
"Widowhood Age and Length of Fertile Union in India." In Szabady et al., eds. (*see* 40): pp. 11-16.

From local studies, estimates of age distribution and remarriage rate for widows and loss of fertile period spent in widowhood.

1611
Angeles, N. de los
"Marriage and Fertility Patterns in the Philippines." *Philippine Sociological Review* (Quezon City) 13, Oct. 1965: pp. 232-248.

Analysis of fertility and nuptiality trends and regional differentials; religious, cultural, and legal aspects of marriage.

1612
Ardener, E.
Divorce and Fertility: An African Study. Nigerian Social and Economic Studies, 3. The Nigerian Institute of Social and Economic Research. London: Oxford University Press, 1962; 171p.

Continuation of an earlier study of a rural sample of African tribesmen; examines marital stability and its relation to fertility.

1613
Basavarajappa, K.G.
"Changes in Age at Marriage of Females and Their Effect on the Birth Rate in India: A Reply." *Eugenics Quarterly* 15(4), Dec. 1968: pp. 293-295.

A rejoinder to comments made by Talwar (see 1626).

1614
Basavarajappa, K.G. and Belvalgidad, M.I.
"Changes in Age at Marriage of Females and Their Effect on the Birth Rate in India." *Eugenics Quarterly* 14(1), March 1967: pp. 14-26.

Effect on birth rate of a change in proportion of women married.

1615
Berksan, S.
"Marriage Patterns and Their Effect on Fertility in Turkey." In Shorter and Güvenc, eds. (*see* 357): pp. 147-165.

1616
Bumpass, L.
"Age at Marriage as a Variable in Socio-Economic Differentials in Fertility." *Demography* 6(1), 1969: pp. 45-54.

1617
Caldwell, J.C.
"Fertility Decline and Female Chances of Marriage in Malaya." *Population Studies* 17(1), July 1963: pp. 20-32.

Examination of Malayan census data on sex ratios of estimated age of marriage as evidence for the hypothesis that postponement of marriage accounts for observed birth rate decline.

1618
Cumper, G.E.
"The Fertility of Commonlaw Unions in Jamaica." *Social and Economic Studies* (Jamaica) 15(3), Sept. 1966: pp. 189-202.

1619
Day, L.H.
"Patterns of Divorce in Australia and the United States." *American Sociological Review* Apr. 1964: pp. 509-522.

Suggests hypothesis to account for differences observed in incidence, duration of marriage, number of children, and age of spouses.

1620
Kim, Y.
"Age at Marriage and the Trend of Fertility in Korea." In *Proceedings of the World Population Conference, 1965* (*see* 44): pp. 145-148.

Shows an increase in the mean age at marriage and estimates its mean fertility effect.

1621
Leasure, J.W.
"Malthus, Marriage and Multiplication." *Milbank Memorial Fund Quarterly* 41(4), Oct. 1963: pp. 419-435.

Investigation of the reduction in growth that would result from specific increases in mean age at marriage in a population not practicing birth control, illustrated by data for Bolivia and Turkey.

1622
Obaidullah, M.
"On Marriage, Fertility, and Mortality." *Demographic Survey in East Pakistan.* Statistical Survey Research Unit. Part 2, Chapter 2, Dacca: University of Dacca, 1966; 53p.

Survey data to study effect on fertility of family size and type and of mortality.

1623
Okediji, O.O. and Okediji, F.C.
"Marital Stability and Social Structure in an African City." *Nigerian Journal of Economic and Social Studies* (Ibadan) 8(1), Mar. 1966: pp. 151-163.

Relates changes in traditional family structure to divorce as part of a broader sociological study of differential fertility, using survey data and court records.

1624
Palmore, J.A. and Ariffin, B.M.
"Marriage Patterns and Cumulative Fertility in West Malaysia: 1966-1967." *Demography* 6(4), Nov. 1969: pp. 383-401.

On the basis of a large sample survey, age at marriage and multiple marriages are related to age, race, rural background, education, occupation, and other social variables; effects on fertility of age at marriage and multiple marriages are estimated.

1625
Talwar, P.P.
"Adolescent Sterility in an Indian Population." *Human Biology* 37(3), Sept. 1965: pp. 256-261.
1947 study of adolescent sterility in Calcutta and of the possible effect of later marriage on shortening the reproductive span.

1626
Talwar, P.P.
"A Note on Changes in Age at Marriage of Females and Their Effect on the Birth Rate." *Eugenics Quarterly* 14(4), Dec. 1967: pp. 291-295.
Comments on article by Basavarajappa & Belvalgidad (see 1614).

1627
Van de Walle, E.
"The Relation of Marriage to Fertility in African Demographic Inquiries." *Demography* 2, 1965: pp. 302-308.
Problems of applying Western concepts in studies of the relation of nuptiality and fertility in Africa; compares age-specific fertility rates for monogamous and polygamous marriages and compares mean age at marriage and crude birth rates for Congolese cities.

1628
Van de Walle, E.
"Marriage and Marital Fertility." *Daedalus* 97(2), Spring 1968: pp. 486-501.
Examines historical relationship of nuptiality patterns and fertility decline in Western Europe in the context of Matras's scheme of "strategies of family formation" (see 565).

1629
Wyon, J.B. et al.
"Delayed Marriage and Prospects for Fewer Births in Punjab Villages." *Demography* 3(1), 1966: pp. 209-217.
Long-term trends in marriage age, cohabitation, and fertility.

XIV.B Child-spacing patterns
See also: 461, 490, 529, 593.

1630
Grabill, W.H. and Davidson, M.
"Recent Trends in Childspacing among American Women." *Demography* 5(1), 1968: pp. 212-225.
Examines trends in child spacing and completed family size, 1955-64; socioeconomic status and child-spacing differentials.

1631
Knodel, J.
"Infant Mortality and Fertility in Three Bavarian Villages: An Analysis of Family Histories from the 19th Century." *Population Studies* 22(3), Nov. 1968: pp. 297-318.
Studies the effect of infant mortality and lactation on fertility via birth interval lengths.

1632
Srinivasan, S.K.
"'The Open Birth Interval'" as an Index of Fertility." *Journal of Family Welfare* (Bombay) 13(2), Dec. 1966: pp. 40-44.

XIV.C Fecundability (including postpartum amenorrhea and coital frequency)

See also: 1, 1133, 1260, 1625.

1633
Glass, D.V.
"Human Infertility and Artificial Insemination: The Demographic Background." *The Journal of the Royal Statistical Society* (Series A) 123(2), 1960: pp. 174-181.

Attempts to estimate the incidence of involuntary childlessness in Great Britain; suggests artificial insemination would have small impact on the total proportion childless.

1634
Knodel, J. and Van de Walle, E.
"Breast Feeding, Fertility and Infant Mortality: An Analysis of Some Early German Data." *Population Studies* 21(2), Sept. 1967: pp. 109-131.

Examines ecological correlations for German cities on lactation, infant mortality, and fertility; presents possible explanation for historical differentials in fertility decline.

1635
Tachi, M. and Nakano, E.
"Some Demographic Implications of Postpartum Amenorrhea." English Pamphlet Series, 62. Tokyo: Institute of Population Problems, 1966; 14p.

1636
*Tietze, C.
"Reproductive Span and Rate of Reproduction among Hutterite Women." *Fertility and Sterility* 8(1), Jan.-Feb. 1957: pp. 89-97.

1637
Udry, J.R. and Morris, N.M.
"Seasonality of Coitus and Seasonality of Birth." *Demography* 4(2), 1967: pp. 673-679.

Compares weekly patterns of coital frequency and conception from various sources of U.S. data.

XIV.D Fetal mortality

See also: 255, 432, 703, 1043, 1065, 1302, 1322, 1494.

1638
Bourgeois-Pichat, J.
"Relation between Fetal-Infant Mortality and Fertility." In *Proceedings of the World Population Conference, 1965 (see* 44): pp. 68-72.

How fetal mortality affects fertility and birth intervals, by age of woman under various conditions.

1639
Frederiksen, H. and Brackett, J.W.
"Demographic Effects of Abortion." *Public Health Reports* 83(12), Dec. 1968: pp. 999-1010.

Annual total fertility rates in comparison with estimated rates for pregnancies, legal abortions, and other abortions for periods since World War II for Bulgaria, Hungary, East Germany, and Japan.

1640
Klinger, A.
"Demographic Effects of Abortion Legislation in Some European Socialist Countries." In *Proceedings of the World Population Conference, 1965 (see* 44): pp. 89-91.

Review of abortion history and prevalence; advances the view that the effect of abortion on the birth rate depends on prior history and social structure of the country and is not a direct mechanical relationship.

1641

Newcome, H.B. and Rhynas, P.O.W.
"Childspacing Following Stillbirth and Infant Death." *Eugenics Quarterly* 9(1), Mar. 1962: pp. 23-35.
Very large body of computer-linked vital records for British Columbia used to establish that stillbirths were followed by higher than average birth rate in the following year, but somewhat less than expected rate over the four following years.

1642

Tietze, C.
"The Demographic Significance of Legal Abortion in Eastern Europe." *Demography* 1(1), 1964; pp. 119-125.
Abortion policies and estimates of their effect on the birth rate.

XIV.E Contraception

See also: 136, 1244, 1367, 1500, 1532, 1602, 1604.

1643

Haynes, M.A. et al.
"A Study on the Effectiveness of Sterilizations in Reducing the Birth Rate." *Demography* 6(1), Feb. 1969: pp. 1-11.
Sets of match sterilized and unsterilized couples used to examine the impact of the sterilization program in Kerala, India, on the population growth rate.

1644

Presser, H.B.
"The Role of Sterilization in Controlling Puerto Rican Fertility." *Population Studies* 23(3), Nov. 1969: pp. 343-361.
On basis of survey data, demonstrates that sterilization was the major birth-control method in Puerto Rico by 1965, probably accounting for a substantial part of the fertility decline; relates incidence to current age, age at sterilization, parity, fecundity.

1645

Ryder, N.B. and Westoff, C.F.
"The United States: The Pill and the Birth Rate, 1960-1965." *Studies in Family Planning* 1(20), June 1967: pp. 1-6. [Based on chapter in item 65.]
Rapid adoption of pill probably does not explain very much of the fertility decline in this period in view of discordant age and time patterns of pill use as compared with fertility decline, but degree and tempo of change probably affected by pill.

1646

Stoeckel, J.E. and Choudhury, M.A.
"The Impact of Family Planning on Fertility in a Rural Area of East Pakistan." *Demography* 4(2), 1967: pp. 569-575.
Comparison of pregnancy rates of adopters and nonadopters of conventional contraceptives, 1962-66.

XIV.F Combination of intermediate variables as they affect fertility

See also: 254, 319, 449, 453, 476, 488, 533, 929, 1032, 1493, 1499, 1504, 1508, 1512, 1531, 1534, 1537, 1538.

1647
Agarwala, S.N.
"Social and Cultural Factors Affecting Fertility in India." *Population Review* (Madras) 8(1), Jan. 1964: pp. 73-78.

Effects on fertility of age at marriage, male mortality, age at widowhood, sex preference, and other factors.

1648
Borrie, W.D.
"Recent Trends and Patterns in Fertility in Australia." *Journal of Biosocial Science* 1(1), Jan. 1969: pp. 57-70.

How changes in age structure, nuptiality status, timing of births, and completed family size affect the declining birth rate.

1649
Bourgeois-Pichat, J.
"Social and Biological Determinants of Human Fertility in Non-industrial Societies." *Proceedings of the American Philosophical Society* 111(3), June 1967: pp. 160-163.

Deals in general terms with the role of nuptiality, fecundability, and mortality in determining the range of reproductive levels, as they are affected potentially by varying social conditions.

1650
Day, L.H.
"Differentials in Age of Women at Completion of Childbearing in Australia." *Population Studies* 18(3), Mar. 1965: pp. 251-264.

1954 census data show age at completion of child bearing related to number of children ever born but not to birth intervals or age at marriage.

1651
Freedman, R. and Adlakha, A.L.
"Recent Fertility Declines in Hong Kong: The Role of the Changing Age Structure." *Population Studies* 22(2), July 1968: pp. 181-198.

An attempt to assess the relative importance of changes in the age distribution, proportion married, and marital age-specific fertility on the birth rate decline of Hong Kong for the periods 1961-65 and 1965-66.

1652
Jain, A.K.
"Pregnancy Outcome and the Time Required for Next Conception." *Population Studies* 23(3), Nov. 1969: pp. 421-433.

Based on Taiwan sample survey data, studies the relation between pregnancy outcome and the interval to next pregnancy; considers methodological problems of memory bias and truncation effect.

1653
Nag, M.
Factors Affecting Human Fertility in Non-Industrial Societies: A Cross-Cultural Study. Yale University Publications in Anthropology, 1966. New Haven: Department of Anthropology, Yale University, 1962; 227p.

Uses ethnographic reports on a large number of preindustrial societies to analyze relationships between a large number of variables believed to affect fertility.

1654
Potter, R.G., Jr.
"Some Physical Correlates of Fertility Control in the United States." In *Inter-*

national Population Conference. New York, 1961. London: U.N.E.S.C.O., 1963; pp. 106-116.

Role of fetal mortality, fecundability, and chance in affecting ability of couples to have just the number of children wanted.

1655
Potter, R.G., Jr. et al.
"A Case Study of Birth Interval Dynamics." *Population Studies* 19(1), July 1965: pp. 81-96.

Effect of lactation, fetal mortality, and age of mother on birth intervals in an Indian village population.

1656
Treffers, P.
"Family Size, Contraception, and Birth Rate before and after the Introduction of a New Method of Family Planning." *Journal of Marriage and the Family* 30(2), May 1968: pp. 338-345.

Interpretation of the role of the pill and abortion in affecting birth rate by reducing "the tension between real and ideal family size"; special reference to the Netherlands and the East European countries.

1657
*Whelpton, P.K. and Kiser, C.V.
"The Comparative Influence on Fertility of Contraception and Impairments of Fecundity." In Kiser and Whelpton, eds. (*see* 1512) Vol. 2: pp. 303-358.

Important early empirical analysis of the relative influence of contraception and fecundity in low Western fertility, based on the Indianapolis study.

APPENDIX

ADDITIONAL RECENT PUBLICATIONS

Many new publications about fertility have appeared since the annotated bibliography was completed. There follows here an alphabetical listing by author's name and chronological sequence of 430 such English-language publications, without annotation or classification. These items were selected from two sources:

1. *Population Index* for October–December 1969 through October–December 1971.
2. A computer search of all monographs published in English world-wide which were cataloged by the Library of Congress from 1 June 1970 to 1 April 1972.

Selection was based on the brief annotation in *Population Index* listings. If, on the strength of this description, we would have considered the item for review in the classified bibliography, then we included it here in the appendix.

A1
Acsádi, G. et al.
Family Planning in Hungary. Main Results of the 1966 Fertility and Family Planning (TCS) Study. Studies on Family Planning, 2. Committee for Demography of the Hungarian Academy of Sciences, 31. Budapest: Demographic Research Institute of the Central Statistical Office, 1970; 212p.

A2
Agarwala, S.N.
A Demographic Study of Six Urbanising Villages. Institute of Economic Growth Occasional Papers, 8. Bombay: Asia Publishing House, 1970; 195p.

A3
Agarwala, S.N.
Family Planning Performance in India, 1967-70: A District-wide Study. Bombay: International Institute for Population Studies, 1971; 20p.

A4
Agarwala, S.N.
A Study of Factors Explaining Variability in Family Planning Performance in Different States of India. Bombay: International Institute for Population Studies, 1971; 15p.

A5
Aitken, A. and Stoeckel, J.
"Dynamics of the Muslim-Hindo Differential in Family Planning Practices in Rural East Pakistan." *Social Biology* 18(3), Sept. 1971: pp. 268-276.

A6
American Economic Association.
"Population and Environment in the United States." Papers and Proceedings of the 83rd Annual Meeting of the AEA. *American Economic Review* 61(2), May 1971: pp. 392-417.

A7
Anand, D.
Family Planning through Hospital Care. Monograph Series, 5. New Delhi: Central Family Planning Institute, 1969; 372p.

A8
Angel, J.L.
"Paleodemography and Evolution." *American Journal of Physical Anthropology* 31(3), 1969: pp. 343-353.

A9
Arriaga, E.E.
Mortality Decline and Its Demographic Effects in Latin America. Berkeley: Institute of International Studies, University of California, 1970; 232p.

A10
Arriaga, E.E.
"The Nature and Effects of Latin America's Non-Western Trend in Fertility." *Demography* 7(4), Nov. 1970: pp. 483-501.

A11
Avery, R. and Freedman, R.
"Taiwan: Implications of Fertility at Replacement Levels." *Studies in Family Planning* 1(59), Nov. 1970: pp. 1-4.

A12
Ayala, F.J. and Falk, C.T.
"Sex of Children and Family Size."

Journal of Heredity 62(1), Jan.-Feb. 1971: pp. 57-59.

A13
Bailey, J. and Marshall, J.
"The Relationship of the Post-ovulatory Phase of the Menstrual Cycle to Total Cycle Length." *Journal of Biosocial Science* 2(2), Apr. 1970: pp. 123-132.

A14
Balakrishna, S.
Family Planning: Knowledge, Attitude, and Practice: A Sample Survey in Andhra Pradesh. Hyderabad, India: National Institute of Community Development, 1971; 139p.

A15
Balakrishna, S. and Radhalyer, B.
"Characteristics of Adopters of Family Planning Methods in Punjab: A Discriminant Function Approach." *Behavioural Sciences and Community Development* (Hyderabad) 2(1), Mar. 1969: pp. 14-25.

A16
Balakrishnan, T.R. et al.
"Analysis of Oral Contraceptive Use through Multiple Decrement Life Table Techniques." *Demography* 7(4), Nov. 1970: pp. 459-465.

A17
Banerji, D.
Family Planning in India: A Critique and a Perspective. New Delhi: People's Publishing House, 1971; 85p.

A18
Bang, S.
"Korea: The Relationship between IUD Retention and Check-up Visits." *Studies in Family Planning* 2(5), May 1971: pp. 110-112.

A19
Barlow, R.
The Economic Effects of Malaria Eradication. School of Public Health, Bureau of Public Health Economics, Research Series, 15. Ann Arbor: University of Michigan, 1968; 167p.

A20
Barnett, H.J.
"Population Problems—Myths and Realities." *Economic Development and Cultural Change* 19(4), July 1971: pp. 545-559.

A21
Barrai, I. et al.
"Further Studies on Record Linkage from Parish Books." In *Record Linkage in Medicine: Proceedings of the International Symposium, Oxford, July 1967.* Edited by E.D. Acheson. Edinburgh: Livingstone, 1968.

A22
Barrett, J.C.
"A Monte Carlo Simulation of Human Reproduction." *Genus* (Rome) 25(1-4), 1969; pp. 1-22.

A23
Barrett, J.C.
"An Analysis of Coital Patterns." *Journal of Biosocial Science* 2(4), Oct. 1970: pp. 351-357.

A24
Barrett, J.C.
"Fecundability and Coital Frequency."

Population Studies 25(2), July 1971: pp. 309-313.

A25
Barrett, J.C.
"Use of a Fertility Simulation Model to Refine Measurement Techniques." *Demography* 8(4), Nov. 1971: pp. 481-490.

A26
Bartlett, M.S.
"Age Distributions." *Biometrics* 26(3), Sept. 1970: pp. 377-385.

A27
Bean, L.L. et al.
Population and Family Planning: Manpower and Training. New York: Population Council, 1971; 118p.

A28
Beasley, J.D. et al.
"Evaluation of National Health Programs: IV. Louisiana Family Planning." *American Journal of Public Health* 61(9), Sept. 1971: pp. 1812-1825.

A29
Beasley, J.D. and Frankowski, R.F.
"United States: Utilization of a Family Planning Program in a Metropolitan Area." *Studies in Family Planning* 1(59), Nov. 1970: pp. 7-16.

A30
Ben-Porath, Y.
Fertility in Israel, an Economist's Interpretation: Differentials and Trends, 1950-1970. Memorandum RM-5981-FF. Santa Monica, Calif.: RAND Corporation, 1970; 46p.

A31
Berelson, B.
"The Present State of Family Planning Programs." *Studies in Family Planning* 1(57), Sept. 1970: pp. 1-11.

A32
Berelson, B.
"Population Policy: Personal Notes." *Population Studies* 25(2), July 1971: pp. 173-182.

A33
Berent, J.
"Causes of Fertility Decline in Eastern Europe and the Soviet Union. II. Economic and Social Factors." *Population Studies* 24(2), July 1970: pp. 247-292.

A34
Bernard, R.I.
"IUD Performance Patterns—A 1970 World View." *International Journal of Gynaecology and Obstetrics* 8, Nov. 1970: pp. 926-940.

A35
Bhende, A., ed.
"A Bibliography of IUCD Studies in India." Demographic Training and Research Centre *Newsletter* (Chembur) 31, Jan. 1970: pp. 11-21.

A36
Biggar, J.C. and Butler, E.W.
"Fertility and Its Interrelationship with Population and Socioeconomic Characteristics in a Southern State." *Rural Sociology* 34(4), Dec. 1969: pp. 528-536.

A37
Blake, J.
"Abortion and Public Opinion: The

1960-1970 Decade." *Science* 171(3971), 12 Feb. 1971: pp. 540-549.

A38
Blake, J.
"Reproductive Motivation and Population Policy." *Bioscience* 21(5), 1 Mar. 1971: pp. 215-220.

A39
Blake, R. et al.
Beliefs and Attitudes about Contraception among the Poor. Monograph Series, 1. Chapel Hill: Carolina Population Center, 1968; 37p.

A40
Blake, J. and Donovan, J.J.
Western European Censuses, 1960: An English Language Guide. Population Monograph Series, 8. Berkeley: Institute of International Studies, University of California, 1971; 421p.

A41
Bock, E.W. and Iutaka, S.
"Social Status, Mobility and Premarital Pregnancy: A Case of Brazil." *Journal of Marriage and the Family* 32(2), May 1970: pp. 284-292.

A42
Bogue, D.J., ed.
Further Sociological Contributions to Family Planning Research. Chicago: Community and Family Study Center, University of Chicago, 1970; 459p.

A43
Borrie, W.D.
The Growth and Control of World Population. The Advancement of Science Series. London: Weidenfeld & Nicolson, 1970; 340p.

A44
Bose, A. et al.
Studies in Demography. Chapel Hill: University of North Carolina Press, 1970; 579p.

A45
Bourgeois-Pichat, J.
"Stable, Semi-stable Populations and Growth Potential." *Population Studies* 25(2), July 1971: pp. 235-254.

A46
Brass, W.
"Assessing the Demographic Effect of a Family Planning Programme." *Proceedings of the Royal Society of Medicine* 63, Nov. 1970: pp. 1105-1107.

A47
Brass, W.
Biological Aspects of Demography. London: Taylor and Francis; New York: Barnes & Noble, 1971; 167p.

A48
Brown, R.E.
"Attitudes toward Family Planning among Peri-urban Africans in Uganda." *Tropical and Geographical Medicine* (Haarlem) 22, 1970; pp. 87-100.

A49
Bumpass, L.L. and Westoff, C.F.
The Later Years of Childbearing. Princeton: Princeton University Press, 1970; 168p.

A50
Bumpass, L. and Westoff, C.F.
"The 'Perfect Contraceptive' Population: The Extent and Implications of Unwanted Fertility in the United States Are Considered." *Science* 169(3951), 18 Sept. 1970: pp. 1177-1182.

A51
Burch, T.K. and Shea, G.A.
"Catholic Parish Priests and Birth Control: A Comparative Study of Opinion in Colombia, the United States, and the Netherlands." *Studies in Family Planning* 2(6), June 1971: pp. 121-139.

A52
Callahan, D.J.
Abortion: Law, Choice and Morality. New York and London: Macmillan, 1970; 544p.

A53
Callahan, D.J., ed.
The American Population Debate. Garden City, N.Y.: Doubleday, 1971; 380p.

A54
Carrier, N. and Hobcraft, J.
Demographic Estimation for Developing Societies: A Manual of Techniques for the Detection and Reduction of Errors in Demographic Data. London: Population Investigation Committee, London School of Economics, 1971; 204p.

A55
Carter, H. and Glick, P.C.
Marriage and Divorce: A Social and Economic Study. American Public Health Association, Vital and Health Statistics Monographs Series. Cambridge, Mass.: Harvard University Press, 1970; 451p.

A56
Cartwright, A.
Parents and Family Planning Services. Reports of the Institute of Community Studies Series. London: Routledge & Kegan Paul; New York: Atherton, 1970; 293p.

A57
Cassedy, J.H.
Demography in Early America: Beginnings of the Statistical Mind, 1600-1800. Cambridge, Mass.: Harvard University Press, 1969; 357p.

A58
Chamberlain, N.W.
Beyond Malthus: Population and Power. New York: Basic Books, 1970; 214p.

A59
Chamberlain, W.M.
"Population Control: The Legal Approach to a Biological Imperative." *Ecology Law Quarterly* 1, Winter 1971: pp. 143-172.

A60
Chandrasekaran, C. et al.
"Some Problems in Determining the Number of Acceptors Needed in a Family Planning Programme to Achieve a Specified Reduction in the Birth Rate." *Population Studies* 25(2), July 1971: pp. 303-308.

A61
Chaplin, D.
Population Policies and Growth in Latin America. Lexington, Mass.: Lexington Books, 1971; 287p.

A62
Chaudhury, R.H.
"Differential Fertility by Religious Group in East Pakistan." *Social Biology* 18(2), June 1971: pp. 188-191.

A63
Chen, P.C.
"China's Birth Control Action Programme, 1956-1964." *Population Studies* 24(2), July 1970: pp. 141-158.

A64
Chiang, C.L.
"A Stochastic Model of Human Fertility." *Biometrics* 27(2), June 1971: pp. 345-356.

A65
Cho, L.J. et al.
Differential Current Fertility in the United States. Chicago: Community and Family Study Center, University of Chicago, 1970; 426p.

A66
Chow, L.P.
"Current Fertility in Taiwan." *Industry of Free China* 32, Dec. 1969: pp. 12-26.

A67
Chow, L.P.
"Family Planning in Taiwan, Republic of China: Progress and Prospects." *Population Studies* 24(3), Nov. 1970: pp. 339-352.

A68
Clifford, W.B., II
"Modern and Traditional Value Orientations and Fertility Behavior: A Social Demographic Study." *Demography* 8(1), Feb. 1971: pp. 37-48.

A69
Clignet, R. and Sween, J.
"Social Change and Type of Marriage." *American Journal of Sociology* 75(1), July 1969: pp. 123-145.

A70
Coale, A.J.
"Age Patterns of Marriage." *Population Studies* 25(2), July 1971: pp. 193-214.

A71
Cochrane, S.H.
"Mortality Level, Desired Family Size, and Population Increase: Comment." *Demography* 8(4), Nov. 1971: pp. 537-540.

A72
Cook, S.F. and Borah, W.
Essays in Population History: Mexico and the Caribbean. Berkeley: University of California Press, 1971; 444p.

A73
Coombs, L. and Freedman, R.
"Pre-marital Pregnancy, Childspacing, and Later Economic Achievement." *Population Studies* 24(3), Nov. 1970: pp. 389-412.

A74
Coombs, L.C. and Zumeta, Z.
"Correlates of Marital Dissolution in a Prospective Fertility Study: A Research Note." *Social Problems* 18(1), Summer 1970: pp. 92-102.

A75
Cooper, C.A. and Alexander, S.S., eds.
Economic Development and Population Growth in the Middle East. New York: American Elsevier, 1971; 620p.

A76
Correa, H. and Beasley, J.D.
"Mathematical Models for Decision-making in Population and Family Planning." *American Journal of Public Health* 61(1), Jan. 1971: pp. 138-151.

A77
Cowgill, D.O. et al.
"Sterilization: A Case of Extensive Practice in a Developing Nation." *Milbank Memorial Fund Quarterly* 49(3, Part 1), July 1971: pp. 363-378.

A78
Cross, H.E. and McKusick, V.A.
"Amish Demography." *Social Biology* 17(2), June 1970: pp. 83-101.

A79
Crow, J.F. and Kimura, M.
An Introduction to Population Genetics Theory. New York: Harper & Row, 1970; 592p.

A80
Curran, C.E., ed.
Contraception: Authority and Dissent. New York: Herder and Herder, 1969; 237p.

A81
Curtin, T.R.C.
"The Economics of Population Growth and Control in Developing Countries." *Review of Social Economy* 27(2), Sept. 1969: pp. 139-153.

A82
Cutright, P.
"Illegitimacy: Myths, Causes and Cures." *Family Planning Perspectives* 3(1), Jan. 1971: pp. 26-48.

A83
David, A.S. and Sarma, R.S.S.
Potential Socioeconomic Consequences of Planned Fertility Reduction, North Carolina—a Case Study. Monograph Series. Chapel Hill: University of North Carolina, 1971; 118p.

A84
David, H.P.
Family Planning and Abortion in the Socialist Countries of Central and Eastern Europe: A Compendium of Observations and Readings. International Research Institute, American Institutes for Research. New York: Population Council, 1970; 306p.

A85
David, H.P. and Wright, N.H.
"Abortion Legislation: The Romanian Experience." *Studies in Family Planning* 2(10), Oct. 1971: pp. 205-210.

A86
Davidson, M.
"Social and Economic Variations in Childspacing." *Social Biology* 17(2), June 1970: pp. 107-113.

A87
Davidson, M.
"Expectations of Additional Children

by Race, Parity, and Selected Socio-economic Characteristics, United States: 1967." *Demography* 8(1), Feb. 1971: pp. 27-36.

A88
Davis, W.H., ed.
Readings in Human Population Ecology. Prentice-Hall Biological Science Series. Englewood Cliffs, N.J.: Prentice-Hall, 1971; 251p.

A89
Demko, G.J. and Casetti, E.
"A Diffusion Model for Selected Demographic Variables: An Application to Soviet Data." *Annals of the Association of American Geographers* 60(3), Sept. 1970: pp. 533-539.

A90
Deprez, P., ed.
Population and Economics: Proceedings of Section V [Historical Demography Section] of the Fourth Congress of the International Economic History Association, 1968. Winnipeg: University of Manitoba Press, 1970; 364p.

A91
Dixon, R.B.
"Explaining Cross-cultural Variations in Age at Marriage and Proportions Never Marrying." *Population Studies* 25(2), July 1971: pp. 215-233.

A92
Dollen, C.
Abortion in Context: A Select Bibliography. Metuchen, N.J.: Scarecrow Press, 1970; 150p.

A93
Dow, T.E., Jr.
"Fertility and Family Planning in Africa." *Journal of Modern African Studies* 8(3), Oct. 1970: pp. 445-457.

A94
Dow, T.E., Jr.
"Fertility and Family Planning in Sierra Leone." *Studies in Family Planning* 2(8), Aug. 1971: pp. 153-165.

A95
Dow, T.E., Jr.
"Family Planning Patterns in Sierra Leone." *Studies in Family Planning* 2(10), Oct. 1971: pp. 211-222.

A96
Drakatos, C.G.
"The Determinants of Birth Rate in Developing Countries: An Econometric Study of Greece." *Economic Development and Cultural Change* 17(4), July 1969: pp. 596-603.

A97
Dreijmanis, J.
The Politics of the Soviet Pro-natalist Policy. Occasional Papers in Political Science, 13. Kingston: University of Rhode Island, 1968; 59p.

A98
Eldin, S.N.
Analysis of Data on Fertility, Mortality and Economic Activity of Urban Population in Libya Based on a Household Sample Survey. Memo No. 996, Cairo, United Arab Republic: Institute of National Planning, 1971; 30p.

252

A99
Elliott, R. et al.
"U.S. Population Growth and Family Planning: A Review of the Literature." *Family Planning Perspectives* (Supplement), Oct. 1970: 16p.

A100
Enke, S.
"Economic Value of Preventing Births: Reply to Simon." *Population Studies* 24(3), Nov. 1970: pp. 455-456.

A101
Enke, S. and Leibenstein, H.
"An Exchange of Comments on Leibenstein's Paper, 'Pitfalls in Benefit-cost Analysis of Birth Prevention.'" *Population Studies* 24(1), Mar. 1970: pp. 115-119.

A102
Erhardt, C.L. et al.
"Seasonal Patterns of Conception in New York City." *American Journal of Public Health* 61(11), Nov. 1971: pp. 2246-2258.

A103
Espenshade, T.J.
"A New Method for Estimating the Level of Natural Fertility in Populations Practicing Birth Control." *Demography* 8(4), Nov. 1971: pp. 525-536.

A104
Family Planning Association of India.
Sixth All India Conference on Family Planning: Report of the Proceedings, 30th November to 5th December 1968, Chandigarh. Bombay: 1970; 295p.

A105
Farley, R.
Growth of the Black Population: A Study of Demographic Trends. Markham Sociology Series. Chicago: Markham, 1970; 286p.

A106
Farley, R. and Hermalin, A.I.
"Family Stability: A Comparison of Trends between Blacks and Whites." *American Sociological Review* 36(1), Feb. 1971: pp. 1-17.

A107
Fawcett, J.T.
Psychology and Population: Behavioral Research Issues in Fertility and Family Planning. New York: Population Council, 1970; 149p.

A108
Ferriss, A.L.
Indicators of Change in the American Family. New York: Russell Sage Foundation, 1970; 145p.

A109
Finner, S.L. and Gamache, J.D.
"The Relation between Religious Commitment and Attitudes toward Induced Abortion." *Sociological Analysis* 30(1), Spring 1969: pp. 1-12.

A110
Fish, M. and Thompson, A.A.
"The Determinants of Fertility: A Theoretical Forecasting Model." *Behavioral Science* 15(4), July 1970: pp. 318-328.

A111
Flinn, M.W.
British Population Growth, 1700-1850.
London: Macmillan, 1970; 68p.

A112
Ford, T.R. and DeJong, G.F., eds.
Social Demography. Englewood Cliffs,
N.J.: Prentice-Hall, 1970; 690p.

A113
Forrester, J.W.
World Dynamics. Cambridge, Mass.:
Wright-Allen Press, 1971; 142p.

A114
Freedman, R. et al.
"Hong Kong's Fertility Decline,
1961-68." *Population Index* 36(1), Jan.-
Mar. 1970: pp. 3-18.

A115
Freedman, R. et al.
"Fertility after Insertion of an IUCD in
Taiwan's Family-Planning Program."
Social Biology 18(1), Mar. 1971: pp.
46-54.

A116
Fryer, P., ed.
*British Birth Control Ephemera
1870-1947.* Collis Collections, 1. Syston,
Leicester, Eng.: Barracuda Press, 1969;
42p.

A117
Gaisie, S.K.
"Social Structure and Fertility." *Ghana
Journal of Sociology* (Legon, Accra) 4(2),
Oct. 1968: pp. 88-99.

A118
Gardezi, H.N. and Inayatullah, A.
*The Dai Study; the Dai, Midwife, a Local
Functionary and her Role in Family Plan-
ning.* Lahore: West Pakistan Family
Planning Association, 1969; 106p.

A119
Gendell, M. et al.
"Fertility and Economic Activity of
Women in Guatemala City, 1964." *De-
mography* 7(3), Aug. 1970: pp. 273-286.

A120
Glass, D.V. et al.
*Towards a Population Policy for the Unit-
ed Kingdom.* Supplement to *Population
Studies.* London: Population Investigation Committee, London School of Economics, 1970; 60p.

A121
Glick, P.C.
"Marital Stability as a Social Indicator."
Social Biology 16(3), Sept. 1969: pp.
158-166.

A122
Glick, P.C. and Norton, A.J.
"Frequency, Duration, and Probability
of Marriage and Divorce." *Journal of
Marriage and the Family* 33(2), May
1971: pp. 307-317.

A123
Goldscheider, C.
*Population, Modernization, and Social
Structure.* Boston: Little, Brown, 1971;
345p.

A124
Goldstein, S.
"Religious Fertility Differentials in

Thailand, 1960." *Population Studies* 24(3), Nov. 1970: pp. 325-337.

A125
Golini, A.
"The Influence of Migration on Fertility." *Genus* (Rome) 24(1-4), 1968; pp. 93-108. [English summaries.]

A126
Goode, W.J. et al.
Social Systems and Family Patterns: A Propositional Inventory. Indianapolis: Bobbs-Merrill, 1971; 779p.

A127
Goodman, L.A.
"The Analysis of Population Growth When the Birth and Death Rates Depend upon Several Factors." *Biometrics* 25(4), Dec. 1969: pp. 659-681.

A128
Goodman, L.A.
"On the Sensitivity of the Intrinsic Growth Rate to Changes in the Age-Specific Birth and Death Rates." *Theoretical Population Biology* 2 (3), Sept. 1971: pp. 339-354.

A129
Gould, F.J. and Magazine, M.J.
"A Mathematical Programming Model for Planning Contraceptive Deliveries." *Socio-Economic Planning Sciences* 5(3), June 1971: pp. 255-261.

A130
Goyal, M.M.L.
Studies on Intra-uterine Contraceptive Devices in India: A Bibliography. New Delhi: Central Family Planning Institute, 1970; 22p.

A131
Gray, H.P. and Tangri, S.S., eds.
Economic Development and Population Growth—A Conflict? Studies in Economics Series. Lexington, Mass.: D.C. Heath, 1970; 162p.

A132
Green, L.W. et al.
"Measuring the Extent of Contraceptive Knowledge and Use Not Reported in Interviews." *Pakistan Journal of Family Planning* (Karachi) 3(2), 1969: pp. 7-16.

A133
Greenberg, B.G. et al.
"A New Survey Technique and Its Applications in the Field of Public Health." *Milbank Memorial Fund Quarterly* 48(4, Part 2), Oct. 1970: pp. 39-55.

A134
Greven, P.J., Jr.
"Family Structure in Seventeenth-century Andover, Massachusetts." *William and Mary Quarterly* 23, 1966: pp. 234-256.

A135
Greven, P.J., Jr.
"Historical Demography and Colonial America: A Review Article." *William and Mary Quarterly* (3rd Series) 24(3), 1967: pp. 438-454.

A136
Greven, P.J., Jr.
Four Generations: Population, Land, and

Family in Colonial Andover, Massachusetts. Ithaca, N.Y.: Cornell University Press, 1970; 329p.

A137
Gulati, S.C.
"Impact of Literacy, Urbanization and Sex-ratio on Age at Marriage in India." *Artha Vijñāna* (Poona) 11(4), Dec. 1969: pp. 685-697.

A138
Habakkuk, H.J.
Population Growth and Economic Development since 1750. Leicester, Eng.: Leicester University Press; New York: Humanities Press, 1971; 110p.

A139
Haldar, A.K. and Bhattacharya, N.
"Fertility and Sex-sequence of Children of Indian Couples." *Recherches Economiques de Louvain* 36(4), Nov. 1970: pp. 405-415.

A140
Hall, M.F.
"Male Use of Contraception and Attitudes toward Abortion, Santiago, Chile, 1968." *Milbank Memorial Fund Quarterly* 48(2, Part 1), Apr. 1970: pp. 145-166.

A141
Hall, M.F.
"Family Planning in Santiago, Chile: The Male Viewpoint." *Studies in Family Planning* 2(7), July 1971: pp. 143-147.

A142
Hall, M.F.
"Male Attitudes to Family Planning Education in Santiago, Chile." *Journal of Biosocial Science* 3(4), Oct. 1971: pp. 403-416.

A143
Hall, R.E., ed.
Abortion in a Changing World. Proceedings of an International Conference Convened in Hot Springs, Virginia, 17-20 Nov. 1968 by the Association for the Study of Abortion. Vol. 1. New York: Columbia University Press, 1970; 377p.

A144
Han, S.
"Family Planning in China." *Japan Quarterly* (Tokyo) 17(4), Oct.-Dec. 1970: pp. 433-442.

A145
Harman, A. J.
Fertility and Economic Behavior of Families in the Philippines. Memorandum RM-6385-AID. Santa Monica, Calif.: RAND Corporation, 1970; 84p.

A146
Harter, C.L.
"The Fertility of Sterile and Subfecund Women in New Orleans." *Social Biology* 17(3), Sept. 1970: pp. 195-206.

A147
Harvard Law Review Association.
"Legal Analysis and Population Control: The Problem of Coercion." *Harvard Law Review* 84(8), June 1971: pp. 1856-1911.

A148
Hastings, P.K., ed.
Population Control: A Bibliography of

Survey Data 1938-1970. Williamstown, Mass.: Roper Public Opinion Research Center, 1970; 98p.

A149
Hata, Y. et al.
"The Effect of Long-term Use of Intrauterine Devices." *International Journal of Fertility* 14(3), July-Sept. 1969: pp. 241-249.

A150
Hauser, P.M., ed.
The Population Dilemma. The American Assembly, Columbia University. Englewood Cliffs, N.J.: Prentice-Hall, 1969; 211p.

A151
Hawthorn, G.
The Sociology of Fertility. Themes and Issues in Modern Sociology Series. London: Collier-Macmillan, 1970; 161p.

A152
Heer, D.M. and Boynton, J.W.
"A Multivariate Regression Analysis of Differences in Fertility of United States Counties." *Social Biology* 17(3), Sept. 1970: pp. 180-194.

A153
Heeren, H.J. and Moors, H.G.
"Family Planning and Differential Fertility in a Dutch City." *Journal of Marriage and the Family* 31(3), Aug. 1969: pp. 588-595.

A154
Helbig, D.W. et al.
"IUD Retention in West Pakistan and

Methodology of Assessment." *Demography* 7(4), Nov. 1970: pp. 467-482.

A155
Henin, R.A.
"Marriage Patterns and Trends in the Nomadic and Settled Populations of the Sudan." *Africa* 39(3), July 1969: pp. 238-259.

A156
Hermalin, A.I. and Chow, L.P.
"Motivational Factors in IUD Termination: Data from the Second Taiwan IUD Follow-up Survey." *Journal of Biosocial Science* 3(4), Oct. 1971: pp. 351-375.

A157
Hill, R. and Konig, R., eds.
Families in East and West: Socialization Process and Kinship Ties. International Family Research Seminar, 9th, Tokyo, 1965. The Hague: Mouton, 1970; 630p.

A158
Hirschman, C. and Matras, J.
"A New Look at the Marriage Market and Nuptiality Rates, 1915-1958." *Demography* 8(4), Nov. 1971: pp. 549-569.

A159
Hoem, J.M.
"Concepts of a Bisexual Theory of Marriage Formation." *Statistisk Tidskrift* (Stockholm) (3rd Series) 7(4), 1969; pp. 295-300.

A160
Hoem, J.M.
"Probabilistic Fertility Models of the

Life Table Type." *Theoretical Population Biology* 1(1), May 1970: pp. 12-38.

A161
Hoem, J.M.
"On the Interpretation of the Maternity Function as a Probability Density." *Theoretical Population Biology* 2(3), Sept. 1971: pp. 319-327.

A162
Hoem, J.M.
"On the Interpretation of Certain Vital Rates as Averages of Underlying Forces of Transition." *Theoretical Population Biology* 2(4), Dec. 1971: pp. 454-468.

A163
Hofsten, E.
"Birth Variations in Populations Which Practise Family Planning." *Population Studies* 25(2), July 1971: pp. 315-326.

A164
Holmberg, I.
Fecundity, Fertility and Family Planning: Application of Demographic Micromodels, 1. University of Goteborg, Demographic Institute Reports, 10. Goteborg, Sweden: Almqvist & Wiksell, 1970; 109p.

A165
Hoover, E.M.
"Basic Approaches to the Study of Demographic Aspects of Economic Development: Economic-Demographic Models." *Population Index* 37(2), Apr.-June 1971: pp. 66-75.

A166
Hooz, I.
"The Impact of Population Policy Measures and the Economic Situation on Birth-rates in the Inter-war Period in Hungary." *Acta Juridica Academiae Scientiarum Hungaricae* (Budapest) 12(3-4), 1970: pp. 407-436.

A167
Horvitz, D.G. et al.
Popsim, a Demographic Microsimulation Model. Monograph, 12. Chapel Hill: Carolina Population Center, 1971; 70p.

A168
Husain, I.Z.
"Educational Status and Differential Fertility in India." *Social Biology* 17(2), June 1970: pp. 132-139.

A169
Husain, I.Z.
An Urban Fertility Field: A Report on City of Lucknow. Lucknow: Demographic Research Centre, Lucknow University, 1970; 154p.

A170
Hyrenius, H.
On the Use of Models in Demographic Research. Goteborg, Sweden: Demographic Institute, University of Goteborg, 1970; 81p.

A171
India. Planning Commission. Programme Evaluation Organisation. Social Development Division.
Family Planning Programme in India: An Evaluation. P.E.O. Publication, 71. New Delhi: 1970; 267p.

A172
India. Uttar Pradesh. Planning Research and Action Institute.

Report on Family Planning Communication Action Research Project (Pilot Phase). Lucknow: New Government Press, 1966; 296p.

A173
International Planned Parenthood Federation. Europe and Near East Region.
Social Demography and Medical Responsibility: Proceedings of the Sixth Conference of the International Planned Parenthood Federation, Europe and Near East Region, held in Budapest, September, 1969. London: 1970; 168p.

A174
International Union for the Scientific Study of Population.
International Population Conference: London 1969. Liege: 1971; 4 vols.

A175
Iutaka, S. et al.
"Factors Affecting Fertility of Natives and Migrants in Urban Brazil." *Population Studies* 25(1), Mar. 1971: pp. 55-62.

A176
Jaffe, F.S.
"Estimating the Need for Subsidized Family Planning Services." *Family Planning Perspectives* 3(1), Jan. 1971: pp. 51-55.

A177
Jaffe, F. S.
"Toward the Reduction of Unwanted Pregnancy: Assessment of Current Public and Private Programs." *Science* 174(4005), 8 Oct. 1971: pp. 119-127.

A178
Jain, A. K. et al.
"Demographic Aspects of Lactation and Postpartum Amenorrhea." *Demography* 7(2), May 1970: pp. 255-271.

A179
Jain, P.K.
"Marriage Age Patterns in India." *Artha Vijñāna* (Poona) 11(4), Dec. 1969: pp. 662-684.

A180
James, W.H.
"Testing for Birth-order Effects in the Presence of Birth Limitation or Reproductive Compensation." *Journal of the Royal Statistical Society* (Series C) 18(3), 1969; pp. 276-281.

A181
James, W.H.
"The Incidence of Spontaneous Abortion." *Population Studies* 24(2), July 1970: pp. 241-245.

A182
James, W.H.
"The Incidence of Illegal Abortion." *Population Studies* 25(2), July 1971: pp. 327-339.

A183
James, W.H.
"Social Class and Season of Birth." *Journal of Biosocial Science* 3(3), July 1971: pp. 309-320.

A184
Jamison, E. et al.
The Two-child Family and Population

Growth: An International View. Washington: Bureau of the Census, Government Printing Office, 1971; 38p.

A185
Janowitz, B.S.
"An Empirical Study of the Effects of Socioeconomic Development on Fertility Rates." *Demography* 8(3), Aug. 1971: pp. 319-330.

A186
Jaszmann, L. et al.
"The Age at Menopause in the Netherlands: the Statistical Analysis of a Survey." *International Journal of Fertility* 14(2), Apr.-June 1969: pp. 106-117.

A187
Jerushalmy, J.
"The Relationship of Parents' Cigarette Smoking to Outcome of Pregnancy—Implications as to the Problem of Inferring Causation from Observed Associations." *American Journal of Epidemiology* 93(6), June 1971: pp. 443-456.

A188
Johnson, S.
Life without Birth: A Journey through the Third World in Search of the Population Explosion. London: William Heinemann, 1970; 364p.

A189
Jones, G.W.
The Economic Effect of Declining Fertility in Less Developed Countries. New York: Population Council, 1969; 30p.

A190
Kale, B.D.
Family Planning Enquiry in Dharwar Ta-

luka (Mysore State). Dharwar, India: Demographic Research Centre, Institute of Economic Research, 1966; 195p.

A191
Kale, B.D.
Family Planning Enquiry in Rural Shimoga (Mysore State). Dharwar, India: Demographic Research Centre, Institute of Economic Research, 1966; 152p.

A192
Kale, B.D. and Koteshwar, R.K.
Family Planning Resurvey in Dharwar. Dharwar, India: Demographic Research Centre, Institute of Economic Research, 1969; 129p.

A193
Kamal, W.H. et al.
"A Fertility Study in Al-Amria." *Egyptian Population and Family Planning Review* (Cairo) 1(2), Dec. 1968: pp. 83-100.

A194
Kammeyer, K.C.W.
"A Re-examination of Some Recent Criticisms of Transition Theory." *Sociological Quarterly* 11(4), Fall 1970: pp. 500-510.

A195
Kammeyer, K.C.W.
An Introduction to Population. San Francisco: Chandler, 1971; 196p.

A196
Kangas, L.W.
"Integrated Incentives for Fertility Control: Wider Use of Material Incentives

Should Make Family Planning Programs More Effective." *Science* 169(3952), 25 Sept. 1970: pp. 1278-1283.

A197
Karkal, M.
Annotated Bibliography of Studies on Age at Marriage in India. Bombay: International Institute for Population Studies, 1971; 25p.

A198
Kasarda, J.D.
"Economic Structure and Fertility: A Comparative Analysis." *Demography* 8(3), Aug. 1971: pp. 307-317.

A199
Kato, T. and Takahashi, T.
"Family Planning in Industry: The Japanese Experience." *International Labour Review* (Geneva) 104(3), Sept. 1971: pp. 161-179.

A200
Kelley, A.C.
"Demographic Cycles and Economic Growth: The Long Swing Reconsidered." *Journal of Economic History* 29(4), Dec. 1969: pp. 633-656.

A201
Kelly, W.J.
"Estimation of Births Averted by Family Planning Programs: The Parity Approach." *Studies in Family Planning* 2(9), Sept. 1971: pp. 197-201.

A202
Kennedy, D.M.
Birth Control in America: The Career of Margaret Sanger. Yale Publications in American Studies, 18. New Haven: Yale University Press, 1970; 320p.

A203
Kennett, K.F. and Cropley, A.J.
"Intelligence, Family Size and Socioeconomic Status." *Journal of Biosocial Science* 2(3), July 1970: pp. 227-236.

A204
Keyfitz, N.
"Age Distribution and the Stable Equivalent." *Demography* 6(3), Aug. 1969: pp. 261-269.

A205
Keyfitz, N.
"On the Momentum of Population Growth." *Demography* 8(1), Feb. 1971: pp. 71-80.

A206
Keyfitz, N.
"Migration as a Means of Population Control." *Population Studies* 25(1), Mar. 1971: pp. 63-72.

A207
Keyfitz, N.
"How Birth Control Affects Births." *Social Biology* 18(2), June 1971: pp. 109-121.

A208
Keyfitz, N.
"Linkages of Intrinsic to Age-specific Rates." *Journal of the American Statistical Association* 66(334), June 1971: pp. 275-281.

A209
Keyfitz, N. and Flieger, W.
Population: Facts and Methods of Demography. San Francisco: W.H. Freeman, 1971; 613p.

A210
Kiser, C.V., ed.
"Demographic Aspects of the Black Community: Proceedings of the Forty-third Conference of the Milbank Memorial Fund . . . New York City, 28-30 Oct. 1969." *Milbank Memorial Fund Quarterly* 48(2, Part 2), Apr. 1970: pp. 1-365.

A211
Kiser, C.V.
"Unresolved Issues in Research on Fertility in Latin America." *Milbank Memorial Fund Quarterly* 49(3, Part 1), July 1971: pp. 379-388.

A212
Korea. Ministry of Health and Social Affairs.
The Findings of the National Survey on Family Planning, 1967. Seoul: Planned Parenthood Federation of Korea, 1968; 206p.

A213
Krishnamurty, K.G.
Research in Family Planning in India. Delhi: Sterling Publishers, 1968; 108p.

A214
Krishnan, P.
"A Note on Changes in Age at Marriage of Females and Their Effect on the Birth Rate in India." *Social Biology* 18(2), June 1971: pp. 200-202.

A215
Kruegel, D.L.
"Metropolitan Dominance and the Diffusion of Human Fertility Patterns, Kentucky: 1939-1965." *Rural Sociology* 36(2), June 1971: pp. 141-156.

A216
Kubat, D. and Bosco, S.E.
"Marital Status and Ideology of the Family Size; Case of Young Men in Urban Brazil." *America Latina* (Rio de Janeiro) 12(2), Apr.-June 1969: pp. 17-34.

A217
Kumar, J.
"Demographic Analysis of Data on Illegitimate Births." *Social Biology* 16(2), June 1969: pp. 92-108.

A218
Kumar, J.
"A Comparison between Current Indian Fertility and Late Nineteenth-century Swedish and Finnish Fertility." *Population Studies* 25(2), July 1971: pp. 269-282.

A219
Kunz, P.R. and Brinkerhoff, M.B.
"Differential Childlessness by Color: the Destruction of a Cultural Belief." *Journal of Marriage and the Family* 31(4), Nov. 1969: pp. 713-719.

A220
Kupinsky, S.
"Non-familial Activity and Socio-economic Differentials in Fertility." *Demography* 8(3), Aug. 1971: pp. 353-367.

A221
Lambrechts, E.
"Religiousness, Social Status and Fertility Values in a Catholic Country." *Journal of Marriage and the Family* 33(3), Aug. 1971: pp. 561-566.

A222
Landsberger, M.
"The Life-cycle Hypothesis: A Reinterpretation and Empirical Test." *American Economic Review* 60(1), Mar. 1970: pp. 175-183.

A223
Lapham, R.J.
"Social Control in the Sais." *Anthropological Quarterly* 42(3), July 1969: pp. 244-262.

A224
Lapham, R.J.
"Family Planning and Fertility in Tunisia." *Demography* 7(2), May 1970: pp. 241-253.

A225
Lapham, R.J.
"Morocco: Family Planning Attitudes, Knowledge, and Practice in the Sais Plain." *Studies in Family Planning* 1(58), Oct. 1970: pp. 11-22.

A226
Lapham, R.J.
"Family Planning in Tunisia and Morocco: A Summary and Evaluation of the Recent Record." *Studies in Family Planning* 2(5), May 1971: pp. 101-110.

A227
Lauriat, P.
"The Effect of Marital Dissolution on Fertility." *Journal of Marriage and the Family* 31(3), Aug. 1969: pp. 484-493.

A228
Lazerwitz, B.
"The Association between Religio-ethnic Identification and Fertility among 'Contemporary' Protestants and Jews." *Sociological Quarterly* 11(3), Summer 1970: pp. 307-320.

A229
Lewit, S.
"Outcome of Pregnancy with Intrauterine Devices." *Contraception* 2(1), July 1970: pp. 44-57.

A230
Lippard, V.W., ed.
Macy Conference on Family Planning, Demography and Human Sexuality in Medical Education. New York: Josiah Macy, Jr. Foundation, 1971; 149p.

A231
Liu, P.T. and Chow, L.P.
"A Stochastic Approach to the Estimation of the Prevalalence of IUD: Example of Taiwan, Republic of China." *Demography* 8(3), Aug. 1971: pp. 341-352.

A232
Livi Bacci, M.
A Century of Portuguese Fertility. Princeton: Princeton University Press for the Office of Population Research, 1971; 149p.

A233
Lloyd, P.J.
"Divorce among the Yoruba." *American*

Anthropologist 70(1), Feb. 1968: pp. 67-81.

A234
Lloyd, P.J.
"A Growth Model with Population as an Endogenous Variable." *Population Studies* 23(3), Nov. 1969: pp. 463-478.

A235
Long, L.H.
"Fertility Patterns among Religious Groups in Canada." *Demography* 7(2), May 1970: pp. 135-149.

A236
Long, L.H.
"The Fertility of Migrants to and within North America." *Milbank Memorial Fund Quarterly* July 1970: pp. 297-316.

A237
Maathuis, J.B.
"Family Growth and Family Planning in a Rural Area of Kenya." *Tropical and Geographical Medicine* (Haarlem) 21, 1969; pp. 191-198.

A238
MacLeod, B., ed.
Demography and Educational Planning. Papers from a Conference on Implications of Demographic Factors for Educational Planning and Research, Sponsored by the Ontario Institute for Studies in Education, 9-10 June 1969. Monograph Series, 7. Toronto: Ontario Institute for Studies in Education, 1970; 274p.

A239
Meijer, M.J.
Marriage Law and Policy in the Chinese People's Republic. Hong Kong: Hong Kong University Press, 1971; 369p.

A240
Malaysia. National Family Planning Board.
Proceedings of the Second National Family Planning Seminar on General Consequences of Population Growth, Kuala Lumpur, 16-17 March, 1970. Kuala Lumpur: 1970; 185p.

A241
Marino, A.
"Family, Fertility, and Sex Ratios in the British Caribbean." *Population Studies* 24(2), July 1970: pp. 159-172.

A242
Mathur, M.V. et al.
Fertility Survey of Jaipur City. Jaipur: Department of Economics, University of Rajasthan, 1967; 91p.

A243
Matras, J. and Bachi, R.
"Practice of Contraception among Jewish Maternity Cases in Jerusalem (Changes in the Interval 1960-1966)." *Indian Demographic Bulletin* (Delhi) 1(1), 1968: pp. 51-59.

A244
Matthiessen, P.C.
Some Aspects of the Demographic Transition in Denmark. Copenhagen: Københavns Universitets Fond til Tilvejebringelse af Laeremidler, 1970; 226p.

A245
Maxwell, J.
"Intelligence, Education and Fertility:

A Comparison between the 1932 and 1947 Scottish Surveys." *Journal of Biosocial Science* 1(3), July 1969: pp. 247-271.

A246
Mazur, D.P.
"Correlates of Divorce in the U.S.S.R." *Demography* 6(3), Aug. 1969: pp. 279-286.

A247
McArthur, N.
"Fertility and Marriage in Fiji." *Human Biology in Oceania* (Sydney) 1(1), Feb. 1971: pp. 10-22.

A248
McCalister, D.V. et al.
"Family Planning and the Reduction of Pregnancy Loss Rates." *Journal of Marriage and the Family* 31(4), Nov. 1969: pp. 668-673.

A249
McFarland, D.D.
"On the Theory of Stable Populations: A New and Elementary Proof of the Theorems under Weaker Assumptions." *Demography* 6(3), Aug. 1969: pp. 301-322.

A250
McFarland, D.D.
"Effects of Group Size on the Availability of Marriage Partners." *Demography* 7(4), Nov. 1970: pp. 411-415.

A251
McLaughlin, C.P. and Trainer, E.S.
Qualitative Evaluation of Family Plan-

ning Proposals and Programs: A Systems Approach. Monograph, 12. Chapel Hill: Carolina Population Center, 1971; 70p.

A252
Mehra, L. et al.
A Report on the Oral Pill Pilot Clinics in India. Technical Paper, 9. New Delhi: Central Family Planning Institute, 1970; 24p.

A253
Mendels, F.F.
"Recent Research in Historical Demography." *American Historical Review* 75(4), Apr. 1970: pp. 1065-1073.

A254
Micklin, M.
"Urban Life and Differential Fertility: Specification of an Aspect of the Theory of the Demographic Transition." *Sociological Quarterly* 10(4), Fall 1969: pp. 480-500.

A255
Micklin, M.
"Traditionalism, Social Class, and Differential Fertility in Guatemala City." *America Latina* (Rio de Janeiro) 12(4), Oct.-Dec. 1969: pp. 59-78.

A256
Milner, E., ed.
"The Impact of Fertility Limitation on Women's Life-career and Personality." *Annals of the New York Academy of Sciences* 175, 1970: pp. 783-1065.

A257
Mitra, S.
"Preferences Regarding the Sex of Chil-

dren and Their Effects on Family Size under Varying Conditions." *Sankhyā* (Calcutta) (Series B) 32(1-2), June 1970: pp. 55-62.

A258
Mogey, J.
"Sociology of Marriage and Family Behavior, 1957-1968: A Trend Report and Bibliography." *Current Sociology* (The Hague) 17(1-3), 1969: pp. 1-364.

A259
Monahan, T.P.
"Are Interracial Marriages Really Less Stable?" *Social Forces* 48(4), June 1970: pp. 461-473.

A260
Morocco. Division of Statistics. Secretariat of State for Planning.
"Morocco: Family Planning Knowledge, Attitudes, and Practice in the Rural Areas." *Studies in Family Planning* 1(58), Oct. 1970: pp. 1-6.

A261
Morocco. Division of Statistics. Secretariat of State for Planning.
"Morocco: Family Planning and an Attitude Survey in the Urban Areas." *Studies in Family Planning* 1(58), Oct. 1970: pp. 6-11.

A262
Mosena, P.W. and Stoeckel, J.
"The Impact of Desired Family Size upon Family Planning Practices in Rural East Pakistan." *Journal of Marriage and the Family* 33(3), Aug. 1971: pp. 567-570.

A263
Mukherji, S. and Venkatacharya, K.
"Effect of Induced Abortion on Birth Rate: A Simulation Model." *Indian Journal of Public Health* (Calcutta) 14(1), Jan. 1970: pp. 49-58.

A264
Namboodiri, N.K.
The Changing Population of Kerala. New Delhi: Office of the Registrar General, Ministry of Home Affairs, 1968; 123p.

A265
Namboodiri, N.K.
"A Method for Comparative Analysis of Fertility Dynamics Represented by Sequences of Fertility Schedules." *Demography* 7 (2), May 1970: pp. 155-167.

A266
Namboodiri, N.K.
"On the Relation between Economic Status and Family Size Preferences When Status Differentials in Contraceptive Instrumentalities are Eliminated." *Population Studies* 24(2), July 1970: pp. 233-239.

A267
Narasimha Rao, M. and Mathen, K.K.
Rural Field Study of Population Control, Singur, 1957-1969. Calcutta: All-India Institute of Hygiene and Public Health, 1970; 88p.

A268
Nash, A.E.K.
"Going Beyond John Locke? Influencing American Population Growth." *Milbank Memorial Fund Quarterly* 49(1, Part 1), Jan. 1971: pp. 7-31.

A269
National Academy of Sciences.
Resources and Man. A Study and Recommendations. National Research Council. Committee on Resources and Man. Publication 1703. San Francisco: W.H. Freeman, 1969; 259p.

A270
National Academy of Sciences. Office of the Foreign Secretary.
Rapid Population Growth: Consequences and Policy Implications. Baltimore: Johns Hopkins Press, 1971; 696p.

A271
Neal, A.G. and Groat, H.T.
"Alienation Correlates of Catholic Fertility." *American Journal of Sociology* 73(3), Nov. 1970: pp. 460-473.

A272
Neher, P.A.
"Peasants, Procreation and Pensions." *American Economic Review* 61(3, Part 1), June 1971: pp. 380-389.

A273
Nerlove, M. and Schultz, T.P.
Love and Life between the Censuses: A Model of Family Decision Making in Puerto Rico, 1950-1960. Memorandum RM-6322-AID. Santa Monica, Calif.: RAND Corporation, 1970; 105p.

A274
Newcombe, H.B. and Smith, M.E.
"Changing Patterns of Family Growth: The Value of Linked Vital Records as a Source of Data." *Population Studies* 24(2), July 1970: pp. 193-203.

A275
Newman, P.
" 'Population Pressure' and Economic Growth: An Operational Treatment." *Journal of Development Planning* 2, 1968: pp. 31-57.

A276
Nortman, D.
"Population and Family Planning Programs: A Factbook." *Reports on Population/Family Planning,* June 1971; 48p.

A277
Nour Eldin, S.S.
Analysis of Data on Fertility, Mortality and Economic Activity of Urban Population in Libya Based on a Household Sample Survey. Memorandum, 996. Cairo: Institute of National Planning, 1971; 30p.

A278
Ohadike, P.
"The Possibility of Fertility Change in Modern Africa: A West African Case." *African Social Research* (Lusaka, Zambia) 8, Dec. 1969: pp. 602-614.

A279
Okazaki, Y.
An Analysis of Decline of Birth Rate in Japan. Tokyo: Institute of Population Problems, Ministry of Health and Welfare, 1967; 42p.

A280
Okediji, F.O.
"Socioeconomic Status and Differential Fertility in an African City." *Journal of Developing Areas* 3(3), Apr. 1969: pp. 339-354.

A281

Olusanya, P.O.
"The Problem of Multiple Causation in Population Analysis, with Particular Reference to the Polygamy-Fertility Hypothesis." *Sociological Review* 19, May 1971: pp. 165-178.

A282

Olusanya, P.O.
"Status Differentials in the Fertility Attitudes of Married Women in Two Communities in Western Nigeria." *Economic Development and Cultural Change* 19(4), July 1971: pp. 641-651.

A283

Organization for Economic Cooperation and Development. Development Centre.
Population Programmes and Economic and Social Development. Paris: 1970; 141p.

A284

Orleans, L.A.
"Evidence from Chinese Medical Journals on Current Population Policy." *China Quarterly* 40, Oct.-Dec. 1969: pp. 137-146.

A285

Pakistan. National Research Institute of Family Planning.
Proceedings of the Fifth Biannual Seminar on Research and Family Planning, Lahore, Nov. 7-9, 1968. Karachi: 1969; 160p.

A286

Pakistan. National Research Institute of Family Planning.
Proceedings of the Sixth Biannual Seminar on Research and Family Planning, Karachi, April 23-26, 1969. Karachi: 1970; 289p.

A287

Palmore, J.A. et al.
"Class and Family in a Modernizing Society." *American Journal of Sociology* 76(3), Nov. 1970: pp. 375-398.

A288

Palmore, J.A. et al.
"Interpersonal Communication and the Diffusion of Family Planning in West Malaysia." *Demography* 8(3), Aug. 1971: pp. 411-425.

A289

Parkes, A.S. et al., eds.
"Biosocial Aspects of Human Fertility, Proceedings of the Seventh Annual Symposium of the Eugenics Society, London, September 1970." *Journal of Biosocial Science* (Supplement) 3, 1970; 148p.

A290

Parkes, A. et al.
Towards a Population Policy for the United Kingdom. London: Population Investigation Committee, London School of Economics, 1970; 60p.

A291

Patankar, T.
A Bibliography of Fertility Studies in India. Bombay: Demographic Training and Research Centre (Chembur), 1969; 38p.

A292
Pathak, K.B.
"On Recurrent Patterns of Fecundity."
Interdiscipline 4(4), 1967: pp. 303-307.

A293
Pathak, K.B.
"A Model for Estimating Fecundability
of the Currently Married Woman from
the Data on Her Susceptibility Status—
A Cohort Approach." *Demography* 8(4),
Nov. 1971: pp. 519-524.

A294
Patna University.
*Fertility and Family Planning in a Social
Class of India: A Case Study of Patna,
Bihar.* D.R.C. Research Monograph, 1.
Patna: 1969; 106p.

A295
Paydarfar, A.A.
*Demographic Consequences of Moderni-
zation: A Population Analysis of Iran and
Comparison with Selected Nations.* Silver
Spring, Md.: International Research In-
stitute, 1967; 154p.

A296
Paydarfar, A.A. and Sarram, M.
"Differential Fertility and Socioeco-
nomic Status of Shirazi Women: A Pilot
Study." *Journal of Marriage and the
Family* 32(4), Nov. 1970: pp. 692-699.

A297
Peng, J.Y. et al.
"Medical Correlates of Termination of
Use of Intrauterine Contraceptive Devices in Taichung." *International Journal
of Fertility* 15(2), Apr.-June 1970: pp.
120-126.

A298
Peng, J.Y. et al.
"Taiwan: Medical Correlates of Termi-
nation of Use of Intrauterine Devices."
Studies in Family Planning 1(60), Dec.
1970: pp. 24-27.

A299
Perkin, G.W.
"Nonmonetary Commodity Incentives
in Family Planning Programs." *Studies
in Family Planning* 1(57), Sept. 1970: pp.
12-15.

A300
Phillips, L. et al.
"A Synthesis of the Economic and Demographic Models of Fertility: An
Econometric Test." *Review of Economics
and Statistics* 51(3), Aug. 1969: pp.
298-308.

A301
Podell, L.
Fertility, Illegitimacy, and Birth Control.
New York: Center for Social Research,
Graduate Center, City University of
New York, 1968; 32p.

A302
Pohlman, E.
How to Kill Population. Philadelphia:
Westminster Press, 1971; 169p.

A303
Pohlman, E.
*Incentives and Compensations in Birth
Planning.* Monograph, 11. Chapel Hill:
Carolina Population Center, 1971; 140p.

A304
Polgar, S., ed.
Culture and Population: A Collection of

Current Studies. Monograph, 9. Chapel Hill: Carolina Population Center, 1971; 196p.

A305
Polgar, S. and Rothstein, F.
"Family Planning and Conjugal Roles in N.Y.C. Poverty Areas." *Social Science and Medicine* 4, July 1970: pp. 135-139.

A306
Pollard, A.H.
Demography: An Introduction. Sydney, N.Y.: Pergamon, 1968; 92p.

A307
Pollard, G.N.
"Factors Influencing the Sex Ratio at Birth in Australia, 1902-65." *Journal of Biosocial Science* 1(2), Apr. 1969: pp. 125-144.

A308
Pool, D.I.
"Social Change and Interest in Family Planning in Ghana: An Exploratory Analysis." *Canadian Journal of African Studies* 4(2), Spring 1970: pp. 207-227.

A309
Pool, D.I.
"Ghana: The Attitudes of Urban Males toward Family Size and Family Limitation." *Studies in Family Planning* 1(60), Dec. 1970: pp. 12-17.

A310
Population Council.
"U.S.S.R. Views on Population/Family Planning." *Studies in Family Planning* 1(49), Jan. 1970: pp. 1-16. [Selection of excerpts from articles by Russian authors.]

A311
Population Problems Research Council.
Summary of Tenth National Survey on Family Planning. Population Problems Series, 21. Tokyo: Mainichi Newspapers, 1971; 60p.

A312
Potter, R.G., Jr.
"Births Averted by Contraception: An Approach through Renewal Theory." *Theoretical Population Biology* 1(3), Nov. 1970: pp. 251-272.

A313
Potter, R.G., Jr.
"Inadequacy of a One-method Family-planning Program." *Social Biology* 18(1), Mar. 1971: pp. 1-9.

A314
Potter, R.G., Jr. et al.
"Net Delay of Next Conception by Contraception: A Highly Simplified Case." *Population Studies* 24(2), July 1970: pp. 173-192.

A315
Potter, R.G., Jr. and Masnick, G.S.
"The Contraceptive Potential of Early versus Delayed Insertion of the Intrauterine Device." *Demography* 8(4), Nov. 1971: pp. 507-517.

A316
Pressat, R.
Population. London: C.A. Watts, 1970; 152p.

A317
Presser, H.B.
"The Timing of the First Birth, Female Roles and Black Fertility." *Milbank Memorial Fund Quarterly* 49(3, Part 1), July 1971: pp. 329-361.

A318
Preston, S.H.
"The Birth Trajectory Corresponding to Particular Population Sequences." *Theoretical Population Biology* 1(3), Nov. 1970: pp. 346-351.

A319
Preston, S.H.
"Empirical Analysis of the Contribution of Age Composition to Population Growth." *Demography* 7(4), Nov. 1970: pp. 417-432.

A320
Price, D.O.
Changing Characteristics of the Negro Population. Washington: Bureau of the Census, Government Printing Office, 1970; 267p.

A321
Princeton University. Office of Population Research.
Population Index Bibliography, Cumulated 1935-1968 by Authors and Geographical Areas: Geographical Index. Boston: G.K. Hall, 1971; 5 vols.

A322
Radel, D., ed.
"Population and Family Planning in Rural Africa." *Rural Africana* 14, Spring 1971; 185p.

A323
Rao, M.N. and Mathen, K.K.
Rural Field Study of Population Control, Singur (1957-1969). Calcutta: All-India Institute of Hygiene and Public Health, 1970; 88p.

A324
Rhodes, L.
"Socioeconomic Correlates of Fertility in the Metropolis: Relationship of Individual and Areal Unit Characteristics." *Social Biology* 18(3), Sept. 1971: pp. 296-304.

A325
Ridker, R.
"Savings Accounts for Family Planning, an Illustration from the Tea Estates of India." *Studies in Family Planning* 2(7), July 1971: pp. 150-152.

A326
Ritchey, P.N. and Stokes, C.S.
"Residence Background, Socioeconomic Status, and Fertility." *Demography* 8(3), Aug. 1971: pp. 369-377.

A327
Rogers, E.M.
"Incentives in the Diffusion of Family Planning Innovations." *Studies in Family Planning* 2(12), Dec. 1971: pp. 241-248.

A328
Romaniuk, A.
A Regression Model for Projecting and

Translating Measurements of Cohort Fertility Age Pattern: An Experiment. Population Studies and Projection Series, 6. Ottowa: Dominion Bureau of Statistics, Census Division, Dec. 1970; 19p.

A329
Rosen, B.C. and Simmons, A.B.
"Industrialization, Family and Fertility: A Structural-psychological Analysis of the Brazilian Case." *Demography* 8(1), Feb. 1971: pp. 49-69.

A330
Rosenfield, A.G. and Muangman, D.
"Thailand: Population Seminar for Representatives of the Press, Radio, and Television." *Studies in Family Planning* 1(57), Sept. 1970: pp. 15-19.

A331
Roussel, L.
"France: Family Building by Socio-occupational Groups." *Studies in Family Planning* 1(60), Dec. 1970: pp. 10-12.

A332
Ryder, N.B. and Westoff, C.F.
Reproduction in the United States, 1965. Princeton: Princeton University Press, 1971; 419p.

A333
Sadik, N., ed.
Population Control: Implications, Trends, and Prospects; Proceedings of the Pakistan International Family Planning Conference at Dacca, January 28th to February 4th, 1969. Islamabad: Pakistan Family Planning Council, 1969; 686p.

A334
Safilios-Rothschild, C.
"Sociopsychological Factors Affecting Fertility in Urban Greece: A Preliminary Report." *Journal of Marriage and the Family* 31(3), Aug. 1969: pp. 595-606.

A335
Saw, S.H., ed.
The Demography of Malaysia, Singapore and Brunei: A Bibliography. University of Hong Kong, Centre of Asian Studies, Bibliographies, 1. London: Oxford University Press, 1970; 39p.

A336
Saw, S.H.
Singapore Population in Transition. Philadelphia: University of Pennsylvania Press, 1970; 227p.

A337
Saxena, G.B.
Indian Population in Transition. New Delhi: Commercial Publications Bureau, 1971; 200p.

A338
Schnaiberg, A.
"Rural-urban Residence and Modernism: A Study of Ankara Province, Turkey." *Demography* 7(1), Feb. 1970: pp. 71-85.

A339
Schultz, T.P.
"An Economic Model of Family Planning and Fertility." *Journal of Political Economy* 77, Mar.-Apr. 1969: pp. 153-180.

A340
Schultz, T.P.
Effectiveness of Family Planning in Taiwan: A Methodology for Program Evaluation. Rand Paper P-4253. Santa Monica, Calif.: RAND Corporation, 1969; 73p.

A341
Schultz, T.P.
Population Growth: Investigation of a Hypothesis. Memorandum P-4056-1. Santa Monica, Calif.: RAND Corporation, 1969; 58p.

A342
Schultz, T.P.
The Decline of Fertility and Child Mortality in Central East Pakistan. Rand Paper P-4660. Santa Monica, Calif.: RAND Corporation, 1971; 29p.

A343
Schultz, T.P.
An Economic Perspective on Population Growth. Rand Paper P-4607. Santa Monica, Calif.: RAND Corporation, 1971; 53p.

A344
Schultz, T.P.
Factors Affecting Fertility and Statistical Inference: A Comment. Rand Paper, P-4691-1. Santa Monica, Calif.: RAND Corporation, 1971; 9p.

A345
Schultz, T.P. and DaVanzo, J.
Analysis of Demographic Change in East Pakistan: A Study of Retrospective Survey Data. Memorandum R-564-AID. Santa Monica, Calif.: RAND Corporation, 1970; 72p.

A346
Schultz, T.P. and DaVanzo, J.
Fertility Patterns and Their Determinants in the Arab Middle East. Rand Paper RM-5978-FF. Santa Monica, Calif.: RAND Corporation, 1970; 116p.

A347
Schweitzer, D.G. and Dienes, G.J.
"A Kinetic Model of Population Dynamics." *Demography* 8(3), Aug. 1971: pp. 389-400.

A348
Shapiro, S. and Abramowicz, M.
"Pregnancy Outcome Correlates Identified through Medical Record-based Information." *American Journal of Public Health and the Nation's Health* 59(9), Sept. 1969: pp. 1629-1650.

A349
Sheps, M.C.
"A Review of Models for Population Change." *Review of the International Statistical Institute* (The Hague) 39(2), 1971; pp. 185-196.

A350
Sheps, M.C. et al.
"Truncation Effect in Closed and Open Birth Interval Data." *Journal of the American Statistical Association* 65(330), June 1970: pp. 678-693.

A351
Sheps, M.C. and Menken, J.A.
"A Model for Studying Birth Rates Given Time Dependent Changes in Reproductive Parameters." *Biometrics* 27(2), June 1971: pp. 325-343.

A352
Siegel, E. et al.
"Continuation of Contraception by Low Income Women: A One Year Follow-up." *American Journal of Public Health* 61(9), Sept. 1971: pp. 1886-1898.

A353
Sifman, R.I. et al.
"A Method of Studying Fertility and the Rate of Marriage." *Soviet Sociology* 7(4), Spring 1969: pp. 44-55. [English translation of Russian text in *Vestnik Statistiki* (Moscow) 12, 1967: pp. 11-23.]

A354
Simmons, G.B.
The Indian Investment in Family Planning. New York: Population Council, 1971; 213p.

A355
Simon, J.L.
"Family Planning Prospects in Less-developed Countries, and a Cost-benefit Analysis of Various Alternatives." *Economic Journal* 80(317), Mar. 1970: pp. 58-71.

A356
Simon, J.L.
"The Per-capita-income Criterion and Natality Policies in Poor Countries." *Demography* 7(3), Aug. 1970: pp. 369-378.

A357
Simpson, M.L. and Williamson, D.
"The Completed Family in Monterrey: Fertility, Mobility, and Migration." *Human Mosaic* 3(1), Fall 1968: pp. 81-104.

A358
Singarimbun, M.
The Population of Indonesia, 1930-1968: A Bibliography. London: International Planned Parenthood Federation, 1969; 56p.

A359
Singer, S.F., ed.
Is There an Optimum Level of Population? A Population Council Book. New York: McGraw-Hill, 1971; 426p.

A360
Singh, S.N. and Bhattacharya, B.N.
"A Generalized Probability Distribution for Couple Fertility." *Biometrics* 26(1), Mar. 1970: pp. 33-40.

A361
Sivin, I.
"Fertility Decline and Contraceptive Use in the International Postpartum Family Planning Program." *Studies in Family Planning* 2(12), Dec. 1971: pp. 248-256.

A362
Sly, D.F.
"Minority-group Status and Fertility: An Extension of Goldscheider and Uhlenberg." *American Journal of Sociology* 76(3), Nov. 1970: pp. 443-459.

A363
Smith, T.L. and Zopf, P.E., Jr.
Demography: Principles and Methods. Philadelphia: F.A. Davis, 1970; 610p.

A364
Spencer, G.
"Pre-marital Pregnancies and Ex-nup-

tial Births in Australia, 1911-66: A Comment." *Australian and New Zealand Journal of Sociology* (Melbourne) 5(2), Oct. 1969: pp. 121-127.

A365
Spengler, J.J.
"Population Problem: In Search of a Solution." *Science* 166(3910), 5 Dec. 1969: pp. 1234-1238.

A366
Spengler, J.J.
Population Economics: Selected Essays of Joseph J. Spengler. Durham: Duke University Press, 1972; 536p.

A367
Srinivasan, K.
"Findings and Implications of a Correlation Analysis of the Closed and the Open Birth Intervals." *Demography* 7(4), Nov. 1970: pp. 401-410.

A368
Stoeckel, J.
"Socio-economic Status and Family Planning Knowledge, Attitudes and Practices in Rural East Pakistan." *Social and Economic Studies* (Mona, Jamaica) 19(20), June 1970: pp. 213-225.

A369
Stoeckel, J. and Choudhury, M.A.
"Pakistan: Response Validity in a KAP Survey." *Studies in Family Planning* 1(46), Oct. 1969: pp. 5-9.

A370
Stoeckel, J. and Choudhury, M.A.
"Trends in Pregnancy and Fertility in a Rural Area of East Pakistan." *Journal of Biosocial Science* 2(4), Oct. 1970: pp. 329-335.

A371
Strauss, M.A.
"Social Class, Fertility, and Authority in Nuclear and Joint Households in Bombay." *Journal of Asian and African Studies* 9, Jan. 1969: pp. 61-74.

A372
Stycos, J.M. et al.
Ideology, Faith, and Family Planning in Latin America: Studies in Public and Private Opinion on Fertility Control. A Population Council Book. New York: McGraw-Hill, 1971; 418p.

A373
Stycos, J.M. and Marden, P.G.
"Honduras: Fertility and an Evaluation of Family Planning Programs." *Studies in Family Planning* 1(57), Sept. 1970: pp. 20-24.

A374
Sundaram, C.
A Follow-up Study of Sterilised Male Industrial Workers in Bombay. Publication Series, 3. Bombay: Family Planning Association of India, 1969; 72p.

A375
Sweet, J.A.
"Family Composition and the Labor Force Activity of American Wives." *Demography* 7(2), May 1970: pp. 195-209.

A376
Sweezey, A.
"The Economic Explanation of Fertility

Changes in the United States." *Population Studies* 25(2), July 1971: pp. 255-267.

A377
Tabbarah, R.B.
"Toward a Theory of Demographic Development." *Economic Development and Cultural Change* 19(2), Jan. 1971: pp. 257-267.

A378
Tachi, M. and Muramatsu, M., eds.
Population Problems in the Pacific: New Dimensions in Pacific Demography: Proceedings of the Congress Symposium No. 1 and Divisional Meeting of Section VIII No. 5, 11th Pacific Science Congress Tokyo, 22 Aug.-10 Sept. 1966. Tokyo: Conveners of the Congress Symposium No. 1, The Eleventh Pacific Science Congress, 1971; 510p.

A379
Tarver, J.D.
"Gradients of Urban Influence on the Educational, Employment, and Fertility Patterns of Women." *Rural Sociology* 34(3), Sept. 1969: pp. 356-367.

A380
Tarver, J.D. et al.
"Urban Influence on the Fertility and Employment Patterns of Women Living in Homogeneous Areas." *Journal of Marriage and the Family* 32(2), May 1970: pp. 237-241.

A381
Taylor, H.C., Jr. and Berelson, B.
"Comprehensive Family Planning Based on Maternal/Child Health Services: A Feasibility Study for a World Program." *Studies in Family Planning* 2(2), Feb. 1971: pp. 21-54.

A382
Taylor, L.R., ed.
The Optimum Population for Britain; Proceedings of a Symposium Held at the Royal Geographical Society, London, on 25 and 26 September, 1969. London and New York: Published for the Institute of Biology by Academic Press, 1970; 182p.

A383
Tewari, R.N.
Agricultural Development and Population Growth: An Analysis of Regional Trends in U.P. [Uttar Pradesh]. Delhi: Sultan Chand, 1970; 226p.

A384
Thorat, S.S. and Fliegel, F.C.
"Some Aspects of Adoption of Health and Family Planning Practices in India." *Behavioural Sciences and Community Development* (Hyderabad) 2(1), Mar. 1968: pp. 1-13.

A385
Tien, H.Y.
"Marital Moratorium and Fertility Control in China." *Population Studies* 24(3), Nov. 1970: pp. 311-323.

A386
Tietze, C. and Lewit, S.
"The IUD and the Pill: Extended Use-effectiveness." *Family Planning Perspectives* 3(2), Apr. 1971: pp. 53-55.

A387
Tsubouchi, Y.
"Changes in Fertility in Japan by Regions: 1920-1965." *Demography* 7(2), May 1970: pp. 121-134.

A388
United Arab Republic. Cairo Demographic Centre.
Demographic Measures and Population Growth in Arab Countries. Research Monograph Series, 1. Cairo: 1970; 352p.

A389
United Nations. Commissioner for Technical Co-operation.
Family Planning Evaluation Mission to Ceylon. ST/SOA/SER.R/14. New York: 1971; 80p.

A390
United Nations. Department of Economic and Social Affairs.
Human Fertility and National Development: A Challenge to Science and Technology. E.71.II:A.12. New York: 1971; 140p.

A391
United Nations. Department of Economic and Social Affairs.
Population and Family Planning in Iran. ST/SOA/SER.R/13. New York: 1971; 140p.

A392
United Nations. Economic Commission for Asia and the Far East.
"Report of the Working Group on Communications Aspects of Family Planning Programmes and Selected Papers, Held at Singapore, 5-15 Sept. 1967." E.68.II.F.17. *Asian Population Studies Series* 3, Nov. 1968; 164p.

A393
United Nations. Economic Commission for Asia and the Far East.
"Report of the Regional Seminar on Evaluation of Family Planning Programmes, Bangkok, Thailand, 24 Nov.-12 Dec. 1969." E.70.II.F.20. *Asian Population Studies Series* 5, 1970; 95p.

A394
United Nations. Population Commission.
Report on the Technical Meeting on Methods of Analysing Fertility Data for Developing Countries (Budapest, 14-25 June 1971). E/CN.9/241. New York: 1971; 56p.

A395
United Nations. Programme of Technical Cooperation.
An Evaluation of the Family Planning Programme of the Government of India. TAO/IND/50.ST/SOA/SER.R/11. New York: 1969; 109p.

A396
University of Chicago. Community and Family Study Center.
R.F.F.P.I. [Rapid Feedback for Family Planning Improvement]. *Family Planning Research Manual* (Series). Chicago: 1970.

A397
Van Keep, P.A.
"Ideal Family Size in Five European Countries." *Journal of Biosocial Science* 3(3), July 1971: pp. 259-265.

A398
Veevers, J.E.
"Childlessness and Age at First Marriage." *Social Biology* 18 (3), Sept. 1971: pp. 292-295.

A399
Veevers, J.E.
"Differential Childlessness by Color: A Further Examination." *Social Biology* 18(3), Sept. 1971: pp. 285-291.

A400
Venkatacharya, K.
"Postponement of Age at Marriage and Its Short-term Impact on Fertility." *Journal of Institute of Economic Research* (Dharwar) 4(2), July 1969: pp. 50-68.

A401
Venkatacharya, K.
"Some Recent Findings on 'Open Birth Intervals.'" *Artha Vijñāna* (Poona) 11(3), Sept. 1969: pp. 372-379.

A402
Venkatacharya, K.
"Some Implications of Susceptibility and Its Application in Fertility Evaluation Models." *Sankhyā* (Calcutta) (Series B) 32(1-2), June 1970: pp. 41-54.

A403
Venkatacharya, K.
"A Model to Estimate Births Averted Due to IUCDs and Sterilizations." *Demography* 8(4), Nov. 1971: pp. 491-505.

A404
Vielrose, E.
"Birth Rates in the Sudan." *Africana Bulletin* 1, 1964; pp. 95-104.

A405
Vig, O.P.
"Demographic Effectiveness of Sterilization Programme in India." *Artha Vijñāna* (Poona) 12(3), Sept. 1970: pp. 398-405.

A406
Vincent, C.E. et al.
"Familial and Generational Patterns of Illegitimacy." *Journal of Marriage and the Family* 31(4), Nov. 1969: pp. 659-667.

A407
Votey, H.L., Jr.
"The Optimum Population and Growth: A New Look. A Modification to Include a Preference for Children in the Welfare Function." *Journal of Economic Theory* 1(3), Oct. 1969: pp. 273-290.

A408
Wajntraub, G.
"Fertility after Removal of the Intrauterine Ring." *Fertility and Sterility* 21(7), July 1970: pp. 555-557.

A409
Waller, J.H.
"Differential Reproduction: Its Relation to IQ Test Score, Education, and Occupation." *Social Biology* 18(2), June 1971: pp. 122-136.

A410
Walsh, B.M.
"Marriage Rates and Population Pres-

sure: Ireland, 1871 and 1966." *Economic History Review* (2nd Series) 23(1), Apr. 1970: pp. 148-162.

A411
Walsh, B.M.
Religion and Demographic Behaviour in Ireland. Dublin: Economic and Social Research Institute, 1970; 50p.

A412
Walsh, B.T.
Economic Development and Population Control: A Fifty-year Projection for Jamaica. Praeger Special Studies in International Economics and Development. New York: Frederick A. Praeger, 1970; 134p.

A413
Ward, R.J.
"Alternative Means to Control Population Growth." *Review of Social Economy* 27(2), Sept. 1969: pp. 121-138.

A414
Weller, R.H.
"Role Conflict and Fertility." *Social and Economic Studies* (Jamaica) 18(3), Sept. 1969: pp. 263-272.

A415
Weller, R.H. and Sly, D.F.
"Modernization and Demographic Change: A World View." *Rural Sociology* 34(3), Sept. 1969: pp. 313-326.

A416
Westoff, L.A. and Westoff, C.F.
From Now to Zero: Fertility, Contraception and Abortion in America. Boston: Little, Brown, 1971; 358p.

A417
Williamson, J.B.
"Subjective Efficacy and Ideal Family Size as Predictors of Favorability toward Birth Control." *Demography* 7(3), Aug. 1970: pp. 329-339.

A418
Wishik, S.M. et al.
"Estimation of Fertility Change in Pakistan by Retrospective Quasi-cohort Analysis of Group-specific Fertility Patterns." *American Journal of Public Health* 61(6), June 1971: pp. 1080-1088.

A419
Wolfers, D.
"The Singapore Family Planning Program: Further Evaluation Data." *American Journal of Public Health and the Nation's Health* 60(12), Dec. 1970: pp. 2354-2360.

A420
Wolfers, H.
"Psychological Aspects of Vasectomy." *British Medical Journal* 5730, 31 Oct. 1970: pp. 297-300.

A421
Wolff, R.J. et al.
A Study of Knowledge, Attitude and Practice Relative to Family Planning among Indigenous Women in Guam, 1969. Honolulu: Population and Family Planning Unit, School of Public Health, University of Hawaii, 1970; 68p.

A422
Wood, C. and Suitters, B.
The Fight for Acceptance: A History of Contraception. Aylesbury: Medical and Technical Publishing, 1970; 238p.

A423
World Health Organization. Scientific Group on Developments in Fertility Control.
Development in Fertility Control: Report of a WHO Scientific Group. Technical Report Series No. 424. Geneva: 1969; 36p.

A424
Wright, N.H.
"Vital Statistics and Census Tract Data Used to Evaluate Family Planning." *Public Health Reports* 85(5), May 1970: pp. 383-389.

A425
Wright, N.H.
"Ceylon: The Relationship of Demographic Factors and Marital Fertility to the Recent Fertility Decline." *Studies in Family Planning* 1(59), Nov. 1970: pp. 17-20.

A426
Wu, H.Y.
"A Demographic Study on the Relationships of Nuptiality, Child Mortality, and Attitude toward Fertility to Actual Fertility in Hsueh-Chia Township in Taiwan. I. Relationship of Marriage Cohort and Marriage to Actual Fertility." *Journal of the Formosan Medical Association* (Taipei) 69, 28 May 1970: pp. 243-255.

A427
Wyon, J.B. and Gordon, J.E.
The Khanna Study: Population Problems in the Rural Punjab. Cambridge, Mass.: Harvard University Press, 1971; 437p.

A428
Zaidan, G.C.
The Costs and Benefits of Family Planning Programs. World Bank Staff Occasional Papers, 12. Baltimore: Johns Hopkins Press for International Bank for Reconstruction and Development, 1971; 52p.

A429
Zatuchni, G.I., ed.
Post-partum Family Planning: A Report on the International Program. A Population Council Book. New York: McGraw-Hill, 1971; 477p.

A430
Zelnik, M. and Kantner, J.F.
"United States: Exploratory Studies of Negro Family Formation—Factors Relating to Illegitimacy." *Studies in Family Planning* 1(60), Dec. 1970: pp. 5-9.

GEOGRAPHICAL INDEX

1231, 1238, 1239, 1255, 1258, 1262, 1264, 1268, 1269, 1285, 1509, 1521, 1526, 1528, 1531, 1610, 1613, 1615, 1624, 1626, 1629, 1643, 1647, 1655

Indonesia 383, 401, 1148

Iran 513, 740

Ireland 347, 484

Israel 626, 628, 978, 979, 1171, 1199, 1200, 1225, 1246

Italy 457, 589, 960, 1063, 1464

Ivory Coast 1276

Jamaica 356, 374, 391, 406, 587, 997, 998, 1472, 1530, 1618

Japan 70, 110, 358, 441, 451, 560, 582, 631, 681, 690, 739, 871, 932, 933, 934, 1035, 1038, 1057, 1065, 1067, 1137, 1417, 1429, 1432, 1459, 1476, 1533, 1577, 1587, 1635, 1639

Kenya 720, 1208, 1418

Korea 353, 388, 408, 409, 562, 739, 740, 763, 820, 835, 870, 904, 905, 1211, 1317, 1513, 1514, 1620

Latin America 26, 27, 38, 69, 75, 108, 134, 145, 350, 354, 412, 542, 545, 693, 695, 739, 811, 837, 986, 1094, 1112, 1123, 1129, 1130, 1160, 1334, 1383, 1398, 1518, 1519, 1520, 1552, 1570

Lebanon 1538

Malaysia 389, 417, 418, 739, 836, 912, 1106, 1516, 1617, 1624

Malta 1517

Mexico 555, 569, 585, 745, 1014, 1039, 1141, 1335, 1386, 1523

Micronesia 185, 411, 421, 423

Morocco 740, 753

Nepal 734, 1387

Netherlands 439, 987, 1345, 1568, 1656

New Zealand 442, 1026

Nigeria 424, 525, 571, 572, 573, 623, 1024, 1203, 1426

Norway 362, 454, 1131, 1289

Pakistan 143, 157, 158, 159, 167, 191, 209, 223, 282, 299, 309, 321, 349, 378, 381, 404, 415, 428, 526, 579, 634, 676, 724, 727, 739, 740, 746, 747, 750, 754, 785, 788, 790, 793, 798, 800, 818, 834, 843, 858, 869, 879, 882, 883, 884, 899, 900, 909, 931, 958, 1002, 1005, 1017, 1240, 1290, 1294, 1403, 1622, 1646

Peru 580, 599, 1107, 1117, 1121, 1124, 1125, 1136, 1210, 1313

Philippines 511, 554, 702, 1022, 1412, 1423, 1424, 1500, 1522, 1611

Poland 376, 1029

Puerto Rico 138, 260, 348, 426, 464, 517, 522, 564, 577, 601, 602, 633, 739, 767, 821, 880, 881, 1045, 1046, 1073, 1181, 1247, 1510, 1511, 1547, 1644

Rhodesia 1102

Romania 1055, 1265

Roman Empire 471, 478, 486

Scotland 1115, 1307, 1457

Singapore 413, 729, 739, 867, 913

Spain 1147, 1561, 1562

South Africa 556, 976, 1077, 1201, 1428, 1461

South Asia 28, 1415, 1429

Sweden 153, 367, 464, 487, 1040, 1059, 1096, 1289, 1304, 1318, 1331, 1584

Sudan 1042, 1043

Taiwan 130, 135, 161, 361, 394, 395, 563, 739, 763, 796, 805, 813, 814, 826, 847, 848, 857, 861, 889, 890, 893, 897, 902, 907, 911, 924, 926, 927, 928, 1091, 1146, 1252, 1253, 1254, 1321, 1376, 1465, 1499, 1507, 1508, 1652

Thailand 76, 309, 335, 399, 739, 760, 828, 855, 876, 896, 901, 930, 948, 999, 1152